THE CSIRO LOW-CARB DIET

EASY 100

As Australia's national science agency, we solve the greatest challenges through innovative science and technology. For more than a century we have worked together with industry, government, universities and research organisations to turn big ideas into disruptive solutions. Solutions for food security and quality; clean energy and resources; health and wellbeing; resilient and valuable environments; innovative industries; and a secure Australia and region. CSIRO is at the forefront of nutritional science and lifestyle research in Australia. Our research involves the complex relationship between the health of individuals, populations, and the environment. We have a track record of translating scientific findings into a variety of practical and easy-to-follow nutrition and exercise programs that support Australians to improve their health.

THE CSIRO LOW-CARB DIET

EASY 100

RECIPES BASED ON SCIENCE TO AID WEIGHT LOSS, MANAGE TYPE 2 DIABETES AND IMPROVE OVERALL HEALTH

PROFESSOR GRANT BRINKWORTH
AND **DR PENNIE TAYLOR**

MACMILLAN
Pan Macmillan Australia

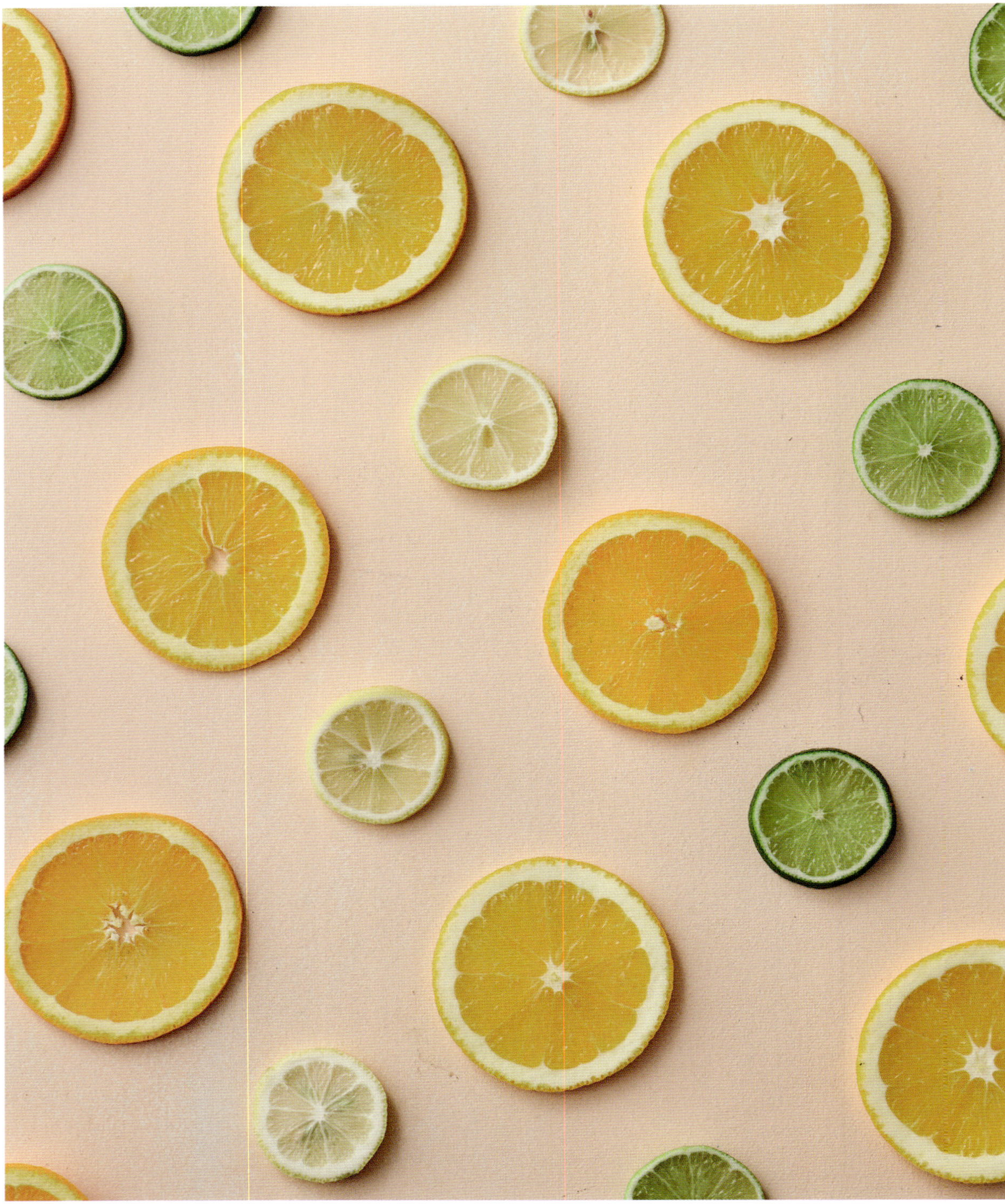

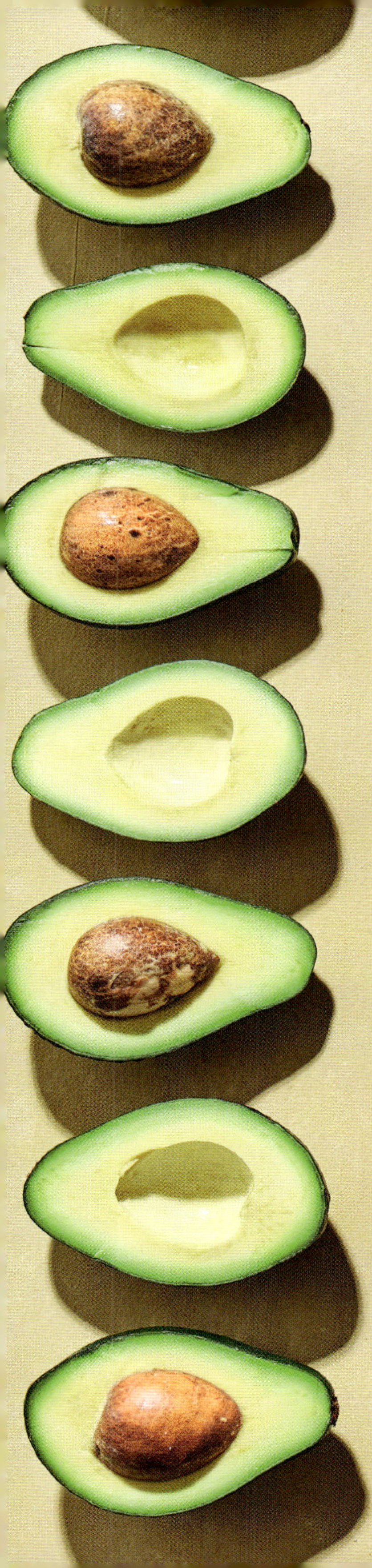

Contents

About the authors

PROFESSOR GRANT BRINKWORTH

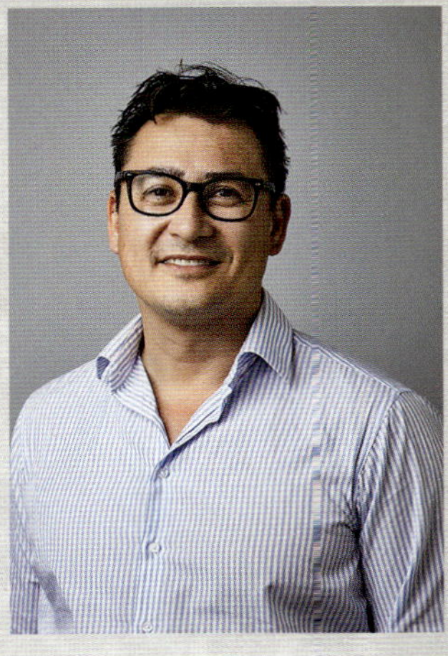

Professor Grant Brinkworth is a Senior Principal Research Scientist at CSIRO and international leader in clinical nutrition and health research. He has a PhD in nutrition and exercise science and more than 20 years' experience leading large-scale clinical studies evaluating the effects of diets, foods, exercise and lifestyle interventions on human health, performance and functionality in healthy and clinical populations. This includes understanding the role and influence of dietary and lifestyle factors for optimising human health, including the prevention and treatment of chronic diseases such as diabetes. Combined with his qualifications and expertise in business management and commercialisation across the academic research, industry and healthcare sectors, Professor Brinkworth is developing, testing and translating effective nutrition and lifestyle solutions and health service models with integration of healthcare technologies and devices for wide-scale adoption and management of obesity, metabolic health and type 2 diabetes. He has published more than 100 peer-reviewed scientific papers and is the co-author and founder of the number-one bestselling CSIRO Low-carb Diet book series, which has been adopted into clinical practice guidelines and product solutions for improving weight and diabetes management. Professor Brinkworth is an Adjunct Research Professor at the University of South Australia and the University of Sydney, and has supervised many post-graduate students in the areas of nutrition, exercise and metabolism.

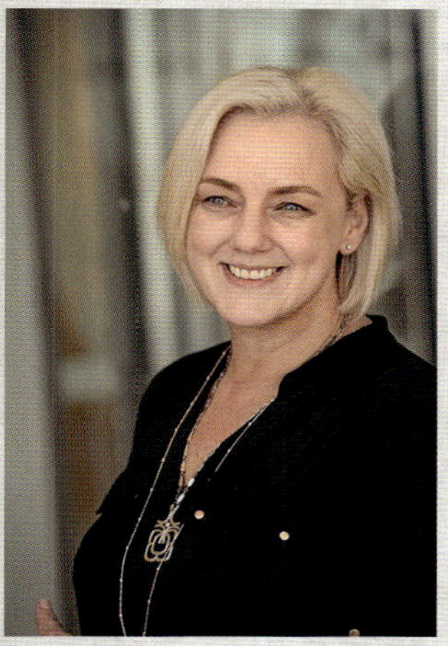

DOCTOR PENNIE TAYLOR

Doctor Pennie Taylor is a Clinical Dietitian and Research Scientist at CSIRO. She has a PhD from the University of Adelaide, School of Medicine, exploring dietary factors and the integrated role of emerging health technologies, including Real Time Continuous Glucose Monitoring (RT-CGM) for obesity, type 2 diabetes and lifestyle management. With extensive experience working across nutrition research and the Australian healthcare system, she has gained excellent knowledge of the clinical health and wellbeing issues facing our Australian population. From her CSIRO nutrition research and clinical trial intervention positions, she brings a sound understanding of diet and specialised food design and the translation of science into the development of community health and chronic disease programs – specialising in obesity, type 2 diabetes and metabolic weight-loss surgery. Adding her private practice experience, she has a deep understanding of how research and evidence links within the healthcare systems frameworks for chronic disease and lifestyle management. Dr Taylor has published more than 30 peer-reviewed scientific papers and is the co-author of the number-one bestselling book *The CSIRO Low-carb Diet*, as well as *CSIRO Low-carb Every Day*, *CSIRO Low-carb Diet Quick & Easy*, *The CSIRO Low-carb Diabetes Diet & Lifestyle Solution*, *CSIRO Healthy Gut Diet* and *CSIRO Gut Care Guide*. Dr Taylor continues to enjoy working with industry and government partners to translate science into clinical and community outcomes, with a particular interest in utilising health technology and novel foods to optimise self-management strategies for improved health and wellbeing across all life and health stages.

Recipe developer

MEG YONSON

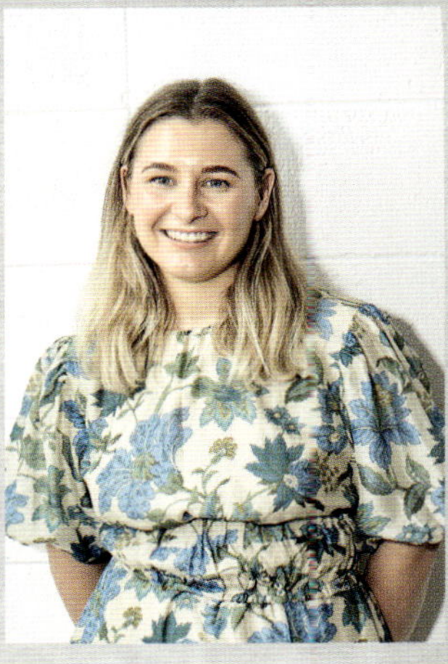

Meg Yonson is a recipe developer, food stylist and creative director. She has a bachelor of Nutritional Medicine. Meg combines her health and nutritional studies with an understanding of global food trends and design to create highly engaging food content that spans across print and digital platforms. Meg co-owns Studio Maybe, a food and lifestyle photo studio in Sydney.

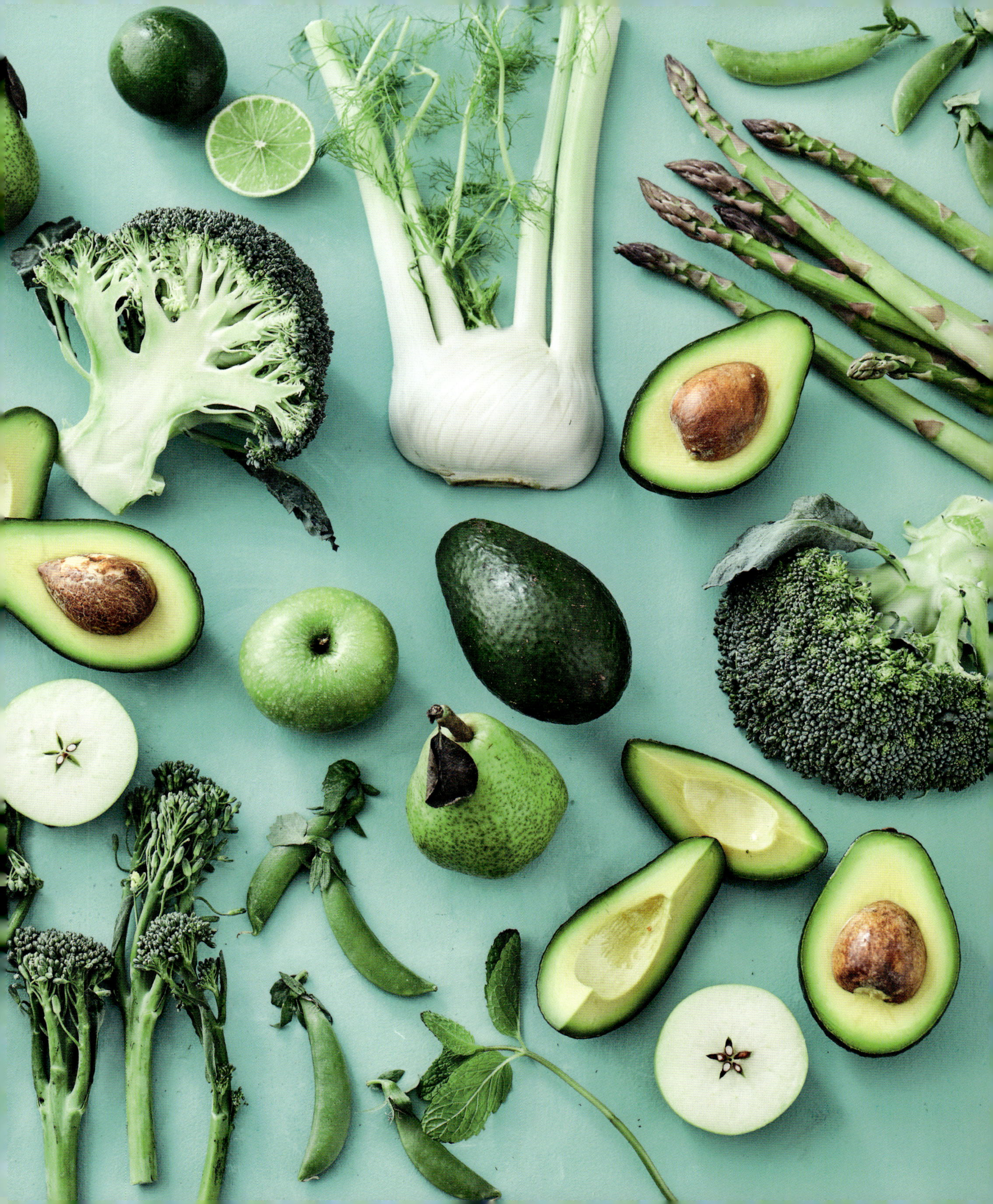

Introduction

We all want to live a long, healthy life without disease or health issues that prevent us from enjoying an active lifestyle and the fun things in life.

Our diet and nutritional status (including carrying excess body weight) are core factors that determine our health and risk of developing major non-communicable diseases, including heart disease and type 2 diabetes. But with so many food, ingredients and dietary options readily available and promoted, combined with confusing or mixed messages – often not grounded in strong scientific evidence – it can be difficult to make good choices confidently, which will deliver improved health and wellbeing.

To help cut through this 'noise' and assist Australians with improving their diet quality and health, we used the latest scientific evidence and principles of healthy eating, and performed rigorous clinical trials, to develop and test the CSIRO Low-carb Diet. This has enabled us to provide Australians with a comprehensive guide, which science has shown to effectively improve diet quality and health status, better manage body weight, and reduce the risk of chronic diseases, such as heart disease and type 2 diabetes, which affect so many people today.

The CSIRO Low-carb Diet is a prescriptive, nutritionally complete eating and lifestyle plan, which clinical research has shown to be highly effective in achieving sustained long-term weight loss, reducing risk factors for heart disease and improving metabolic health.

The high popularity of the CSIRO Low-carb Diet book series, including the *CSIRO Low-carb Diabetes Diet & Lifestyle Solution*, has helped many Australians improve their health and better manage chronic diseases like type 2 diabetes, often with less medication. This has created demand from our readers seeking more recipe and meal options to help align their changing lifestyles and food preferences.

The CSIRO Low-carb Diet Easy 100 is a companion book, which provides a suite of new creative recipes that focus on providing more vegetarian options, incorporating new and unfamiliar foods available in supermarkets today, and remaining consistent with the scientific principles and nutrition benchmarks of the CSIRO Low-carb dietary approach used in our book series.

We hope this book will provide you with a short-cut guide, and motivation, creativity, and inspiration to start or to continue your renewed lifestyle journey to make you healthier, feel better and to get the most out of life.

The CSIRO Low-carb Diet is a nutritionally complete eating and lifestyle plan.

WHO WE ARE AND WHY WE DO WHAT WE DO

CSIRO is Australia's national science agency and is at the forefront of nutrition science and lifestyle research. Our mission is to research and understand the latest scientific principles and concepts for optimal health and wellbeing and to translate this knowledge and our research findings into easy-to-follow, practical, evidence-based solutions that Australians can use to improve their health.

We are passionate about addressing Australia's major national challenges and creating effective solutions to these problems.

A key health issue and research priority for the Australian Government and CSIRO has been to address the dramatic rise in obesity levels over the past 30 years and the rapidly rising incidence of type 2 diabetes, which have reached epidemic levels worldwide. In Australia, approximately two-thirds of adults are overweight or obese and an estimated 1.2 million have type 2 diabetes, accounting for over 85% of all diabetes cases, with a further estimated 2 million having pre-diabetes and at high risk of developing type 2 diabetes. Globally, approximately 483 million adults live with type 2 diabetes and, without sufficient action and effective solutions, the number is expected to rise to 580 million by 2030, and 705 million by 2045.

The reason why it is so important to urgently arrest the major public health issue of obesity is that being obese increases the risk of type 2 diabetes, which is a condition that causes an inability to effectively control blood glucose (sugar) levels. Type 2 diabetes is a condition where a person has blood glucose levels that are high on average but can also experience extreme highs and lows that can fluctuate throughout the day. This unfavourable blood glucose profile is associated with a significantly increased risk of a number of health complications, including heart disease; stroke; eye, kidney and blood vessel disease; nerve damage; foot problems and limb amputation; gum disease; and mental health problems, including depression and Alzheimer's disease. Recent evidence has also shown that people with type 2 diabetes and poor blood glucose control have increased risk of infections, and a higher chance of poor outcomes from infection, including COVID-19. Still more, obesity and type 2 diabetes negatively affect people's general feeling of overall wellbeing and quality of life, including a lack of energy, restricted mobility, and capacity to work, which impacts their ability to undertake activities of daily living. This is why we are so passionate about helping Australians improve their weight status and metabolic health and to reduce their risk of, and improve the management of, type 2 diabetes.

What can we do to improve our health?

While there are some non-modifiable risk factors that determine our risk of obesity and type 2 diabetes, including our age, gender, family history and ethnicity, there are several non-modifiable risk factors that we *can* change to reduce our health risk. Importantly, diet and lifestyle choices remain at the top of this list. Indeed, improved diet and increased physical activity remain the first treatment for obesity and type 2 diabetes. Research consistently shows this is an effective strategy to reduce body weight and improve blood glucose control in individuals who are overweight or obese and/or with poor blood glucose control, including pre-diabetes and type 2 diabetes.

Informed by a large body of research, we also know that all dietary approaches are not equal; some achieve better results than others. But with so much confusion out there and with many approaches not grounded in strong scientific evidence, our role at CSIRO is to conduct rigorous controlled scientific studies and to use the latest scientific principles and nutrition knowledge to create, test, substantiate and translate effective dietary approaches that will optimise health improvements.

A diet low in carbohydrate and higher in proportions of protein and fat is effective for reducing the risk of type 2 diabetes and heart disease.

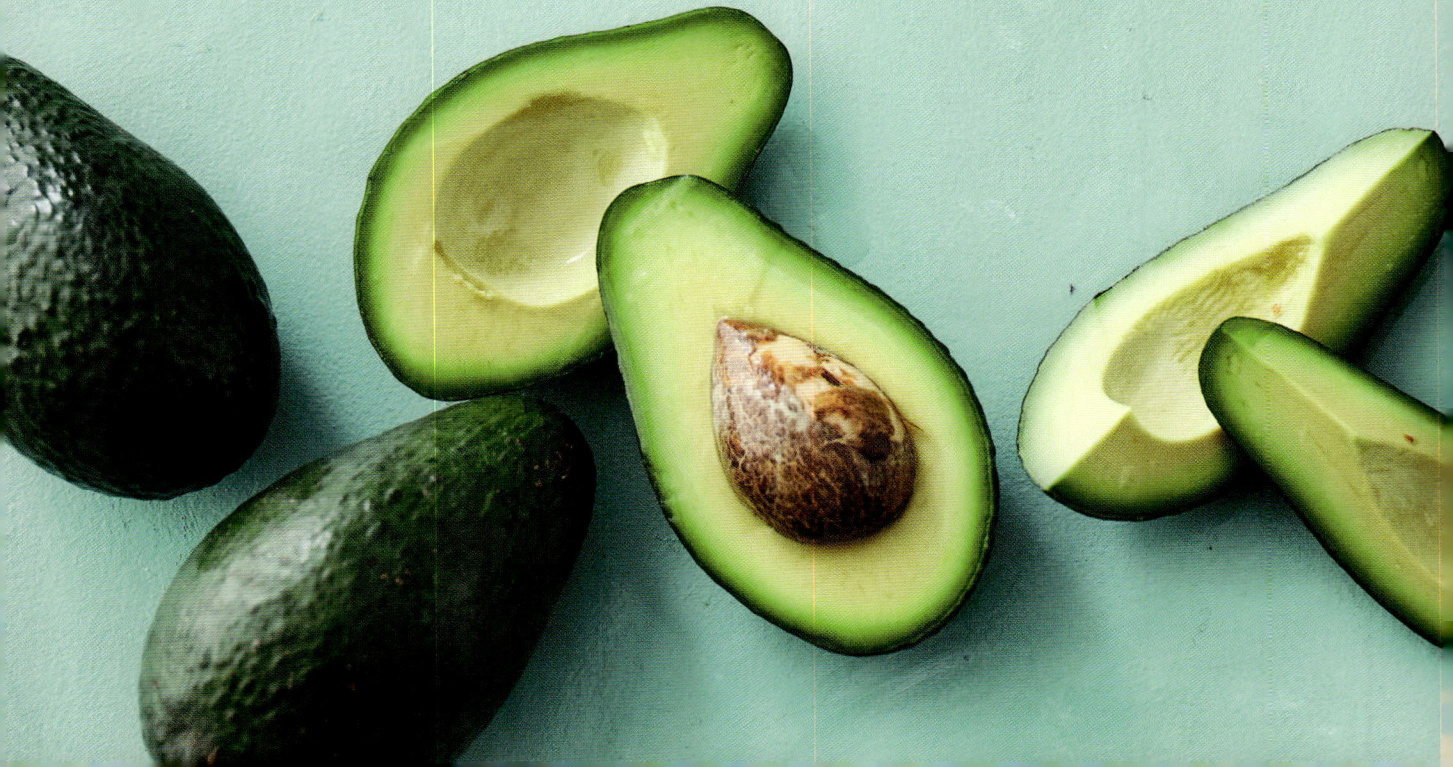

Why a low-carb diet is beneficial

For so many years we were told that a traditional high-carbohydrate, moderate-protein, low-fat diet was the most appropriate and, in many cases, the only dietary approach for healthy eating, weight control and type 2 diabetes management. In fact, some health professionals and public health messages still promote this dietary approach as the only dietary approach to be considered. Despite this long-standing message, research shows that a high-carbohydrate, low-fat approach is often only associated with modest weight loss and reduction in risk factors for type 2 diabetes and heart disease, and that many patients find these recommendations difficult to follow.

Over the years, nutrition research has evolved and advanced our understanding of dietary factors that influence weight management, blood glucose control and risk factors of metabolic and heart disease. Research now shows there is no 'one-size-fits-all' dietary approach for the management and treatment of obesity and type 2 diabetes, and that a variety of different dietary approaches can be effective and necessary in order to tailor diet approaches for individual needs, preferences and health goals. Moreover, contrary to what we have been told for so long, research has also shown that, compared to a traditional high-carbohydrate, moderate-protein, low-fat diet, a diet low in carbohydrate and higher in proportions of protein and fat is at least as, if not more so, effective for improving many health factors, which reduces the risk of type 2 diabetes and heart disease. This is making us rethink how we tackle and manage these major health challenges in our society today.

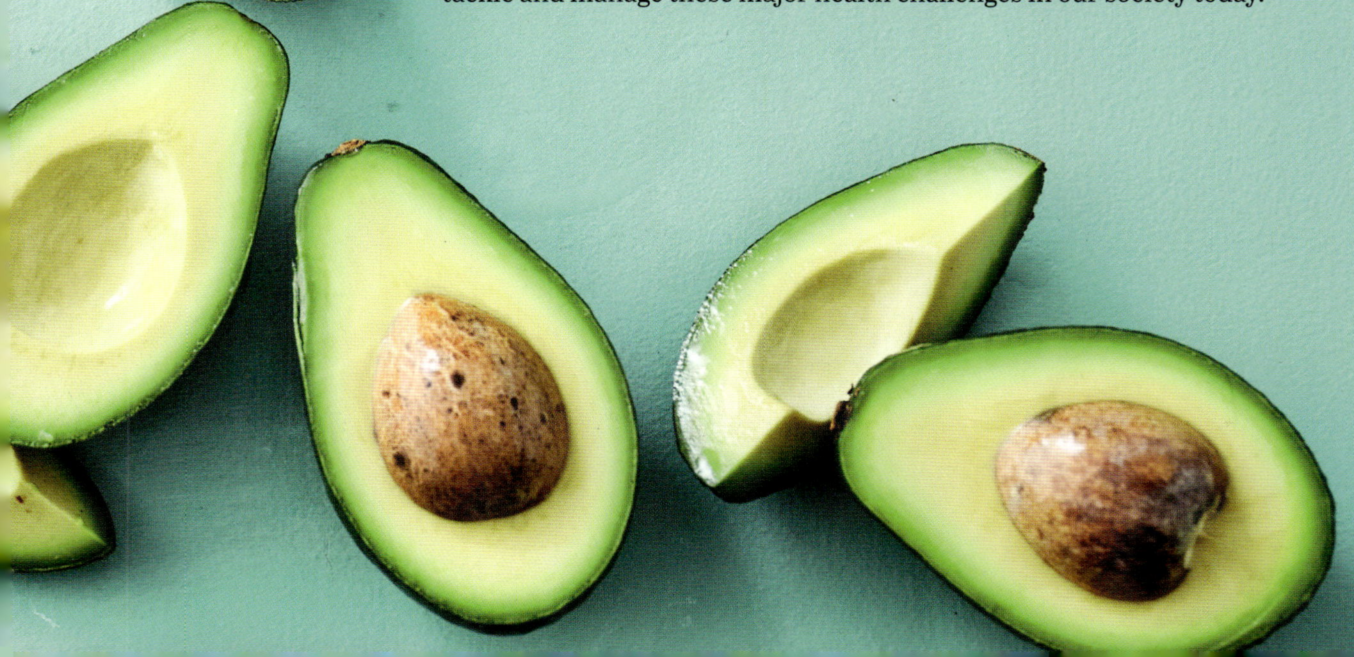

The CSIRO Low-carb Diet research trial

In 2012, we conducted a randomised controlled clinical trial. In this study, 115 adults who were overweight or obese with type 2 diabetes were randomised to one of two groups who were assigned to follow a particular dietary approach for 2 years.

Group 1 followed an energy-reduced diet, which was low in carbohydrate but included good-quality, low glycaemic index (GI), high-fibre foods, high in protein and unsaturated fat, and low in saturated fat. In other words, the CSIRO Low-carb Diet. Of the total daily energy allowance:

- 14% of total energy came from carbohydrates (aiming for 50–70 grams of carbohydrate per day)
- 28% was from protein, and
- the remaining 58% was from fat (with less than 10% from saturated fat).

Group 2 followed a diet that prescribed the same amount of energy, however:

- it was high in unrefined good-quality carbohydrates, preference to refined carbohydrate (53% of total energy equating to 200–300 grams of carbohydrate each day)
- with low to moderate protein (17% of total energy)
- and low in fat (30% of total energy, with less than 10% saturated fat).

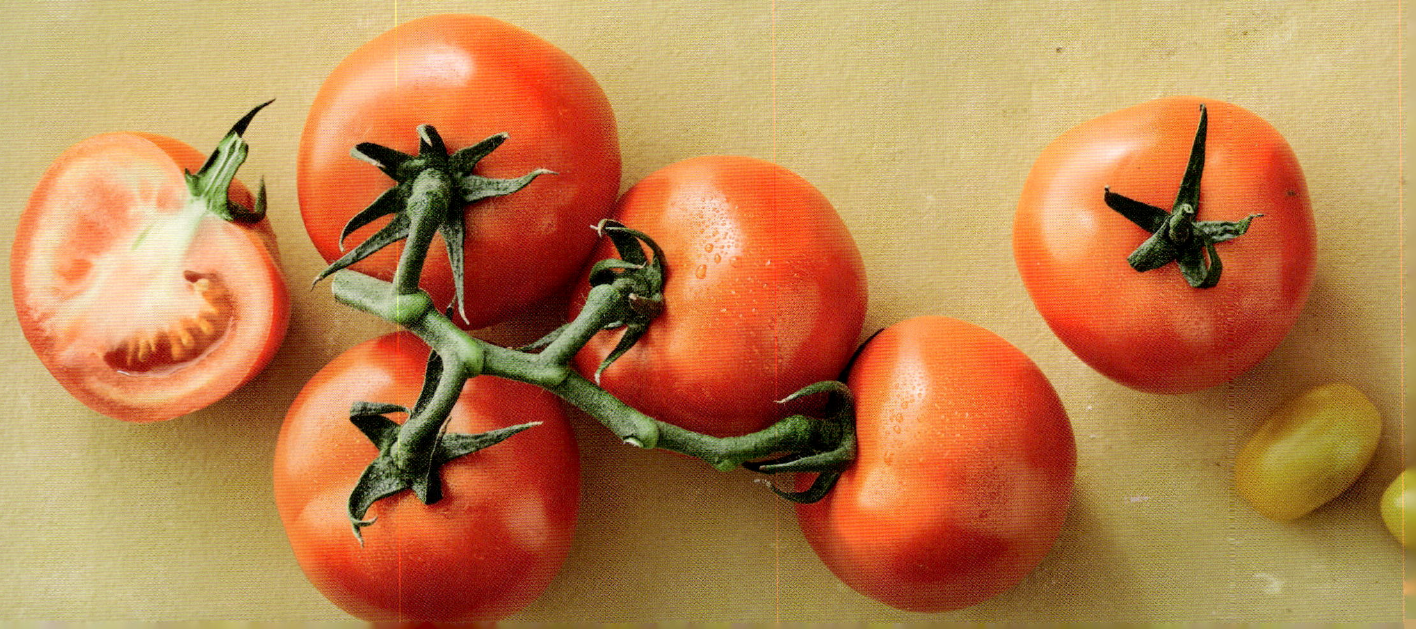

The high-carbohydrate, moderate-protein, low-fat approach followed by group 2 has traditionally been recommended by leading health authorities for the management of obesity and type 2 diabetes.

Both groups also participated in the same structured exercise program, undertaking 60 minutes of combined aerobic and resistance exercise, three times per week.

Before and after the intervention, each participant underwent a comprehensive health assessment to determine which diet approach worked better.

Results of the clinical trial showed that, after 2 years, the number of people who completed the trial remained similar in both groups. Both diet approaches also achieved sustained and similar long-term results:

- weight loss, with an average 7% (7 kg) reduction in body weight
- clinically relevant reductions in blood pressure, fasting blood glucose levels and glycosylated haemoglobin (HbA1c) levels – a routine clinical measure of blood glucose levels and control
- reductions in blood levels of low-density lipoprotein – LDL ('bad') cholesterol levels
- improved mood and quality of life with similar effects on mental function and performance.

Both diets also did not affect clinical markers of renal (kidney) function, and blood levels of important nutrients – including folate, beta-carotene, vitamins B12, D and E, copper, zinc, selenium, calcium, magnesium, sodium, potassium, iron, ferritin and transferrin saturation – remained within normal ranges on both diets, indicating that both diets were nutritionally complete.

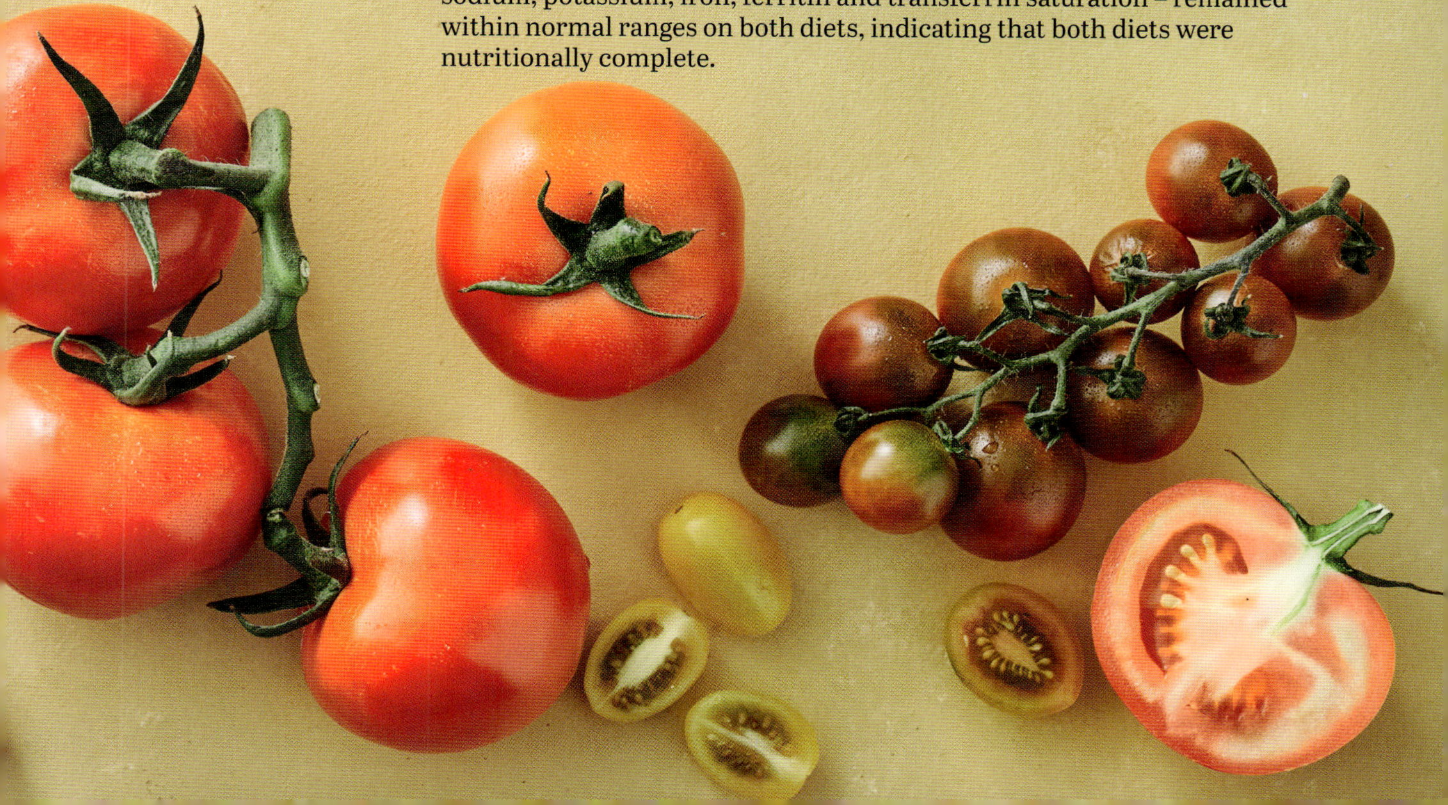

THE CSIRO LOW-CARB DIET ADVANTAGE

In addition to the common health improvements that occurred with both diets, compared to the traditional high-carbohydrate, low-fat diet, the CSIRO Low-carb Diet achieved greater improvements in several important health outcomes including:

- greater reductions in blood glucose variability – i.e., a more stable blood glucose profile throughout the day – which means a lower risk of excessively high blood glucose levels (hyperglycaemia) and low blood glucose levels (hypoglycaemia), thereby lowering the risk of health complications associated with diabetes
- greater reductions in the requirements for diabetes medication to control blood glucose levels – which means reduced medication costs and fewer medication side effects
- greater improvements in blood cholesterol profile, with greater reductions in blood triglyceride levels and increases in high-density lipoprotein – HDL ('good') cholesterol levels – which means greater improvements in heart health and lower risk of heart disease.

The results of this 2-year study showed that the CSIRO Low-carb Diet was not only effective in sustaining long-term weight loss, but magnified the health benefits typically observed with losing weight by providing superior benefits for improving blood glucose control, lowering risk factors for heart disease and reducing diabetes medication requirements. The CSIRO Low-carb Diet was also able to deliver these benefits without any negative effects on other important aspects of health, including brain function and kidney health, and the diet remained nutritionally complete – meaning it provided adequate amounts of essential vitamins, minerals and trace elements.

This research clearly shows that the CSIRO Low-carb Diet is an effective all-in-one solution, which simultaneously improves the health markers that doctors and health professionals use to assess diabetes and health risk and management, and that the improvements that can be achieved are greater than what can be achieved with a traditional high-carbohydrate, moderate-protein, low-fat diet.

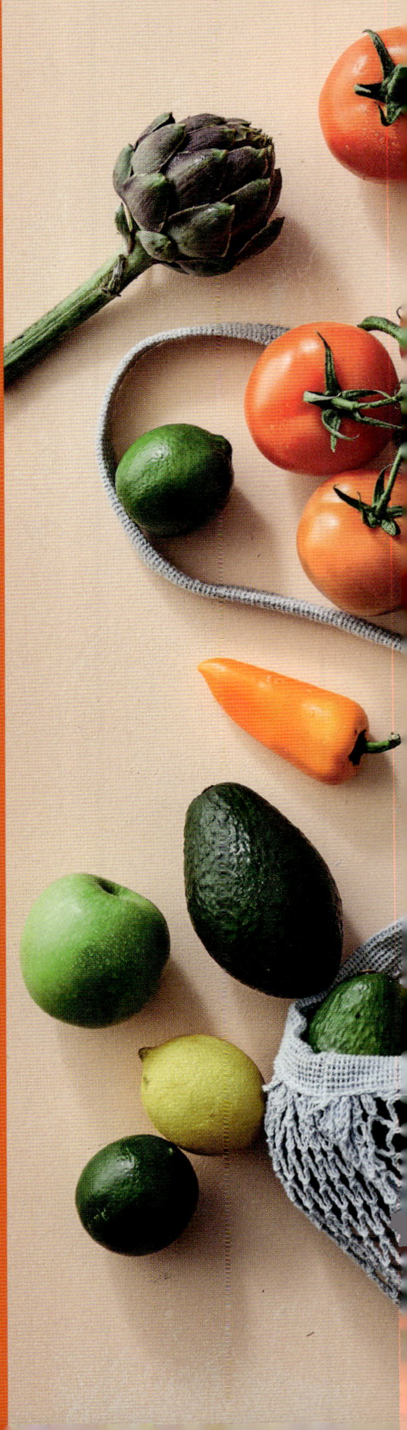

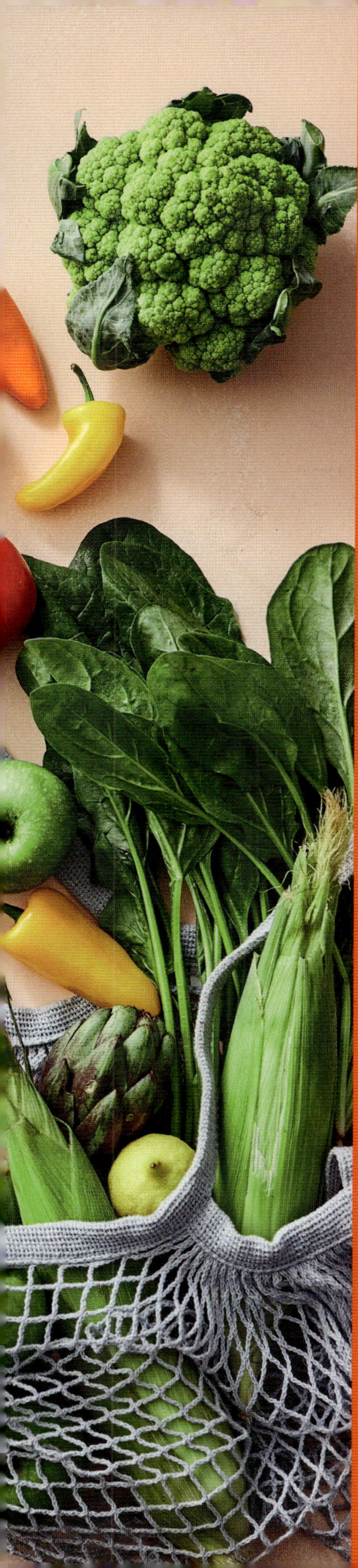

In support of our research, clinical trials from many other independent laboratories around the world have shown similar beneficial effects of a low-carbohydrate diet. Collectively, this large body of evidence suggests that in individuals with type 2 diabetes, compared to consuming a traditional high-carbohydrate, low-fat diet, low-carbohydrate diets have superior advantages for:

- improving weight loss
- reducing HbA1c levels, indicating improved blood glucose control
- reducing diabetes medication requirements
- improving blood lipid profile by reducing triglyceride levels (high levels increase the risk of heart disease) and increasing HDL ('good') cholesterol levels (low levels increase the risk of heart disease), with no differential responses in LDL ('bad') cholesterol levels.

Emerging evidence further suggests that, compared to a traditional high-carbohydrate, low-fat diet, a low-carbohydrate diet can be a more effective strategy to achieve remission of type 2 diabetes. This is when a person previously diagnosed with type 2 diabetes improves and lowers their blood glucose levels to a point no longer in the range where they could be classified as having diabetes. This increased likelihood of achieving diabetes remission is partly why low-carbohydrate diets are gaining so much attention and popularity, not only among individuals suffering from pre-diabetes or type 2 diabetes, but also with members of their healthcare team, including GPs and practising dietitians.

In addition, the growing scientific evidence base supporting the effectiveness of low-carbohydrate diets to improve health and the management and remission of type 2 diabetes, is also driving a shift in clinical practice guidelines of leading health authorities around the world. In recent years, the American Diabetes Association, Diabetes Australia, Diabetes UK and Diabetes Canada have all released position statements and/or updated their guidelines to acknowledge and support the role of low carbohydrates as part of an individualised approach in the management of type 2 diabetes. Moreover, the Australian Government Department of Health Australian National Diabetes Strategy 2021–2030 has stated that remission of type 2 diabetes in adults can be achieved with dietary interventions including low-carbohydrate diets, and have endorsed the need to consider offering these alternative dietary interventions to people with type 2 diabetes aiming for remission.

Why does the CSIRO Low-carb Diet work?

Overall, the CSIRO Low-carb Diet works so well because it is a select combination of foods proven to provide health benefits by:

- focusing on good-quality carbohydrates (low-glycaemic index/GI and high in fibre) and limiting the total amount of high-carb foods
- increasing the amount of 'healthy' unsaturated fats
- keeping the amount of 'unhealthy' saturated fats low
- increasing the amount of quality protein
- remaining nutritionally complete and providing adequate amounts of essential vitamins, minerals, dietary fibre and trace elements
- focusing on including low-energy, nutrient-dense whole foods
- limiting intake of high-energy, nutrient-poor discretionary foods.

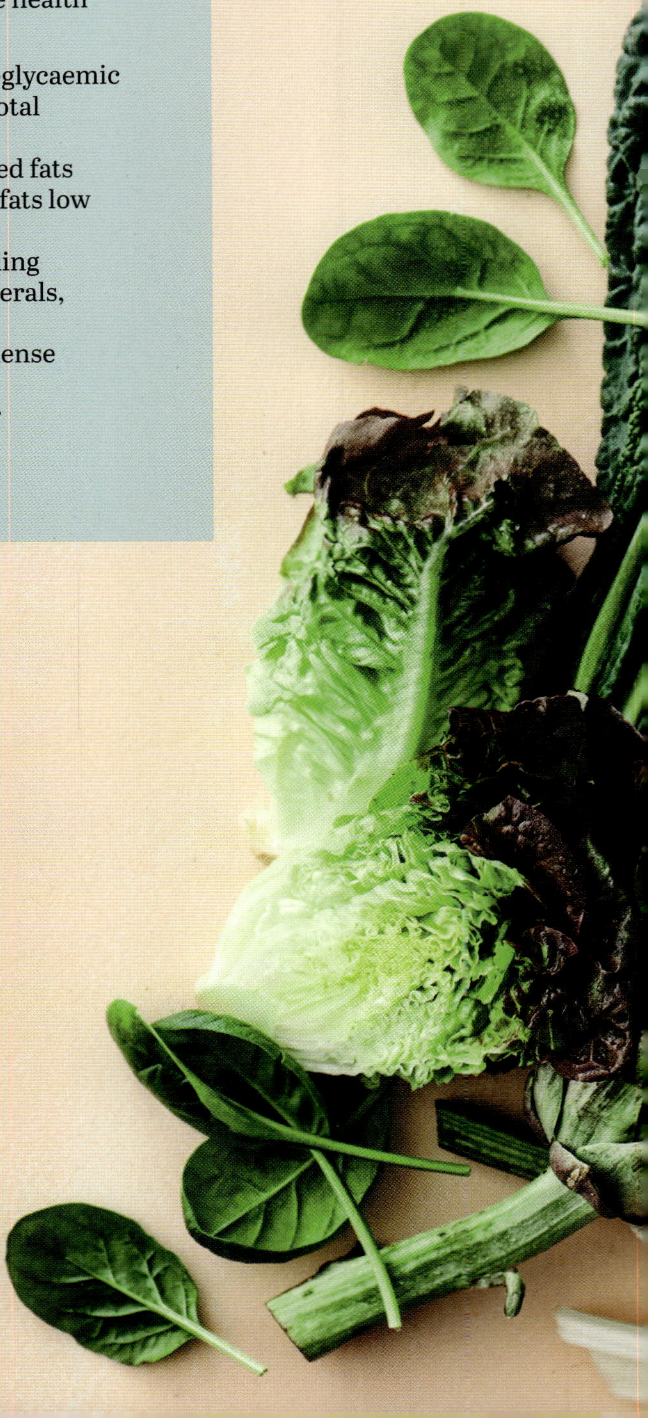

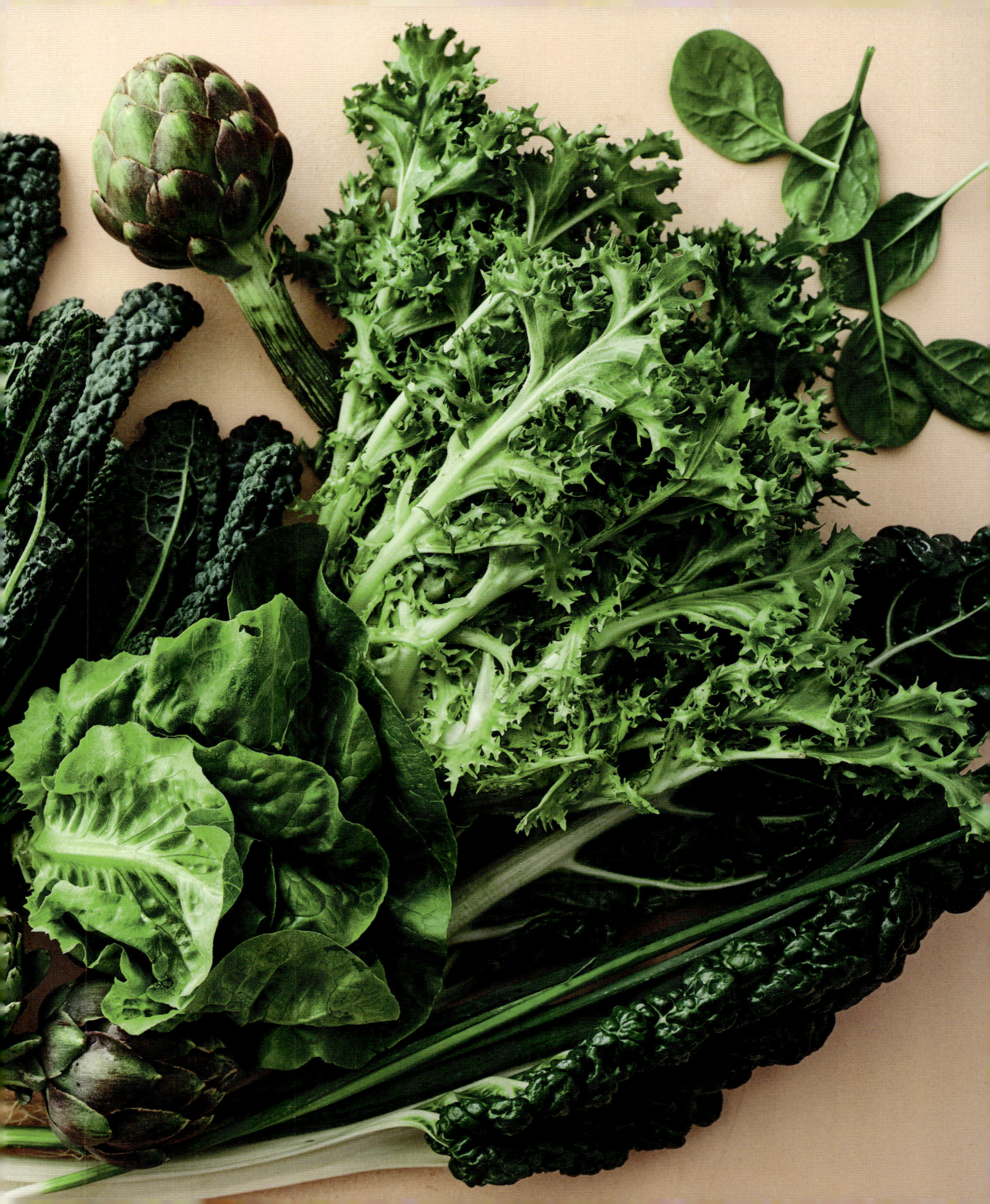

An easy-to-follow diet and lifestyle program

Due to the significance of these research findings, the enormous health improvements that can be achieved with low-carbohydrate diets, and the popular demand from both health professionals and the public to use these scientific evidence–based principles to improve health outcomes, we translated our proven CSIRO Low-carb Diet and lifestyle approach into a comprehensive, easy-to-follow, self-help book series. With the publication of this volume, the series has now grown to six books.

The CSIRO Low-carb Diet books provide:

- a comprehensive overview of how scientific nutrition principles have evolved over time and the latest scientific evidence behind why this eating approach provides important health benefits
- a simple prescriptive guide of how to follow the CSIRO Low-carb Diet using our unique and purpose-designed food unit system, including a comprehensive list of common food ingredients and education about which foods and how much to choose to personalise a plan for an individual's weight management goals and food preferences. This includes more than 500 delicious and nutritious recipes, from breakfast, lunches and mains, to spice blends, sauces and dressings, beverages and snacks
- fully illustrated home-based exercise plan of combined aerobic and resistance exercise training to complement and enhance the benefits of the diet plan.

These books and this evidenced-based eating and lifestyle approach have had an enormous uptake by Australians and have helped so many people reduce their weight and improve their health. This has included helping Australians maintain a healthier weight and to dramatically reduce the risk factors for diabetes and heart disease that health professionals aim to achieve in their patients, and to achieve these benefits often with less medication.

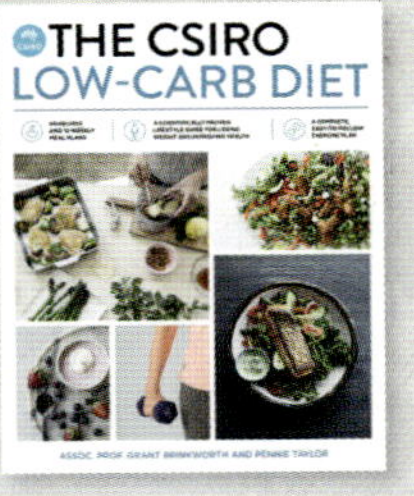

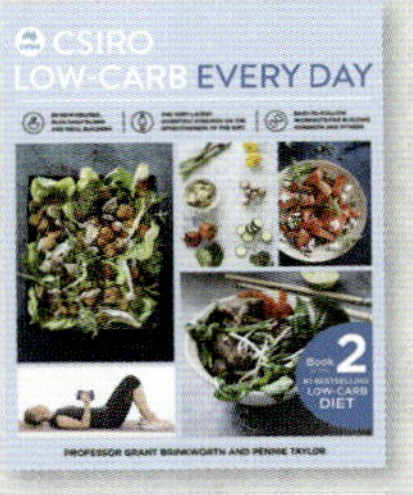

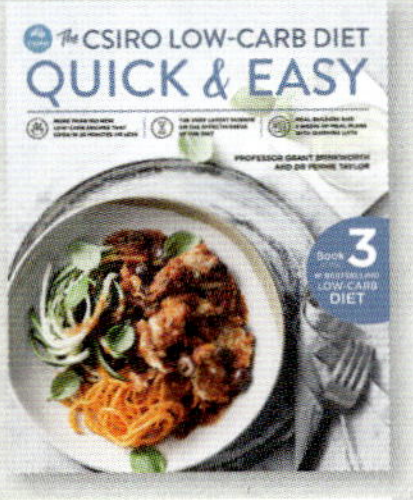

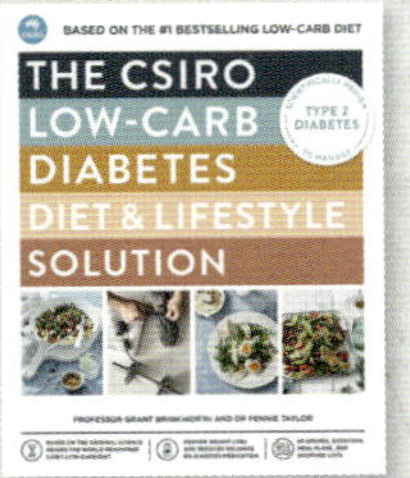

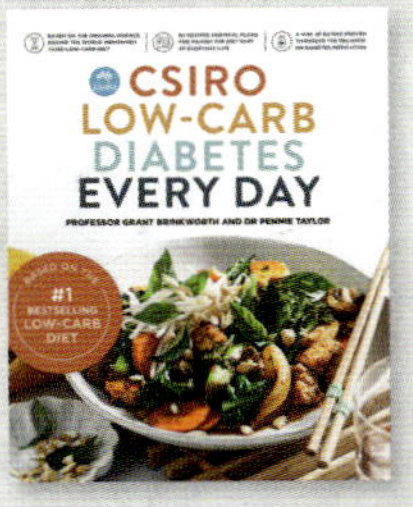

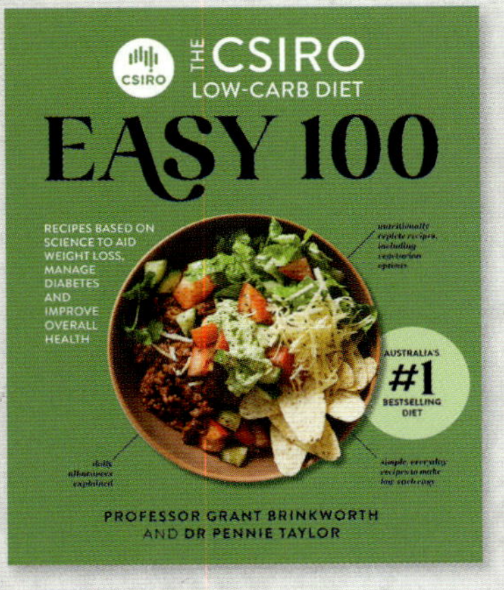

What's new in this book?

We listened to your feedback

The recipes in this book include:

More vegetarian options

Freezable recipes

Recipes for one or two people

Drinks and snacks

Recipes for entertaining

Due to the strong demand and increasing public interest in the use of the CSIRO Low-carb Diet to improve health, there have been increasing requests for more recipes to expand our already existing recipe catalogue, which will add even more flexibility and variety, and make it easier to follow and gain the benefits of the CSIRO Low-carb Diet.

In response, *The CSIRO Low-carb Diet Easy 100* provides a collection of 100 new recipes, all creatively designed to provide enhanced flavour and taste, but to remain consistent with the CSIRO Low-carb Diet food and nutrient specifications.

With evolving food preferences and increasing interest and demand for vegetarian-based recipes, we have also specifically focused on providing more vegetarian recipes to complement those in our previous CSIRO Low-carb Diet books. Followers of the CSIRO Low-carb Diet have also asked for freezable recipe options, as well as solutions when cooking for one or two people, or when entertaining, plus snacks and beverages, so this book addresses those requests.

All recipes use easy-to-access foods available from local markets and supermarkets and have a unit tally for each food group and a carbohydrate flag to help you select recipes for the day, at a glance. This will help you to focus on achieving your 50 grams of daily carbohydrate targets and to make sure you reach your food units for the day so your daily intake has all the essential vitamins, minerals and fibre your body needs for good health (for more information, see page 27).

To help plan and prepare ahead in adopting the CSIRO Low-carb Diet, we understand that having the right foods and ingredients regularly on your shopping list is as important as having the right kitchen utensils and equipment for preparing meals. For this reason, we have also provided lists of what food items we suggest you keep in your kitchen pantry, as well as what equipment to have on hand, which will help you to achieve success and your health goals.

Daily food guide: what foods you can eat

The CSIRO Low-carb Diet provides a flexible eating plan focused on good-quality carbohydrates to help you achieve a low-carbohydrate, high-protein and high healthy fat intake in proportions for good health. The plan remains grounded within the core principles of healthy eating, which emphasise consuming low-energy, nutrient-dense whole foods, all of which can be easily found at your local supermarket.

To make it simple for you, we have listed all foods that can be used as part of your plan and grouped these into five different food groups and outlined how much of each food is equivalent to 1 food unit (a serve size = 1 food unit). This information is summarised in the Daily food guide on pages 24–25.

It is a good idea to first become familiar with the information in the Daily food guide, which will assist you with your shopping and meal planning. A good tip to remember is that, when planning your meals and recipes, you can include smaller amounts of each food from within the same food group to make up 1 full food unit. For example, within the Lean meat, fish, poultry, eggs and tofu category, 100 g (raw weight) of lean meat (chicken, turkey, pork, beef, lamb, kangaroo; fresh or tinned fish or seafood) is equivalent to 1 full unit. This means that you could have 100 g of chicken to achieve 1 unit, or alternatively have 50 g of turkey (equivalent to 0.5 units), 25 g of lamb (equivalent to 0.25 units) and 25 g of seafood (equivalent to 0.25 units), which would also achieve 1 unit.

The simple nature of the plan is that, provided you are consuming the correct number of total food units of each food group every day that corresponds to the number of food units for your energy level (see Food units for your energy level on page 27), you will maintain a daily low-carbohydrate intake of 50 grams each day, as well as receiving all your key nutrients required for good health.

The Daily food guide shows you how much of each allowable food = 1 serve (1 food unit).

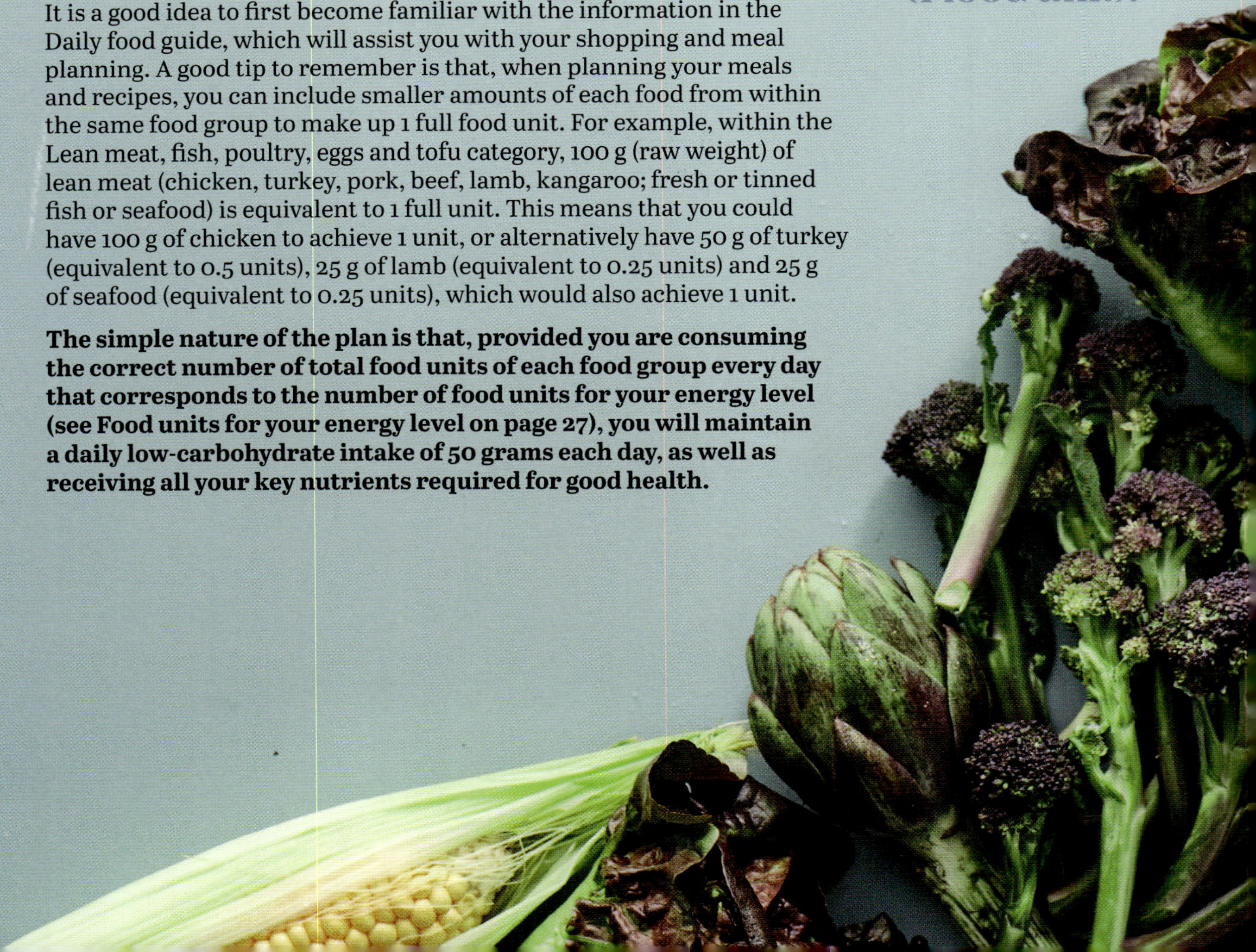

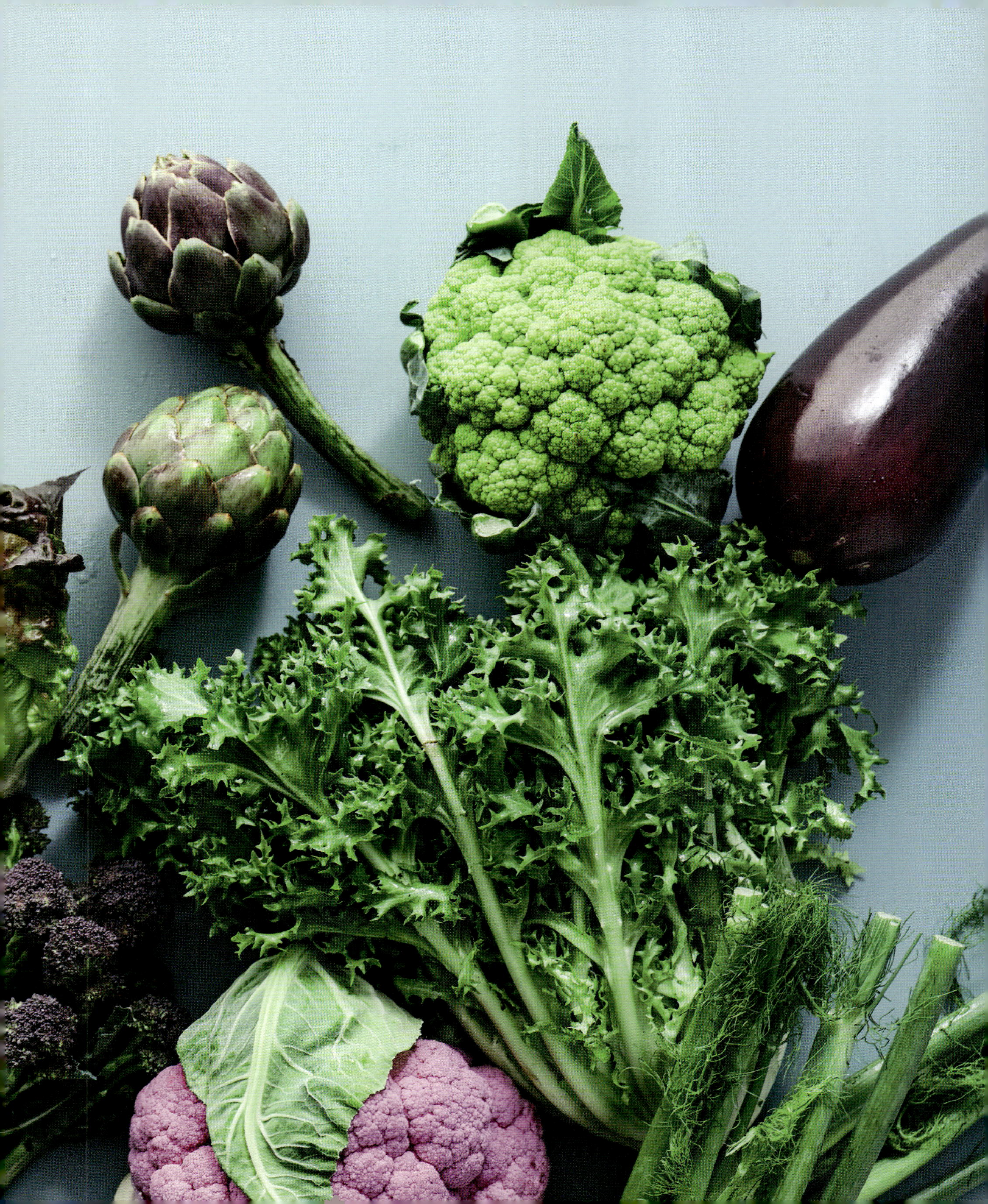

DAILY FOOD GUIDE

Food groups for the diet	Amount of food per 1 food unit
Bread, cereals, legumes, starchy vegetables We recommend using low-GI, wholegrain and resistant starch–rich varieties	**High-soluble-fibre, low-GI cereals** 30 g suitable breakfast cereals (e.g. All-Bran, All-Bran Fibre Toppers, All-Bran Wheat Flakes, Hi-Bran and/or Weet-Bix Protein), untoasted natural muesli with nuts (no fruit), plain rolled oats **Breads** 35 g multigrain bread, seeded breads, dark rye 1 thin (30 g) slice fruit bread ½ (35 g) wholemeal pita bread (e.g. mountain bread wrap) ½ small (25 g) wholemeal scone 3 Ryvitas or 4 rye Cruskits 4 × Vita-Weats 9 Grains 1 slice Herman Brot low-carb bread 25 g wholemeal or wholegrain breadcrumbs **Legumes** 30 g uncooked (dry) or 90 g cooked, drained lentils 25 g uncooked (dry) or 80 g cooked, drained chickpeas or red kidney beans 35 g uncooked (dry) or 100 g cooked, drained cannellini beans or four-bean mix **Low-GI, high-starch vegetables** 100 g white potato 100 g sweet potato 70 g corn **Grains and other** 15 g wholemeal plain or self-raising flour, including wholemeal wheat flour, cornflour, rice flour, arrowroot, chickpea flour (besan), green banana flour, tapioca starch, almond meal, baking powder, buckwheat groats (uncooked) 20 g uncooked commercial low-GI rice 25 g uncooked commercial soba noodles 30 g uncooked commercial low-GI pasta 20 g uncooked (dry) or 40 g cooked quinoa or couscous 20 g uncooked (dry) freekeh 20 g low-salt corn chips
Dairy When choosing dairy alternatives, select types with 'added calcium' on the label	200 ml plain skim milk, low-fat cow's milk, calcium-enriched soy milk, almond milk, macadamia milk 180 ml full-fat milk 18 g full-fat milk powder 20 g skim milk powder 150 ml reduced-fat evaporated milk 100 g plain unflavoured yoghurt or plain lactose-free soy yoghurt 20 g cheddar, haloumi, parmesan, Swiss, goat's or feta cheese 55 g ricotta or cottage cheese 25 g mozzarella, bocconcini or reduced-fat cream cheese
Lean meat, fish, poultry, eggs, tofu	100 g (raw weight) lean meat or fish: fresh or tinned fish or seafood, chicken, turkey, pork, beef, lamb, kangaroo 2 × 55 g whole eggs 100 g tofu (firm or silken), tempeh or textured vegetable protein (TVP) where soy provides at least 90% of protein source

Low–moderate carbohydrate vegetables Be careful to observe smaller serving sizes. Additional moderate-carbohydrate vegetables and low-carbohydrate fruits have been added to provide greater flexibility in your daily choices.	**Low-carbohydrate vegetables (choose at least 3 units per day)** 150 g uncooked or frozen (raw), or 75 g cooked (or raw salad vegetables) of any of the following: artichoke (high-resistant starch), asparagus, bean sprouts, bok choy, broccoli, broccolini, cabbage (mustard and Chinese), chillies, choy sum, cucumber, cumquat, gai lan (Chinese broccoli), garlic, grapefruit, kale, lemon, lettuce (all varieties), lime, loquat, mushrooms, nori, rocket, silverbeet, spinach (English and baby), tomatoes, witlof (endive), zucchini (and zucchini noodles/zoodles) and fresh herbs and spices 150 ml tomato passata (no added sugar or salt) 75 g tinned tomatoes (no added salt) **Moderate-carbohydrate vegetables (maximum of 2 units per day)** 150 g uncooked or frozen (raw), 75 g cooked (or raw salad vegetables) of any of the following: bamboo shoots, broad beans, brussels sprouts, cabbage, capsicum (all colours), carrot, cauliflower (and cauliflower rice), celery, eggplant, fennel, green beans, leek, micro greens, onion, parsnip, radish, spring onion, snow peas, sugar snap peas, shallots, swede, turnip 100 g cooked edamame 75 g uncooked or frozen (raw) beetroot, green peas, pumpkin 10 g sun-dried tomatoes 80 g raw or frozen mixed berries, including strawberry, blueberry, raspberry, blackberry, mulberry
Healthy fats	5 g (1 teaspoon) oil – olive, grapeseed, flaxseed (linseed), sunflower, macadamia, sesame, chilli 5 g (1 teaspoon) tahini 5 g (1 teaspoon) cashew butter and other nut butters (sugar free) 5 g (1 teaspoon) oil-based pesto 5 g (1 teaspoon) oil-based curry paste 20 g (1 tablespoon) hummus 5 g (1 teaspoon) margarine – Nuttelex or olive oil–based or canola-based margarine 20 g whole-egg mayonnaise 20 g avocado 10 g unsalted nuts or seeds – almonds, brazil nuts, flaxseed (linseed) flakes, macadamias, pecans, pine nuts, pumpkin seeds (pepitas), pistachios, poppy seeds, sesame seeds, walnuts 10 g almond meal 20 g olives 10 g coconut flakes
Indulgence foods Use these foods sparingly	**Limit to 2 units a week** 150 ml wine 20 g chocolate 40 g store-bought low-fat dips 10 Arnott's Shapes 1 × 20 g packet of chips 10 Pringles ½ slice of pizza 35 g hot chips
Condiments/other These items are free to use daily	Artificial sweeteners, cacao nibs, capers, clear soup, coconut flakes, curry powder, diet jelly, diet topping, espresso, fish sauce, ginger, harissa, herbal teas (sugar-free), hoisin sauce, hot sauce, kombucha (sugar-free), matcha, mustard powder or creams, nori sheets, oil-free dressings, soda water, soy sauce, sriracha, stock cubes, tamari, tomato salsa, vanilla extract/paste/beans, Vegemite, vinegar (including white, red wine, rice wine, apple cider), stevia, za'atar

Daily food units: how much to eat per day

The table opposite shows you how many units of each food group you should consume per day for each energy level. Obviously as the energy levels increase, the number of food units within each food group also increases to provide that additional energy and nutrient requirements.

In order to know which energy level is best for you, you will need to do a few simple calculations (see page 28).

TIP: If you feel you need more or less energy than is allowed for your level, you can move up and down in the levels until you experience your desired changes. Seeking support and speaking to your GP about seeing your local dietitian for guidance can also be beneficial.

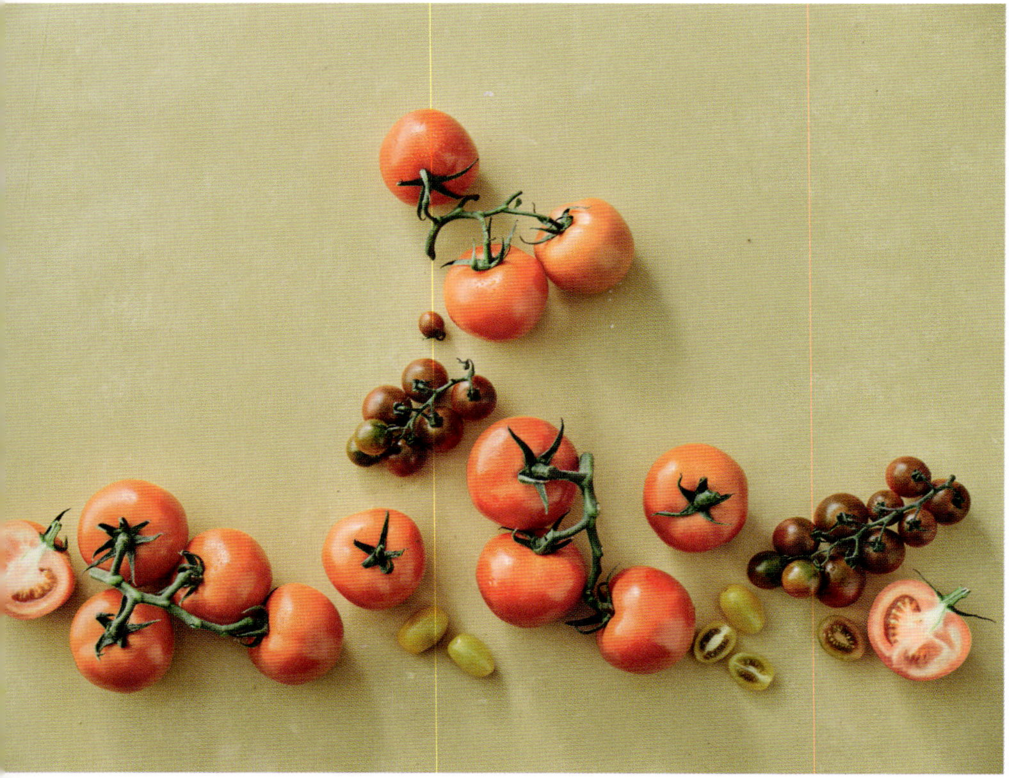

FOOD UNITS FOR YOUR ENERGY LEVEL

The table below shows you the different food groups, how many units of that food group you should eat per day for your energy level, and the key nutrients provided.

Eating the correct amount of food units for your energy level will ensure you maintain a daily carbohydrate intake of 50 grams each day, as well as receiving the key nutrients required for good health.

Food groups for the diet	Level 1 (6000 kJ/day)	Level 2 (7000 kJ/day)	Level 3 (8000 kJ/day)	Level 4 (9000 kJ/day)	Key nutrients provided
Breads, cereals, legumes, starchy vegetables	1.5 units	1.5 units	1.5 units	1.5 units	Slow-release, low-GI carbohydrates, folate, fibre and B-group vitamins.
Dairy	3 units	3 units	3.5 units	4 units	Protein, calcium, vitamin B12 and zinc. Dairy (except most cheeses) also contains carbohydrates.
Lean meat, fish, poultry, eggs, tofu *	1 unit lunch 1.5 units dinner	1 unit lunch 2 units dinner	1 unit lunch 2.5 units dinner	1.5 units lunch 2.5 units dinner	Protein, zinc and vitamin B12. Red meats are highest in iron, fish in omega-3 fatty acids and pork in thiamin.
Low–moderate carb vegetables	At least 5 units (maximum 2 units from moderate-carb vegetables)	At least 5 units (maximum 2 units from moderate-carb vegetables)	At least 5 units (maximum 2 units from moderate-carb vegetables)	At least 5 units (maximum 2 units from moderate-carb vegetables)	Minimal carbohydrates, and plenty of fibre, folate, vitamins A, B6 and C, magnesium, beta-carotene and antioxidants.
Healthy fats	10 units	11 units	14 units	15 units	Vitamins A, E and K, antioxidants and omega-3 and omega-6 fats.
Indulgences (optional)	2 units per week	2 units per week	2 units per week	2 units per week	Limited beneficial nutrients. Most contain added sugars, alcohol and/or saturated fats.
Optional carbohydrate extras	2 extras per day	2 extras per day	2 extras per day	2 extras per day	Carbohydrates. They also contribute vitamins and minerals as they come from your core food units.

* For flexibility you can use ½ unit of this food group at breakfast, keeping in mind you will need to reduce your lunch or dinner portion by ½ unit.

CALCULATE YOUR ENERGY LEVEL

Before you start the CSIRO Low-carb Diet, it's vital to determine your estimated daily energy requirements to determine which energy level would be the most appropriate for you and how many food units from each food group you should be consuming each day. This involves calculating your basal metabolic rate (BMR) and multiplying it by your daily activity factor. Once you calculate your specific energy requirements, you will not only ensure that the energy level of your diet plan is tailored to your personal needs, so you can attain and maintain a healthy body weight, but you will know how much of each food group you should eat in order to achieve the right energy and nutrient balance for your body size and exercise levels.

Determine your daily kilojoule (energy) requirements

The calculation on the opposite page was used in our scientific trial to personalise the diet to each participant's energy needs. It estimates your daily kilojoule requirements to keep your weight stable. Simply follow the steps.

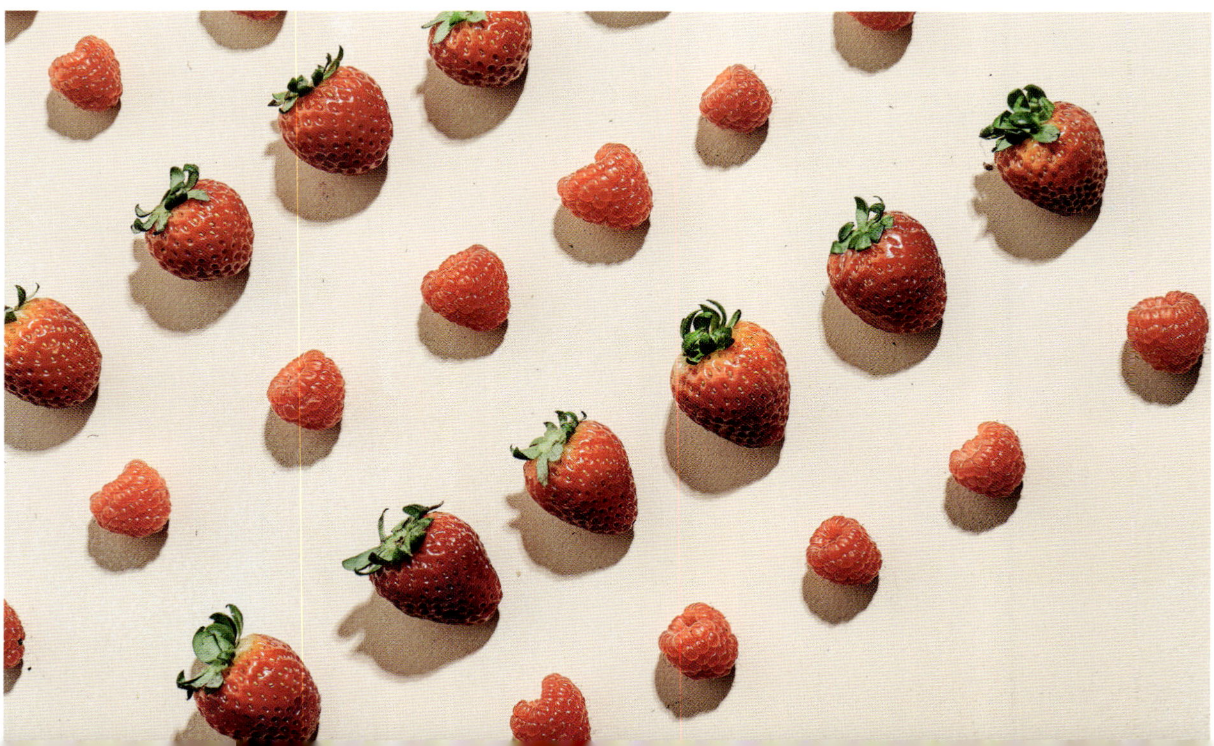

1 Calculate your basal metabolic rate

First, by using the table below, calculate your BMR, or basal metabolic rate.

	BMR equation	
Age (years)	**Women**	**Men**
18–29	(62 × weight in kilograms) + 2036	(63 × weight in kilograms) + 2896
30–59	(34 × weight in kilograms) + 3538	(48 × weight in kilograms) + 3653
60 and over	(38 × weight in kilograms) + 2755	(49 × weight in kilograms) + 2459

Note: There are a few different methods for calculating BMR. We've used the Schofield Equation.

2 Rate your activity factor

		Activity factor	
Activity level	**Description**	**Women**	**Men**
Sedentary	Very physically inactive (work and leisure)	1.3	1.3
Lightly active	Daily activity of walking or intense exercise once or twice a week and a sedentary job	1.5	1.6
Moderately active	Intense exercise lasting 20–45 minutes at least three times a week or an active job with a lot of daily walking	1.6	1.7
Very active	Intense exercise lasting at least 1 hour each day or a heavy, physical job	1.9	2.1
Extremely active	Daily intense activity (i.e. nonstop training, such as an athlete in training) or a highly demanding physical job (e.g. armed forces)	2.2	2.4

3 Multiply your BMR by your activity factor

This figure will allow you to estimate your total daily kilojoule requirements in order to maintain your current weight. Check the table on page 27 to find your corresponding energy level.

Sample calculation for Kim, 56 years old, female weighing 82 kilograms with an activity level of 'lightly active':

BMR **= (34 × weight in kilograms) + 3538**
= (34 × 82) + 3538
= 6326 kJ per day

To calculate her total daily kilojoule requirements, Kim multiplies her BMR by her activity factor:

Total daily energy requirement **= 6326 × 1.5**
= 9489 kilojoules per day

Note: If Kim wanted to continue to maintain their current body weight, rounding down to the 9000 kJ/day (Level 4) meal plan would be ideal. If your activity level changes or weight loss occurs, it is always good practice to revisit this calculation for relevant energy needs.

MAINTAINING OR LOSING WEIGHT

If you're a healthy weight, there's no need to reduce your energy intake, so the number you're left with now is your **daily kilojoule requirement**, and you can use this number to choose the correct level for you of the CSIRO Low-carb Diet by checking the Food units for your energy level table on page 27. See also How to assess your body weight status on page 258 to find out if you are overweight or obese.

If you need to lose weight, calculate your estimated daily kilojoule requirement as follows.

In order to reduce your weight by about 0.5 kilograms each week, you'll need to reduce your energy intake by 2000 kilojoules per day. Once you've calculated your total daily kilojoule requirements, subtract 2000 from this number to determine how many kilojoules to eat each day to achieve this rate of weight loss and, therefore, which of the four energy levels to choose.

To reduce your weight by about 1 kilogram each week, you'll need to reduce your energy intake by 4000 kilojoules per day. Calculate your total daily kilojoule needs and subtract 4000. This will tell you how many kilojoules to eat each day to achieve this rate of weight loss and, therefore, which of the four energy levels to choose.

Note: If your chosen level isn't working, you can move between levels until you start to see the changes you desire. Many people hit a weight-loss plateau after an initial drop in weight. If this happens, you can switch to a lower level until you reach your target weight. Your dietitian and exercise physiologist can also help you to overcome a plateau.

NOW THAT YOU:

1. have calculated and determined your desired energy requirements
2. identified the energy level within the energy level table that tells you how many units of each food category should be consumed each day
3. know which foods are categorised into each food group and how much food is equal to 1 food unit

. . . you are now ready to go. By eating the correct number of food units within each food category for your desired energy level means you are following the CSIRO Low-carb Diet. It is that simple.

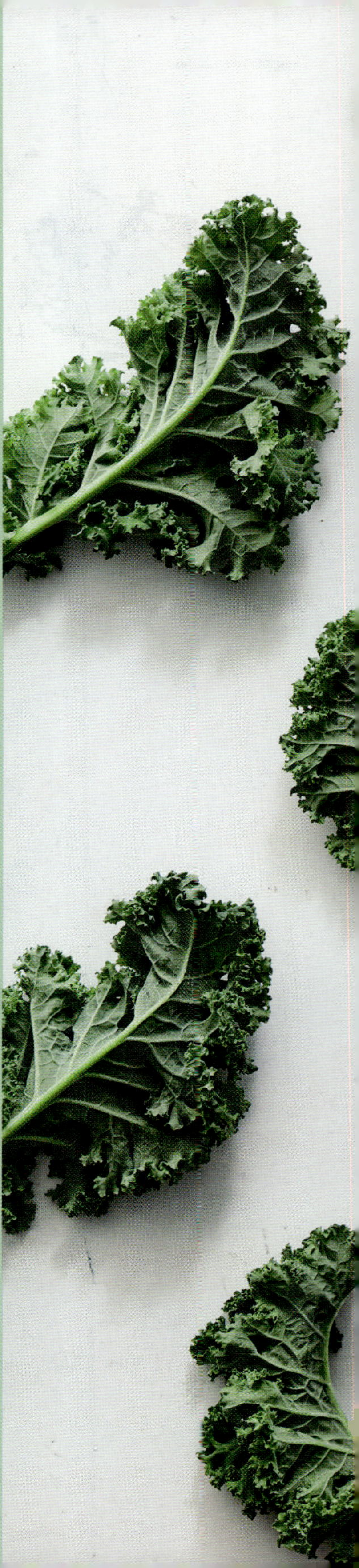

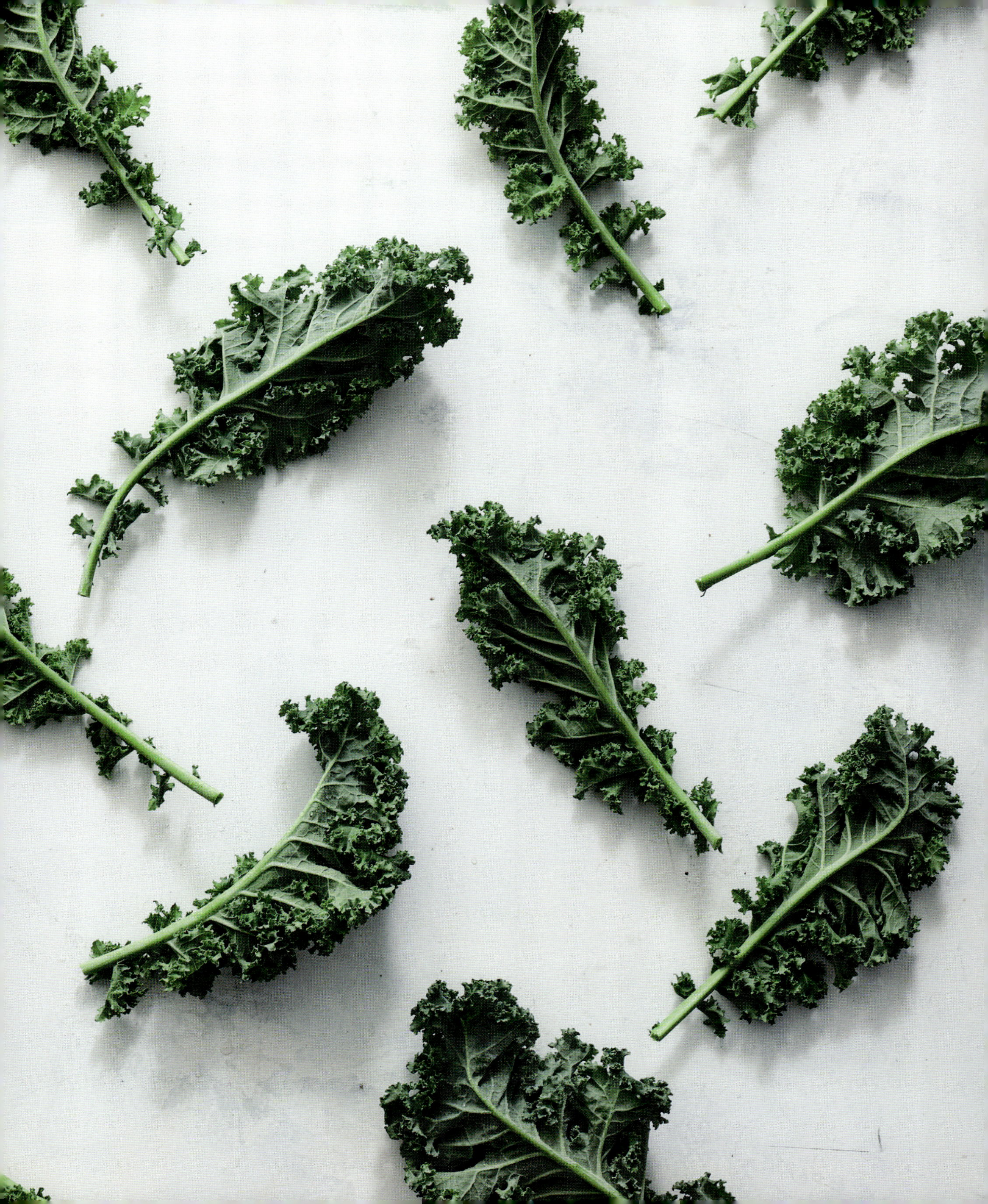

Optional carbohydrate extras

It has been our experience through clinical trials and feedback received from people following the CSIRO Low-carb Diet, that it is best to start with the base structure of the diet plan (as outlined on the previous pages, without any optional carbohydrate extras). This will provide you with 50 grams of total carbohydrate per day, provided you are consuming the food units in the required amounts for your chosen energy level.

Over time, as you become more confident and knowledgeable about how this dietary approach benefits you, and how to use the food units effectively, you may find you need greater flexibility based on your food preferences, exercise levels or that you just desire to have a little more carbohydrate in your diet. If you are using this diet to reduce your body weight, it could also be at a stage where you just want to maintain your new lower body weight. If this is you, there is the option to increase your daily carbohydrate intake by 20 grams, or 2 carbohydrate extras (10 g of carbohydrate per carbohydrate extra) to reach a target of 70 grams of total carbohydrate per day.

We have included a list of these carbohydrate 'extras' (see opposite) to guide you in making selections in the right type and amount of these added extras so you can adjust your carbohydrate intake yourself.

Our research suggests that these 'extras' are best used as snacks between meals, especially if you are finding yourself hungry at 3pm, or are exercising and need a small snack to 'replenish' you. However, if you decide to add these to meals, add them to meals that are already lowest in carbohydrate. You can identify these meals by looking at the carbohydrate flag on the recipes. Also, it is best to add these to the part of the day where you are most active – for many this is between breakfast and dinner, not late at night.

Remember: Adding the 20 g or 2 serves of carbohydrate extras per day is completely OPTIONAL.

Please see the recipes Banana tahini pancakes on page 221 and Espresso banana smoothie on page 228 for examples on how to use your optional carb extras.

Check the effect of carb extras

To find out if adding the carbohydrate 'extras' is right for you and not making your blood levels spike dramatically, you should measure your blood glucose levels 2 hours after eating, to assess the effect of these extras on your blood glucose control. It is also important to monitor your weight. If you start to regain body weight, it could mean that you do not really need the carbohydrate 'extras' in your day.

1 serving = 1 carb extra (10 grams of carbohydrate or less)

Fruit	
Apples	50 g
Apricots, dried	20 g
Apricots, fresh	2 medium
Bananas	40 g
Blueberries, frozen or fresh	60 g
Cherries	60 g
Dates, dried	2
Figs, dried	20 g
Kiwifruit	1
Mixed fruit, dried	10 g
Orange	100 g
Pear	50 g
Raspberries, frozen or fresh	100 g
Strawberries	200 g
Sultanas	10 g
Vegetables	
Corn kernels, tinned, cooked	40 g
Green peas, fresh, cooked, no added fat	120 g
Pumpkin, uncooked	120 g
Sweet potato, peeled, baked, no added fat	50 g
Dairy	
Reduced-fat evaporated milk (e.g. Carnation)	100 ml
Reduced-fat Greek-style yoghurt	75 g
Skim milk	100 ml

Bread, grains, crackers	
Quinoa, uncooked	15 g
Quinoa, cooked, no added fat	48 g
Couscous, uncooked	10 g
Couscous, cooked, no added fat	40 g
Corn cakes/thins, multigrain	2 cakes
Vita-Weats, regular	2 biscuits
Rice crackers (e.g. Sakata, Fantastic)	5 crackers
Wholegrain bread	½ regular slice
Mountain bread (wholegrain)	½ regular rectangle
Fruit loaf	½ regular slice
Scone, wholemeal (commercial)	½ small (20 g)
Tortilla, corn	½ small
Beans and legumes	
Cannellini beans, cooked and drained	50 g
Chickpeas, cooked and drained	40 g
Four-bean mix, cooked and drained	40 g
Lentils, cooked and drained	80 g
Lentils, dried	15 g
Red kidney beans, cooked and drained	40 g

The recipes and how to use them

Now that you've worked out your energy level, and have become familiar with the Daily food guide, which includes the types of foods and how much of them you can eat, it's time to put it all together and start planning your meals.

The tasty and easy-to-prepare recipes in *The CSIRO Low-carb Diet Easy 100* have all been designed using foods from the Daily food guide in the recommended portions. To make it easy for you to use these recipes to follow the CSIRO Low-carb Diet eating plan, each recipe indicates the number of food units from each food group in a serve of the recipe.

If you are using a specific recipe, all you need to do is subtract these units from your daily food unit allowances when planning your daily meal intake, to ensure you are eating the correct number of units of each food group for your corresponding energy level; it is that simple. In addition, in most of the recipes we have ensured the carbohydrate amount of all foods combined in each recipe does not exceed 20 grams per serve. The aim is for you to use these details to monitor your daily carbs (50 grams daily) and your daily unit allowance.

In some cases, you may find that you have 'left-over food units', that is, you may not reach all the food units across your day just by using the recipes. Often, healthy fat units, dairy units or vegetable units may not reach your target.

If so, this is not a bad thing as it means that you can use any left-over food units as top-ups to your meals, or as allowable snacks throughout the day. For example, if you have 1 unit of dairy, 2 units of healthy fats and 0.5 units of low–moderate carbohydrate vegetables left over from your day, you can create a dip plate of 20 g hummus (1 unit healthy fat) + sliced cucumber, celery and capsicum sticks (0.5 units low–moderate carb vegetables) + 100 g natural yoghurt (1 unit dairy) + 10 g nuts (1 unit healthy fat). See the sample day on the level 1 diet on pages 36–37.

Devise your own recipes

Check the portion sizes and food units in the Daily food guide to help you to construct a dish that includes the correct amount of ingredients for your personal plan.

Number of food units from each food group per serve

Carbohydrates per serve

UNITS PER SERVE:	
Bread, Cereals, Legumes, Starchy Veg	0
Dairy	0
Lean Meat, Fish, Poultry, Eggs, Tofu	1.5
Low-Moderate Carbohydrate Veg	3
Healthy Fats	3

Chicken with Chimichurri Sauce

CARBS 8 g PER SERVE

SERVES: 4 | PREPARATION: 30 MINUTES + 20 MINUTES–24 HOURS MARINATING | COOKING: 15 MINUTES

2 × 300 g chicken breast fillets, visible fat removed, sliced in half horizontally to make 2 thin steaks
3 zucchini, sliced lengthways

CHIMICHURRI SAUCE
½ cup finely chopped oregano leaves
1 bunch flat-leaf parsley, roughly chopped
5 cloves garlic, crushed
1 teaspoon sweet paprika
½ teaspoon ground cumin
Pinch dried chilli flakes
¼ cup (60 ml) red wine vinegar
2 tablespoons extra virgin olive oil

TOMATO SALAD
500 g tomatoes, cut into wedges
½ small red onion, thinly sliced
1 tablespoon red wine vinegar
1 tablespoon extra virgin olive oil
¼ teaspoon freshly ground black pepper

1. Add all the ingredients for the chimichurri sauce to a food processor and blitz for about 2 minutes until finely chopped and well combined. Allow to sit for 20 minutes, or up to overnight, in the refrigerator to allow the flavours to develop.
2. To make the tomato salad, place all the ingredients in a bowl and toss to combine. Set aside to marinate.
3. Place half the chimichurri sauce in a large bowl with the chicken steaks and toss to coat.
4. Preheat a barbecue grill plate to high or a chargrill pan on the stovetop over high heat. Cook the chicken steaks for 4 minutes on each side, or until cooked through and charred. Set aside to rest, loosely covered with foil. Add the zucchini slices to the barbecue and cook for 2 minutes on each side until charred and softened.
5. Divide the chicken, zucchini and tomato salad between four plates, spoon over the remaining chimichurri sauce and serve.

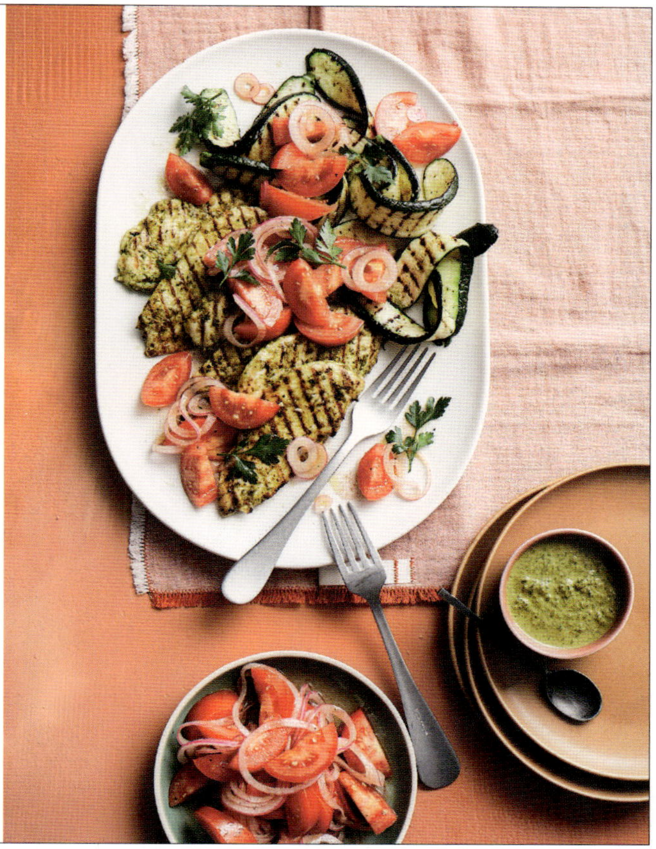

A SAMPLE DAY ON THE DIET FOR LEVEL 1 (6000 KJ)

Daily unit requirements are: Breads, cereals, legumes, starchy veg = 1.5 units | Lean meat, fish, poultry, tofu = 2.5 units | Dairy = 3 units | Low–moderate carbohydrate vegetables = at least 5 units | Healthy fats = 10 units

BREAKFAST

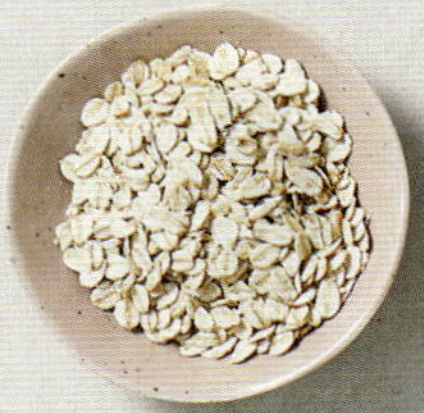

30 g raw oats
(1 unit Breads, cereals, legumes, starchy veg)

+

180 ml full-fat milk
(1 unit Dairy)

+

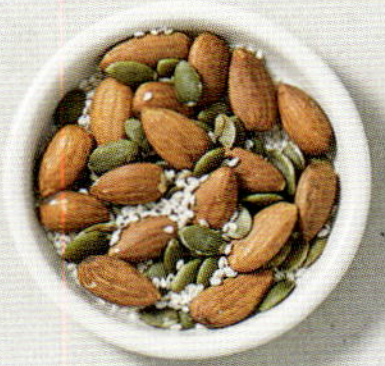

30 g nut and seed mix
(3 units Healthy fats)

+

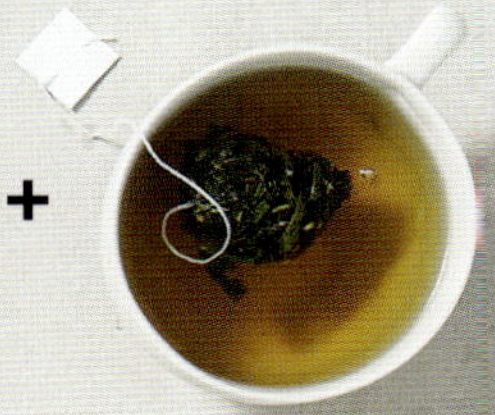

1 cup herbal tea
(no sugar) ('free' item)

LUNCH

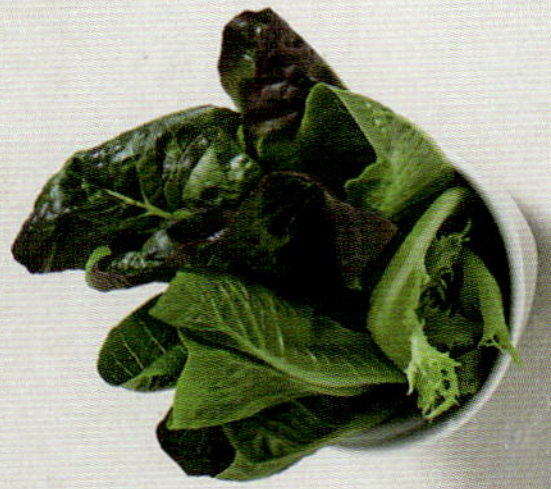

1 cup mixed lettuce
(1 unit Low–moderate carbohydrate veg)

+

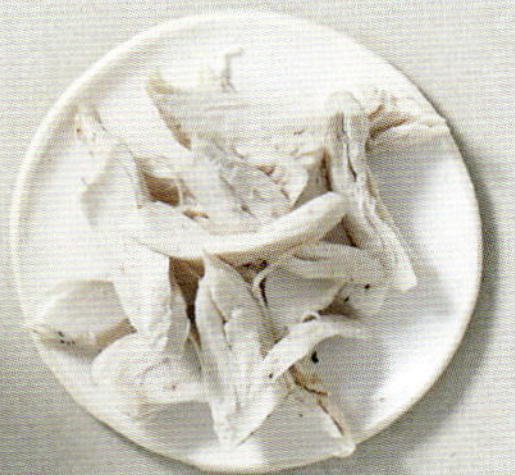

100 g cooked chicken
(1 unit Lean meat, fish, poultry, eggs, tofu)

+

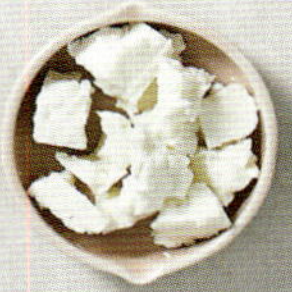

20 g feta cheese
(1 unit Dairy)

+

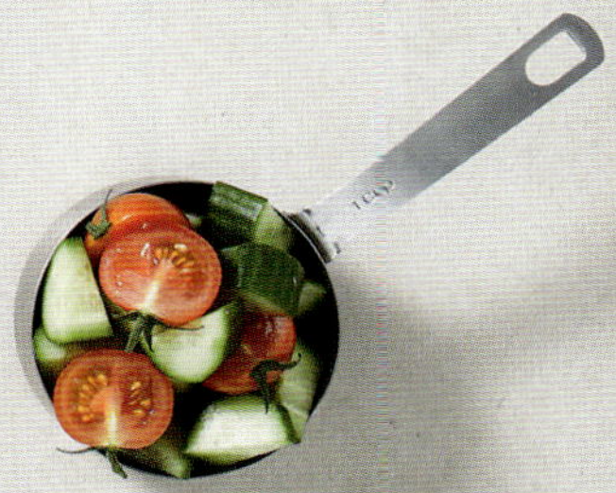

1 cup mixed cucumber and tomato
(1 unit Low–moderate carbohydrate veg)

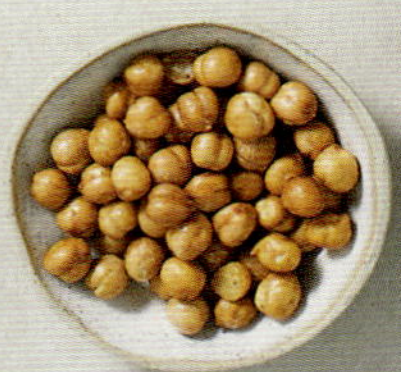

40 g toasted chickpeas
(½ unit Breads, cereals, legumes, starchy veg)

+

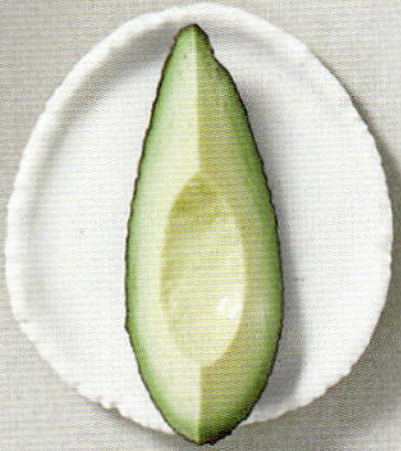

40 g avocado
(2 units Healthy fats)

+

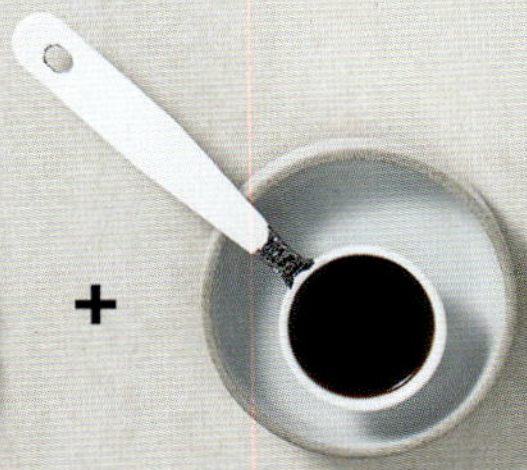

1 tablespoon (20 ml) balsamic vinegar
('free' item)

+

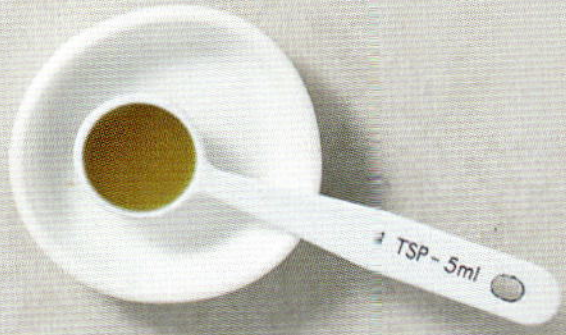

1 teaspoon (5 ml) olive oil
(1 unit Healthy fats)

DINNER

150 g meat, fish, chicken or marinated tofu, grilled to your preference (use a spice rub for flavour) (1.5 units Lean meat, fish, poultry, eggs, tofu)

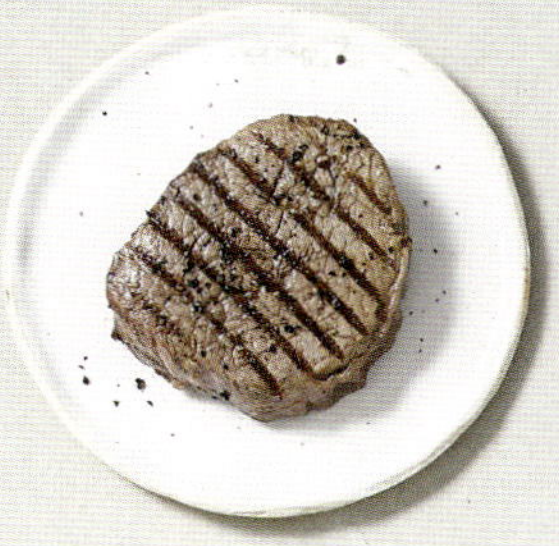

+

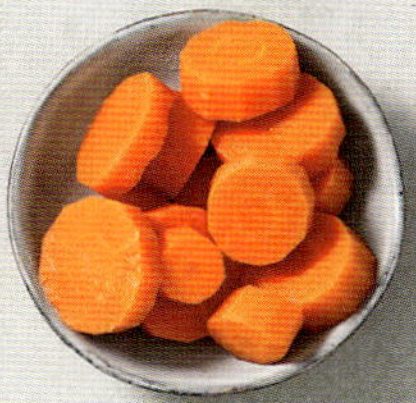

1 cup steamed carrot (1 unit Low–moderate carbohydrate veg)

1.5 cups mixed steamed veg (zucchini, green beans, broccoli) (1.5 units Low–moderate carbohydrate veg)

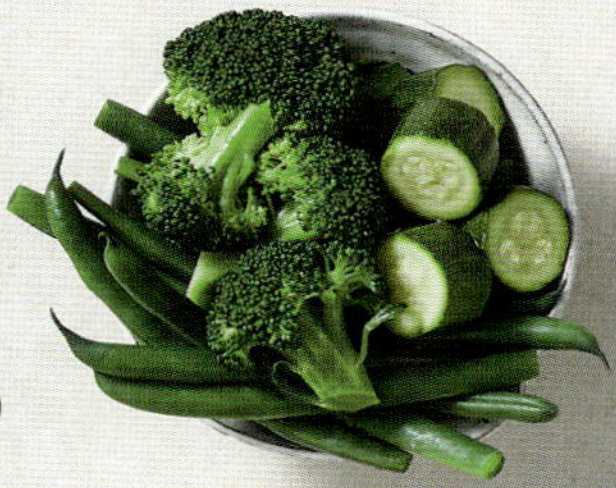

+

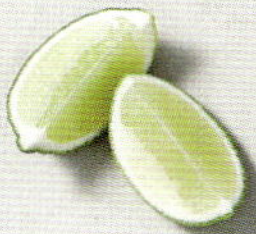

Lime juice, as desired ('free' item)

+

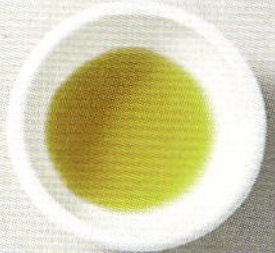

2 teaspoons (10 ml) olive oil for cooking (2 units Healthy fats)

TOTAL UNITS USED

1.5 units Breads, cereals, legumes, starchy veg (full daily allowance used)
2.5 units Lean meat, fish, poultry, tofu (full daily allowance used)
2 units Dairy (from daily allowance of 3 units)
4.5 units Low–moderate carbohydrate vegetables (from daily allowance of 5 units)
8 units Healthy fats (from daily allowance of 10 units)

LEFT OVER FOR UNIT TOP-UPS

1 unit Dairy
2 units Healthy fats
½ unit Low–moderate carbohydrate vegetables

UNIT TOP-UPS

20 g hummus (1 unit Healthy fats)

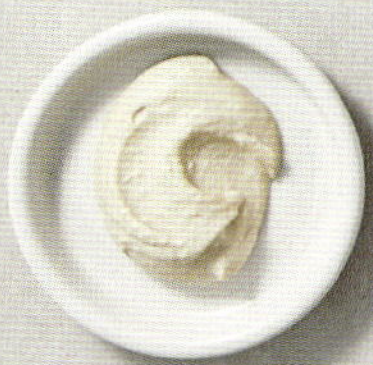

+

Sliced cucumber, celery and capsicum sticks (½ unit Low–moderate carbohydrate veg)

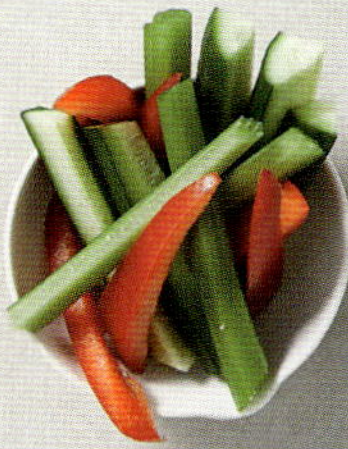

+

100 g natural yoghurt (1 unit Dairy)

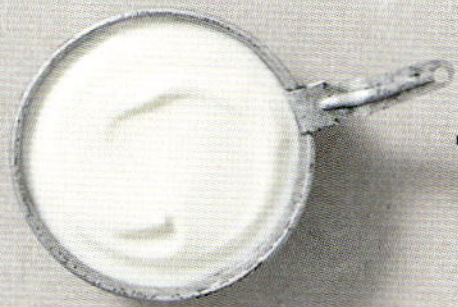

+

10 g nut and seed mix (1 unit Healthy fats)

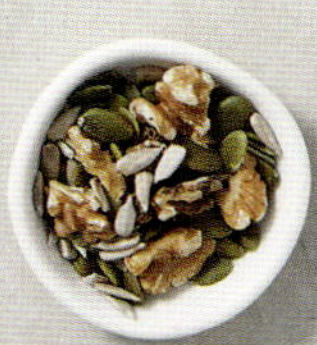

Setting up your CSIRO Low-carb Diet kitchen

If you're someone who can easily pick up new recipes, or even a whole new way of eating, that's great – even better if you are super-organised and have spare time. However, if you are not a natural in the kitchen, or have a busy timetable, here are some ideas to help make starting the CSIRO Low-carb Diet, as well as your continuing journey, a success.

GETTING STARTED

Too often the thoughts 'I am too busy' or 'I don't have the time' are the first barriers. By reading this book you have already jumped the first hurdle to make the commitment to improve your health and lifestyle, so your next step should be to mark in your calendar when you plan to start. Don't make it 'tomorrow' – be realistic. Plan to start in a suitable week, preferably one free of excess commitments and social activities.

You will need a few planning days before you start the diet. Read through the recipes and select a few to cook for, say, the first week (don't forget to bookmark your favourites as you go through). Next, set aside a day to check what ingredients you already have on hand, and what you need to put on your shopping list. Once you've done the shopping, pick a day where you will either have help to prepare and chop ingredients for a whole week or, if you're on your own, for at least two recipes. It's likely that many of the recipes you select will call for the same ingredient. If this is the case, get ahead by prepping the ingredient for the meal you're cooking as well as for the next one.

Store your prepared ingredients separately in clean, airtight containers in the fridge (for up to 3 days) until you are ready to use them. Moving forward, set aside at least one day a week when you can plan and prepare. Sunday is often a great day for planning the week ahead.

It is a good idea to select one recipe that you can portion and freeze. Get in the habit of freezing your left-over portions, or making double quantities for freezing, so you'll have meals to heat and go for your busiest days. Don't forget to label the container with the name of the recipe and the date. Have ziplock bags and airtight containers handy, including microwave-safe ones so you can thaw and heat.

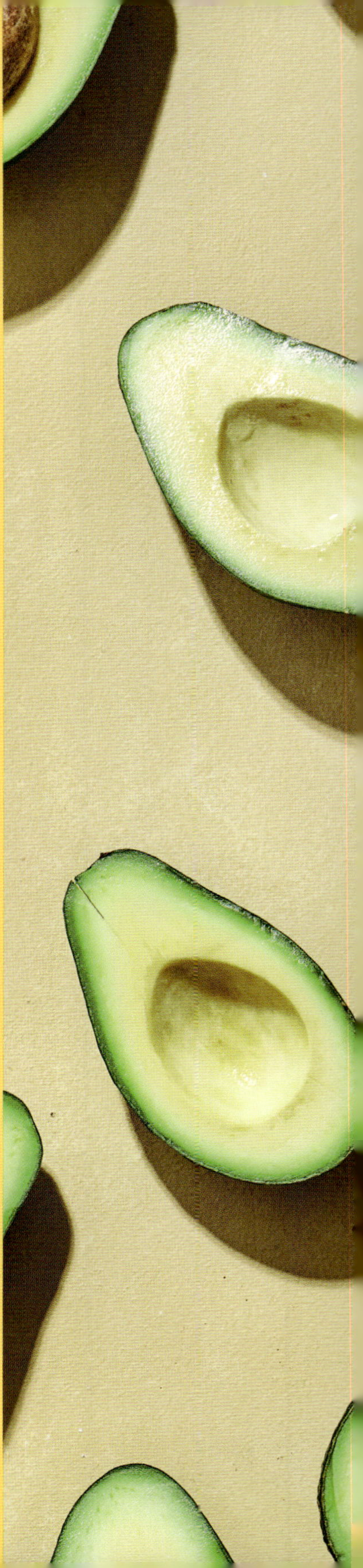

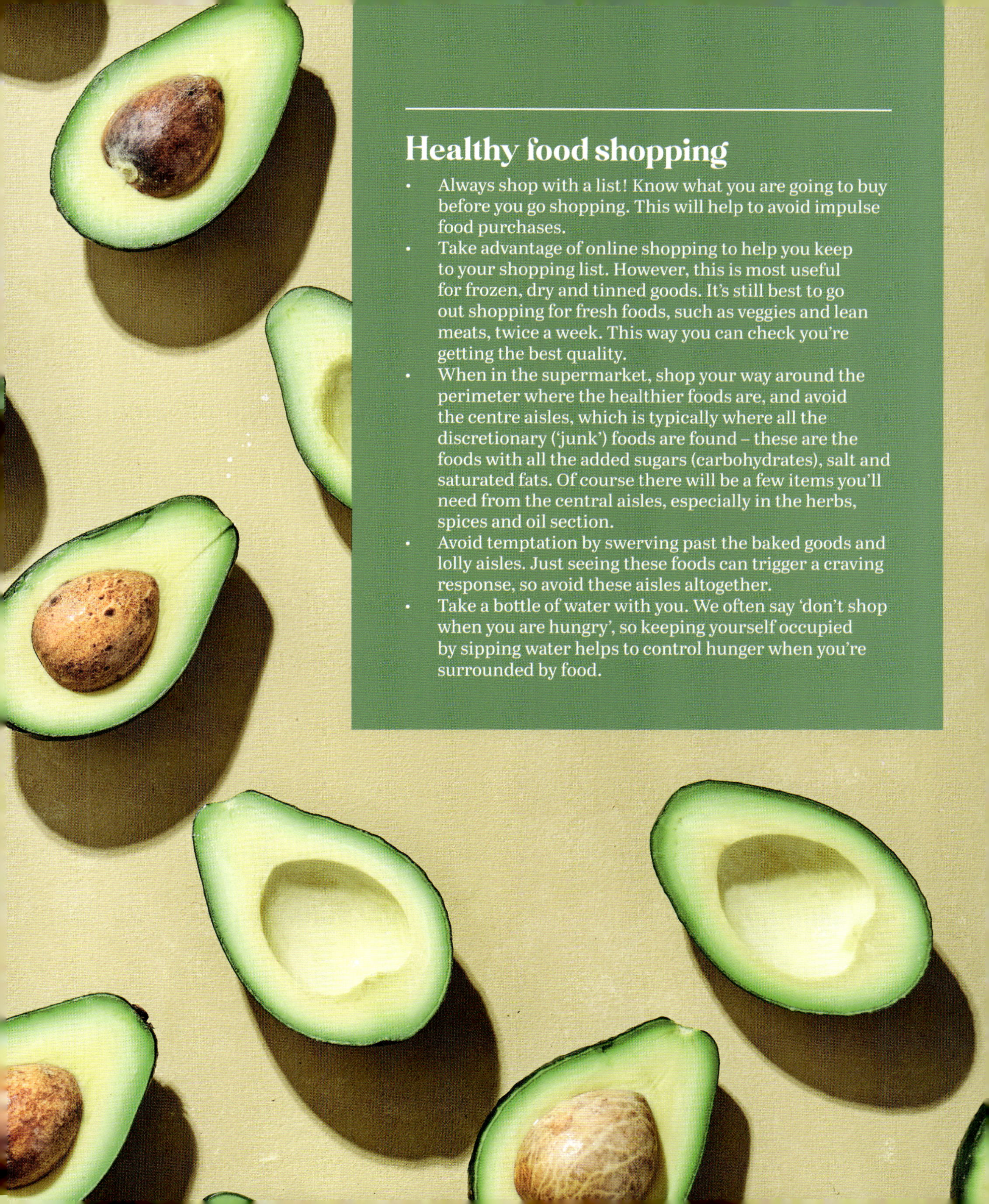

Healthy food shopping

- Always shop with a list! Know what you are going to buy before you go shopping. This will help to avoid impulse food purchases.
- Take advantage of online shopping to help you keep to your shopping list. However, this is most useful for frozen, dry and tinned goods. It's still best to go out shopping for fresh foods, such as veggies and lean meats, twice a week. This way you can check you're getting the best quality.
- When in the supermarket, shop your way around the perimeter where the healthier foods are, and avoid the centre aisles, which is typically where all the discretionary ('junk') foods are found – these are the foods with all the added sugars (carbohydrates), salt and saturated fats. Of course there will be a few items you'll need from the central aisles, especially in the herbs, spices and oil section.
- Avoid temptation by swerving past the baked goods and lolly aisles. Just seeing these foods can trigger a craving response, so avoid these aisles altogether.
- Take a bottle of water with you. We often say 'don't shop when you are hungry', so keeping yourself occupied by sipping water helps to control hunger when you're surrounded by food.

PREPARE YOUR PANTRY

When making major changes to your diet, it doesn't always mean you need to completely clean out your pantry and start from scratch. However, look at the foods you have that don't fit in the new plan and, if you don't want to throw them out, donate them to friends or family. For an at-a-glance guide to the kinds of food you will now be filling your pantry and fridge with, see Stocking your kitchen the CSIRO Low-carb way on pages 42–49.

HAVE THE RIGHT UTENSILS

As you browse through the recipes, you'll see what kitchen equipment you're likely to need. You'll see that the oven, microwave and barbecue are all used. If you don't have a barbecue, you can use a chargrill pan on the stovetop.

Make sure you have the right tools on hand to make meal preparation more efficient and enjoyable. A set of accurate kitchen scales, preferably digital, will be essential for weighing food, as well as accurate cup and spoon measures.

Other useful kitchen equipment:

- mortar and pestle or an electric spice grinder
- food processor
- upright blender and/or stick blender
- wok
- stainless steel bento box/es (optional)
- non-stick frying pan/s
- non-stick baking tray/s
- non-stick muffin tin/s
- jars with lids for storing dressings, spice blends etc.
- microwave-safe containers for freezing
- ziplock bags
- potato masher
- grater (either standard box grater, or an attachment for your food processor)
- spiraliser
- mandoline.

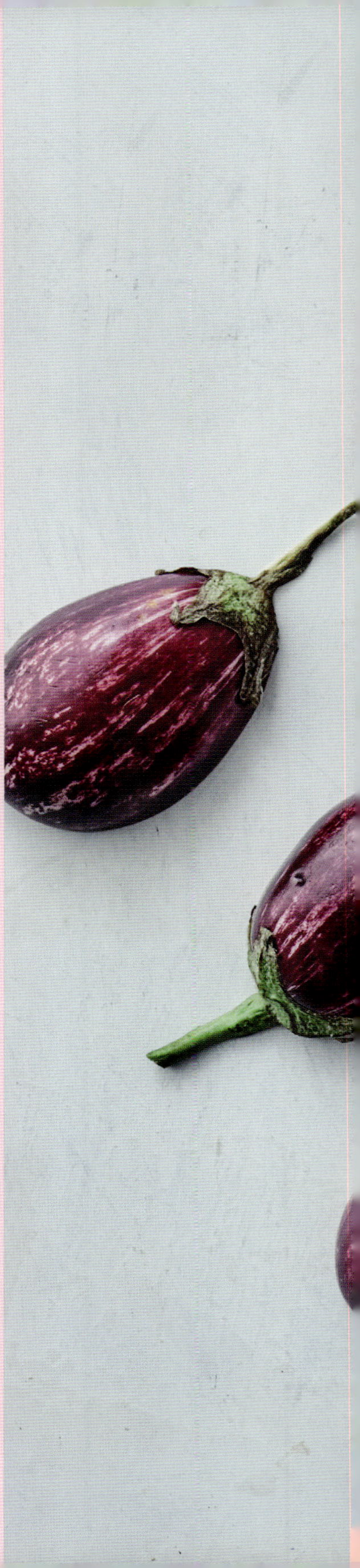

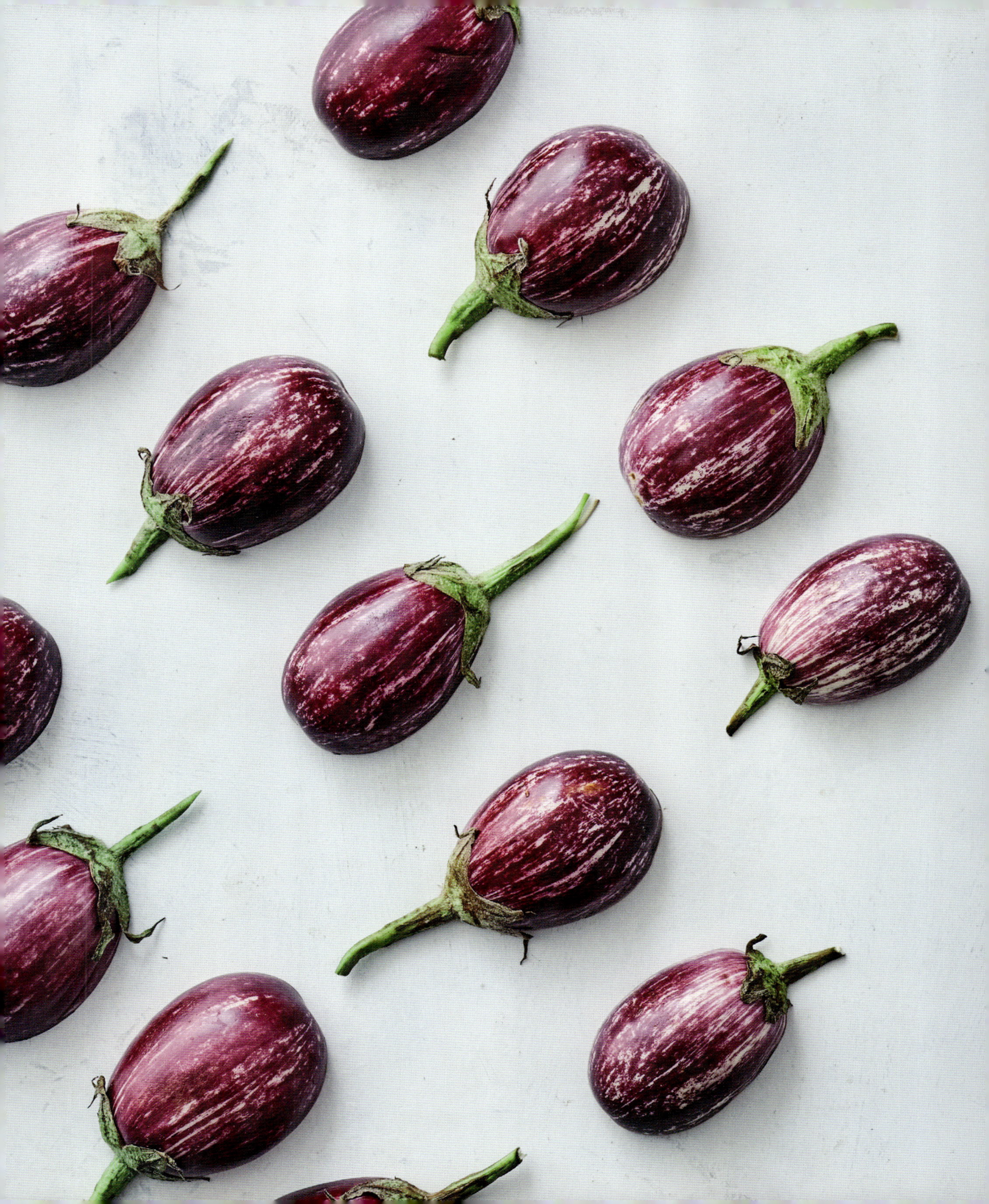

Stocking your kitchen the CSIRO low-carb way

Now that you are eating the CSIRO low-carb way, the contents of your fridge, freezer and pantry might look a little different. To help you sustain this way of eating, here is a guide to the best ingredients to have on hand in your kitchen. For information on the exact ingredients and supermarket items you can use, as well as precise portion sizes, see the Daily food guide on page 24.

BREADS, CEREALS, LEGUMES AND STARCHY VEGETABLES

Most of these items will be stored in the pantry, but your bread and wraps can be frozen for up to 3 months, which is important as these foods will be used least in your day.

Fridge and freezer

- breads – multigrain types
- corn – cobs and kernels

Pantry

- sweet potatoes
- wholegrain bread – wholegrain flat bread, wholegrain pita bread, such as mountain bread wraps
- wholemeal scones
- wholegrain crispbreads – types with seeds are also a good option
- breakfast cereals, such as untoasted natural muesli with nuts but no fruit
- buckwheat groats
- freekeh
- lentils – red and brown, dried or tinned
- quinoa – grains and flakes
- chickpeas, dried or tinned
- red kidney beans, dried or tinned
- cannellini beans, dried or tinned
- four-bean mix, tinned
- green banana flour

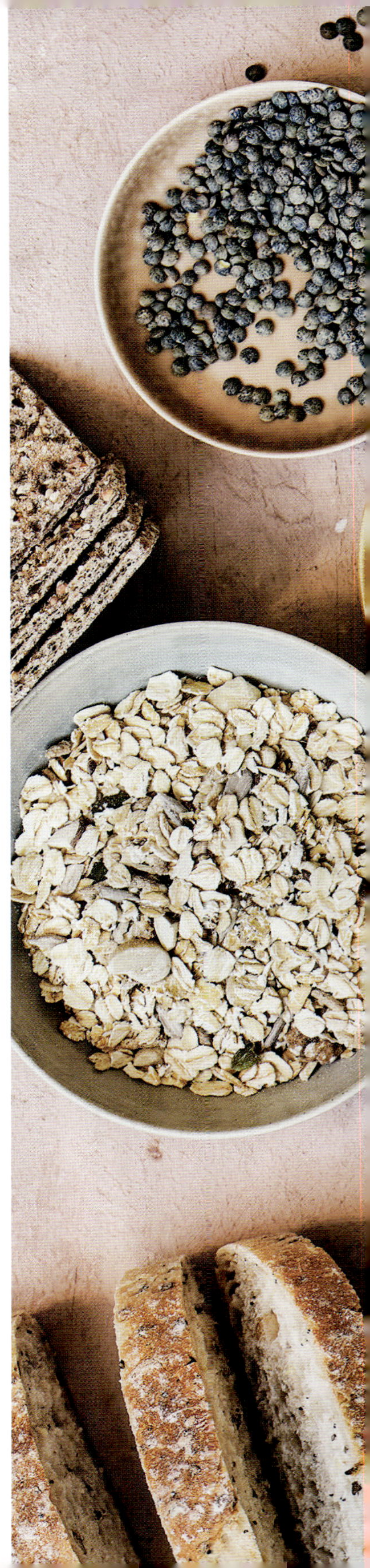

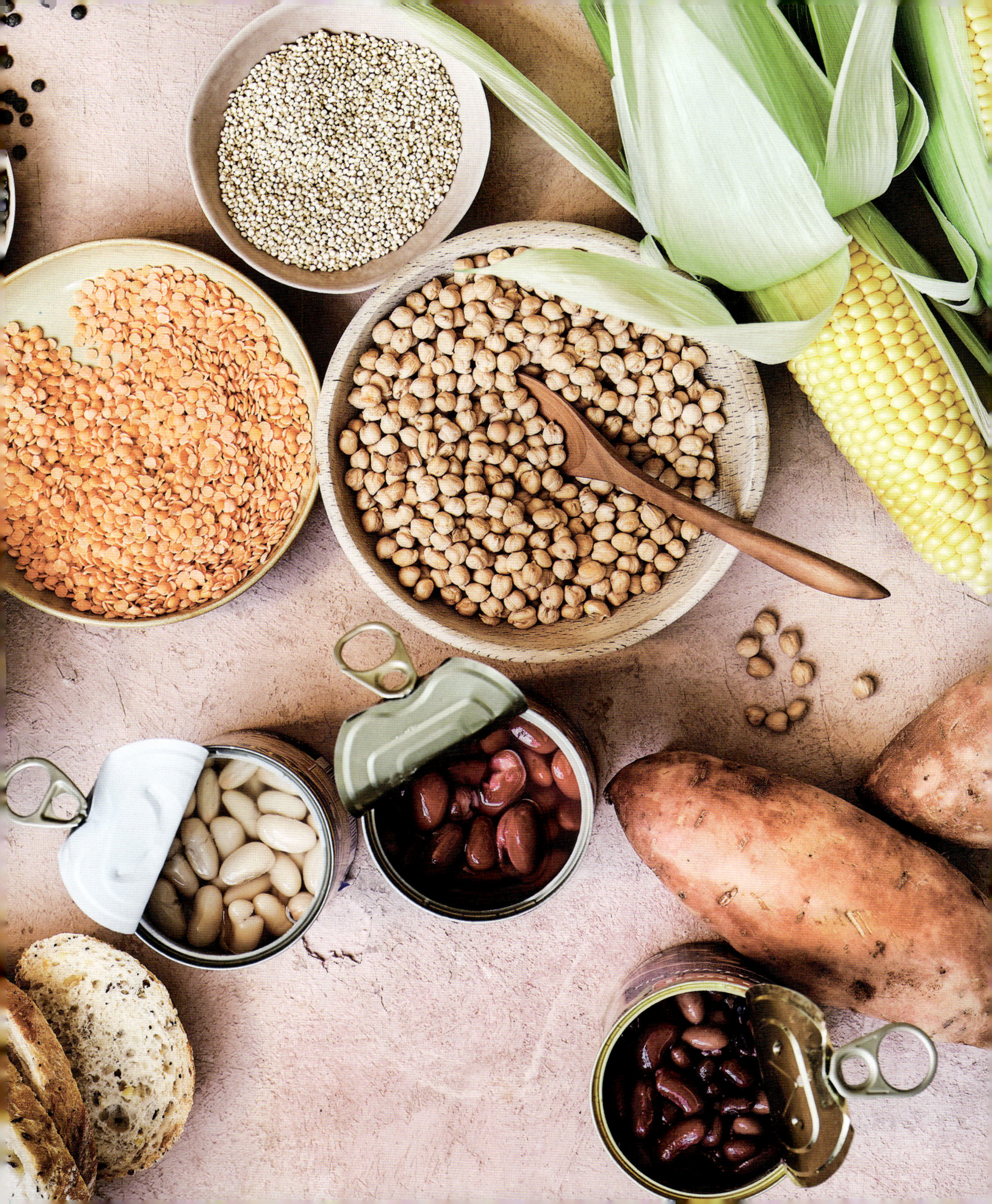

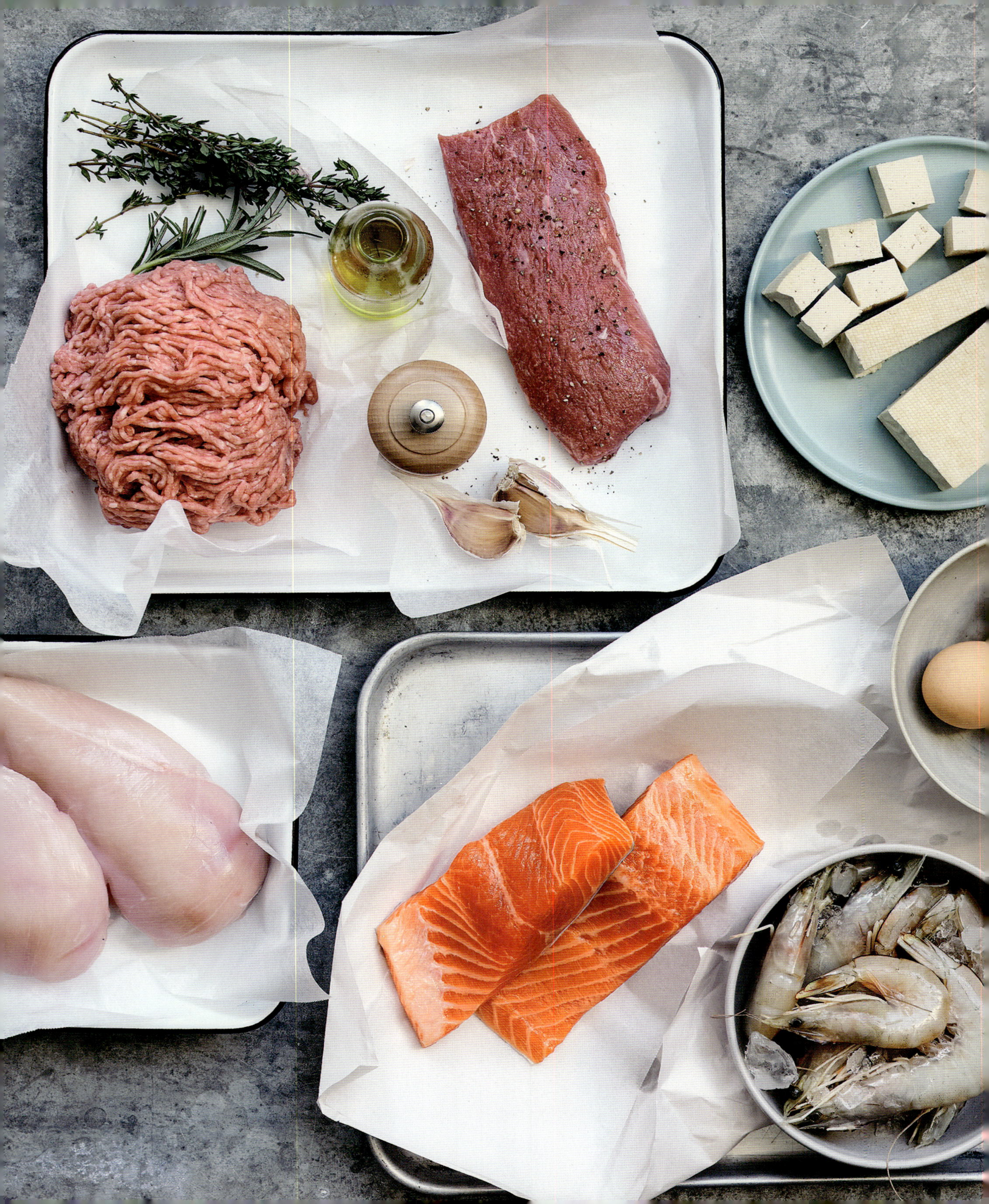

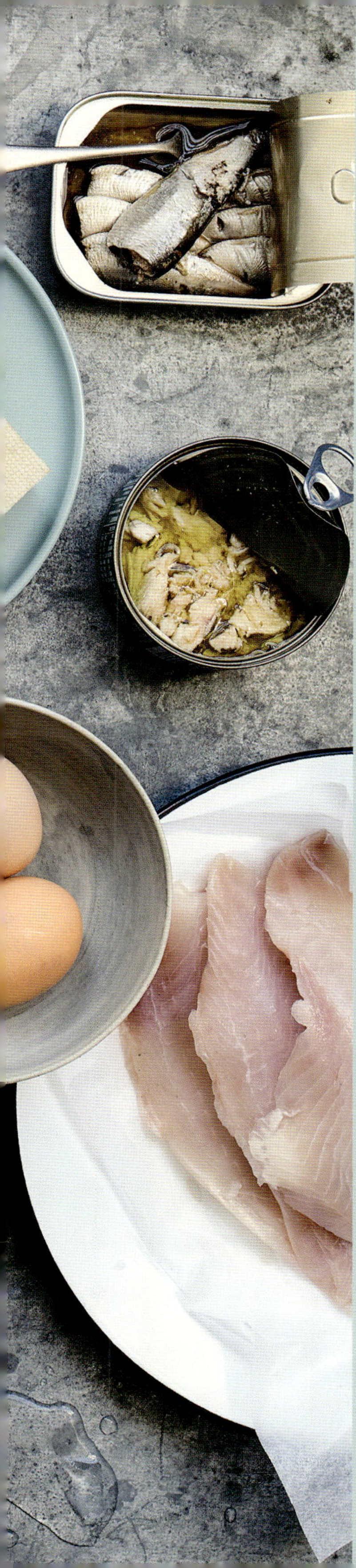

DAIRY

The fridge is where you will be storing most of your dairy items, but Tetra Paks can be stored in the pantry – check the storage instructions on the packet. Milk in cartons can be frozen, but it's best to use it within 1 month. Avoid any dairy products with added sugar or other flavourings.

Fridge and freezer

- full-fat, skim or reduced-fat cow's milk
- calcium-enriched soy milk
- almond milk
- natural yoghurt
- low-fat, lactose-free soy yoghurt
- cheddar
- parmesan
- Swiss cheese
- feta
- ricotta
- cottage cheese
- mozzarella
- bocconcini
- cream cheese

Pantry

- tinned reduced-fat evaporated milk
- Tetra Paks of milk

LEAN MEAT, FISH, POULTRY, EGGS, TOFU

Most of these fresh items will be stored in separate containers, either in the coldest part of the fridge or in the freezer. If you cut up meat or fish into portion-sizes before freezing, this can save time, but be mindful to prepare your foods safely and to store separately to avoid contamination.

Fridge and freezer

- lean fresh white snapper
- lean fresh ocean trout
- fresh flathead
- fresh mackerel
- fresh salmon
- prawns – unpeeled, or raw prawn meat
- chicken – whole, lean breast fillets, lean thigh fillets, marylands, lean mince
- lean turkey mince
- pork – lean mince, lean chops
- beef – lean rump steak, lean mince
- lamb – backstrap, lean mince
- lean kangaroo mince
- free-range 55 g eggs
- firm tofu

Pantry

- tinned tuna in brine
- tinned salmon in oil or tomato
- tinned sardines
- textured vegetable protein (TVP)

LOW-CARBOHYDRATE VEGETABLES

Most vegetables can be frozen, with the exception of those with a high water content, such as cucumber and lettuce. Although it's great to shop regularly for fresh vegetables, keep frozen vegetables on hand for when you don't have time to shop for fresh. Cut vegetables up into portion sizes before freezing. Fresh vegetables are best stored in a cool, dark and dry space – most vegetables last longer away from moisture and heat.

Fridge and freezer

- lettuce – iceberg, cos, butter
- spinach (English and baby)
- kale
- Tuscan kale
- rocket
- broccoli
- broccolini
- Chinese broccoli (gai lan)
- bok choy
- choy sum
- artichokes
- asparagus
- bean sprouts
- Lebanese cucumber
- mushrooms – Swiss brown, button
- tomatoes – regular, cherry, roma
- zucchini
- witlof (endive)
- radicchio
- garlic
- chillies – long green and small red
- watercress

Pantry

- tomato passata (no added sugar or salt)
- tomato paste (no added sugar or salt)
- tinned tomatoes (no added salt)
- tinned artichoke hearts in water

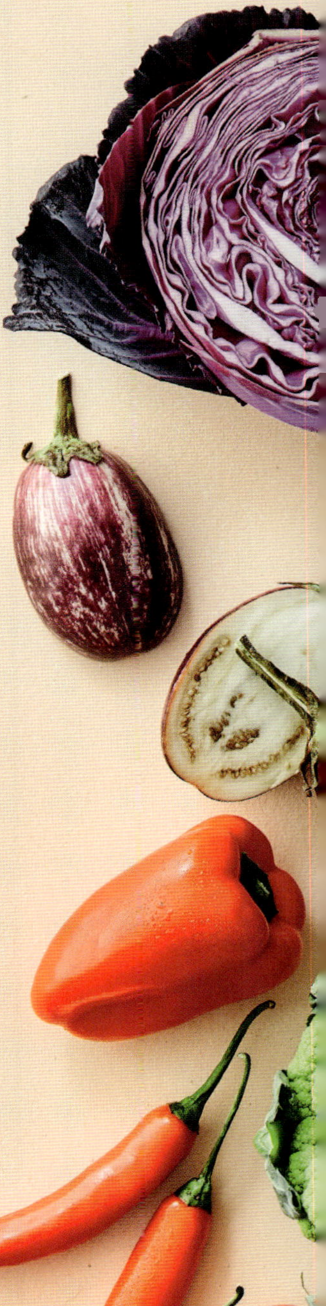

MODERATE-CARBOHYDRATE VEGETABLES

Most vegetables can be frozen, with the exception of those with a high water content, such as celery and radishes. Fresh berries can be frozen, or buy frozen berries with no added sugar.

Fridge and freezer

- cauliflower
- celery
- green beans
- capsicums
- brussels sprouts
- cabbage
- onions – brown, red
- leeks
- spring onions
- golden shallots
- broad beans
- snow peas
- sugar snap peas
- carrots – regular, Dutch
- eggplant
- parsnips
- beetroot
- swede
- turnips
- fennel bulbs
- bamboo shoots
- radishes
- peas
- pumpkin
- baby squash
- lemon
- lime
- grapefruit
- strawberries
- blueberries
- raspberries
- blackberries
- mulberries
- cranberries
- loquats
- cumquats

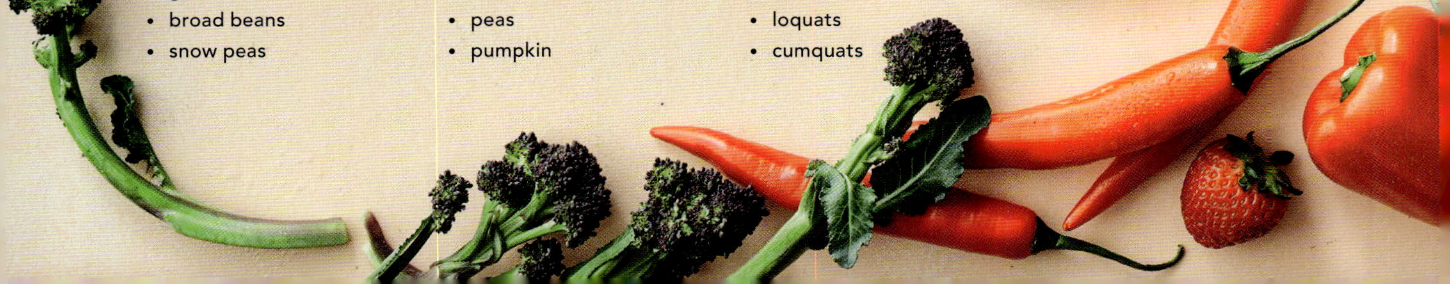

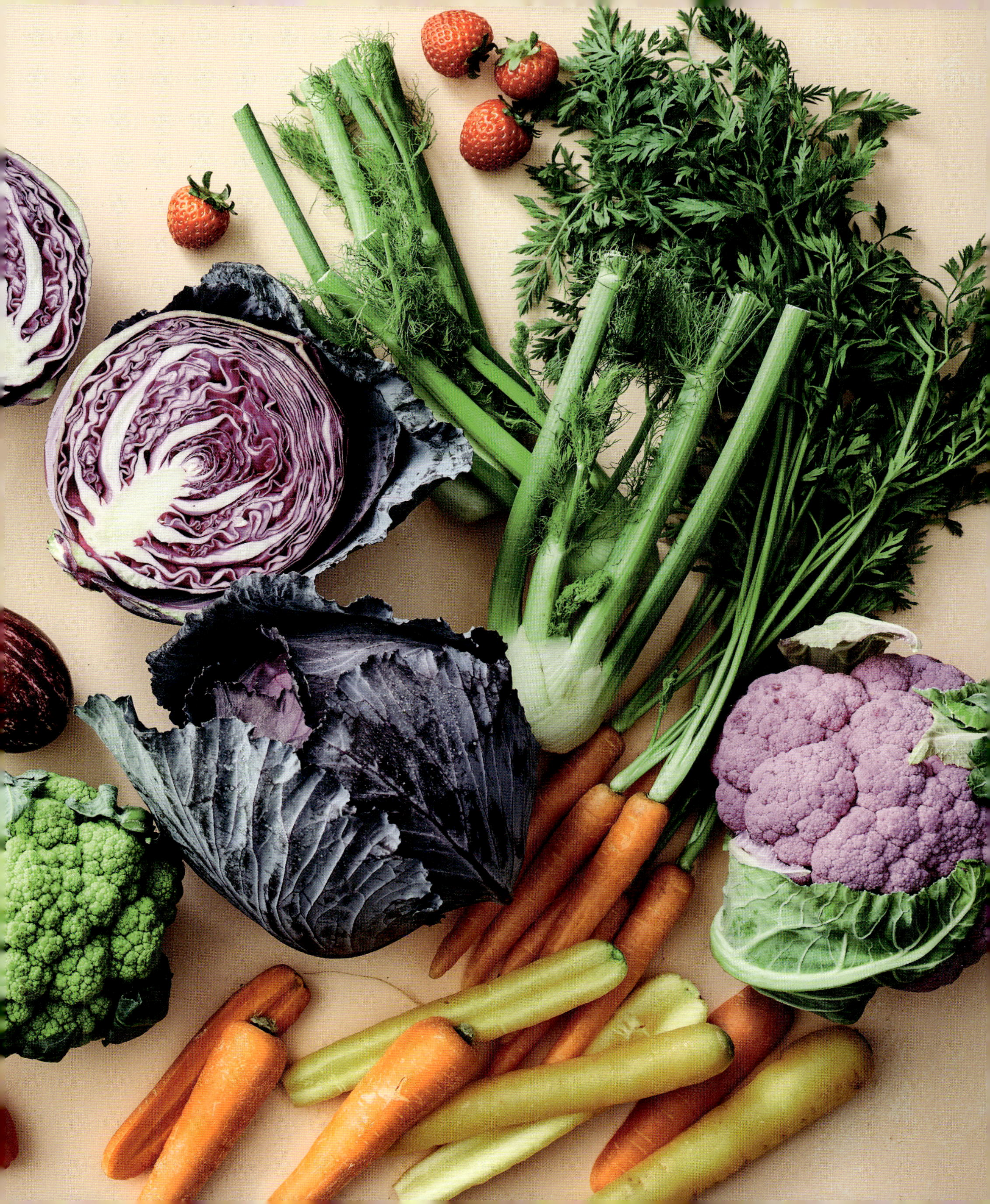

HEALTHY FATS

Dietary fat is an essential part of the CSIRO Low-carb Diet. Choosing mostly healthy fats ensures you are selecting foods that have properties beneficial to the body. You will store most of these in the pantry. Ensure that all nuts are unsalted, and portion-pack them for ready-to-go snacks.

Fridge and freezer

- hummus
- margarine – Nuttelex, olive oil–based or nut-based spread
- olives – kalamata (in oil)
- capers in brine

Pantry

- oils – olive oil, avocado oil, grapeseed oil, flaxseed (linseed) oil, macadamia oil, sesame oil
- curry paste – oil-based
- tahini
- almond butter and other nut butters (sugar free)
- pesto – oil-based
- avocado
- coconut flakes
- chestnuts
- pine nuts
- almonds – whole, slivered, ground
- pecans
- macadamias
- walnuts
- brazil nuts
- pistachio nuts
- hazelnuts
- chia seeds
- flaxseeds (linseeds)
- sesame seeds
- pumpkin seeds (pepitas)

DRINKS

Although plain water is ideal, you could serve it with a squeeze of lemon or lime juice, or perhaps make up a bottle of water and add a slice of citrus or some fruit essence and store it in the fridge. These drinks are also 'free' items (0 units).

Fridge

- unflavoured mineral or soda water

Pantry

- tea – black*, green, herbal, jasmine, lemon, peppermint
- coffee – unsweetened and black*
- fruit essence

*If you prefer to use milk, take this from your daily Dairy allowance

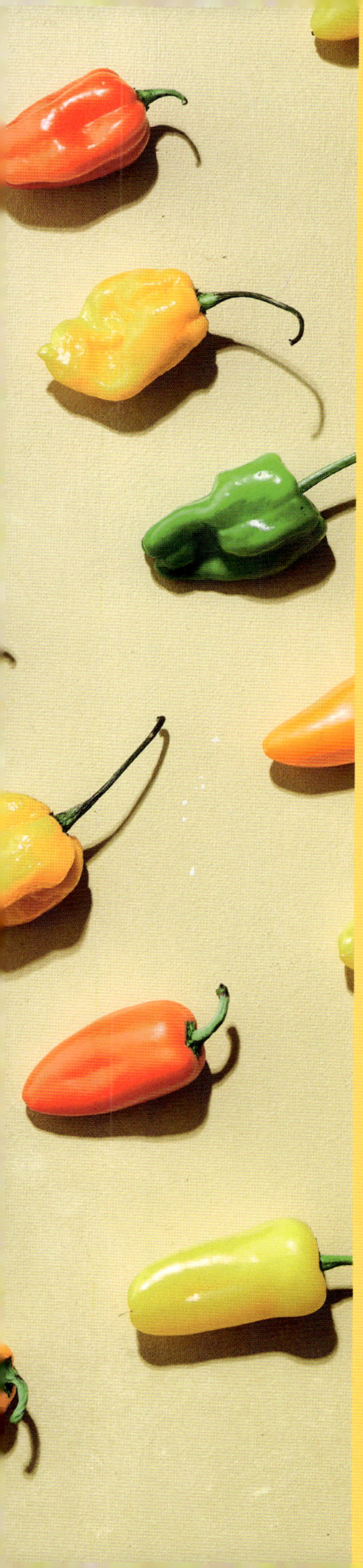

FLAVOUR BUILDERS: HERBS, SPICES, CONDIMENTS AND SAUCES

Considered 'free' items (i.e. they don't count as a food unit), these are the pantry essentials that add the greatest flavour boost to foods. This will become the go-to area of your pantry, where all the flavour lives. You could even pre-blend your own spice mixes, cutting down time when preparing your meals.

Pantry

Spices

- dried chillies
- chilli flakes
- cinnamon – ground and sticks
- fennel seeds
- cumin – seeds and ground
- coriander – seeds and ground
- cardamom – pods and ground
- cloves – whole and ground
- ginger – fresh and ground
- fresh galangal
- turmeric – fresh and ground
- mustard seeds
- shredded coconut
- paprika – sweet, smoked, plain
- sumac
- black peppercorns
- Sichuan peppercorns
- allspice
- curry leaves
- Makrut lime leaves

Fresh or dried herbs

- basil
- flat-leaf parsley
- coriander
- tarragon
- marjoram
- sage
- dill
- thyme
- oregano
- mint
- chives
- lemongrass
- garlic powder
- rosemary
- bay leaves
- mixed dried herbs

Condiments

- mustard – Dijon, wholegrain, powder
- hot sauce
- reduced-salt tamari
- reduced-salt soy sauce
- rice wine vinegar
- red wine vinegar
- white wine vinegar
- balsamic vinegar
- apple cider vinegar
- lemon juice – concentrated
- lime juice – concentrated
- nori sheets

Seek advice and support from your healthcare team

Now that you are ready to go, we recommend that if you are going to change your lifestyle in any way, including our lifestyle and dietary approach, that you should do this in close consultation with your healthcare team, particularly if you are taking diabetes medication.

One of the key benefits shown repeatedly by scientific research is that a low-carb diet is very effective in improving blood glucose control and reducing diabetes medication requirements. This is a good thing as it means you are improving your blood glucose control with less medication, meaning reduced costs and side effects.

This is why following a low-carb diet plan in close consultation with your healthcare professional is important, as it means they can monitor and adjust your medication requirements as necessary to ensure it is at the correct level. Taking too much medication can cause your blood glucose levels to fall too low, which can be quite dangerous.

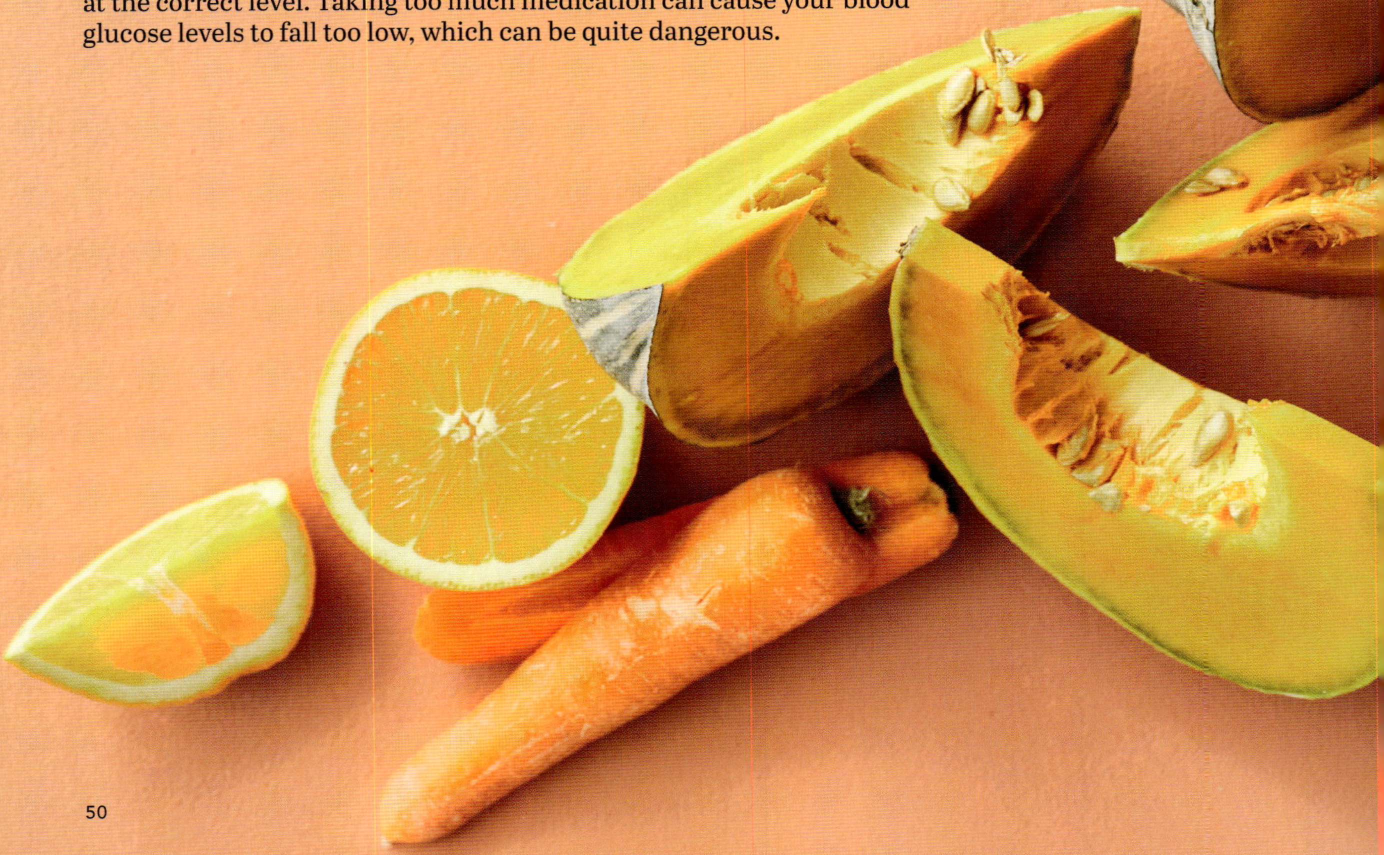

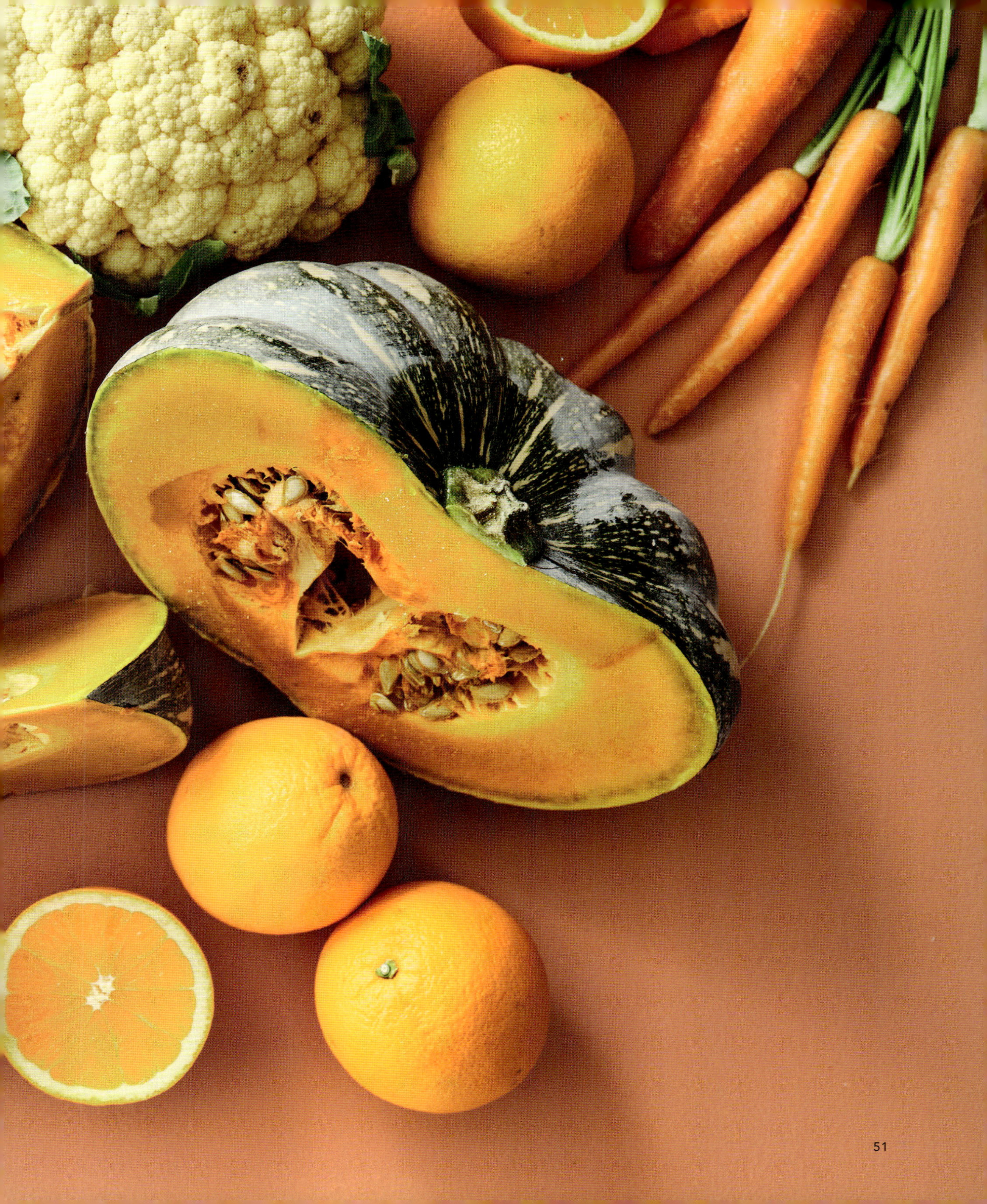

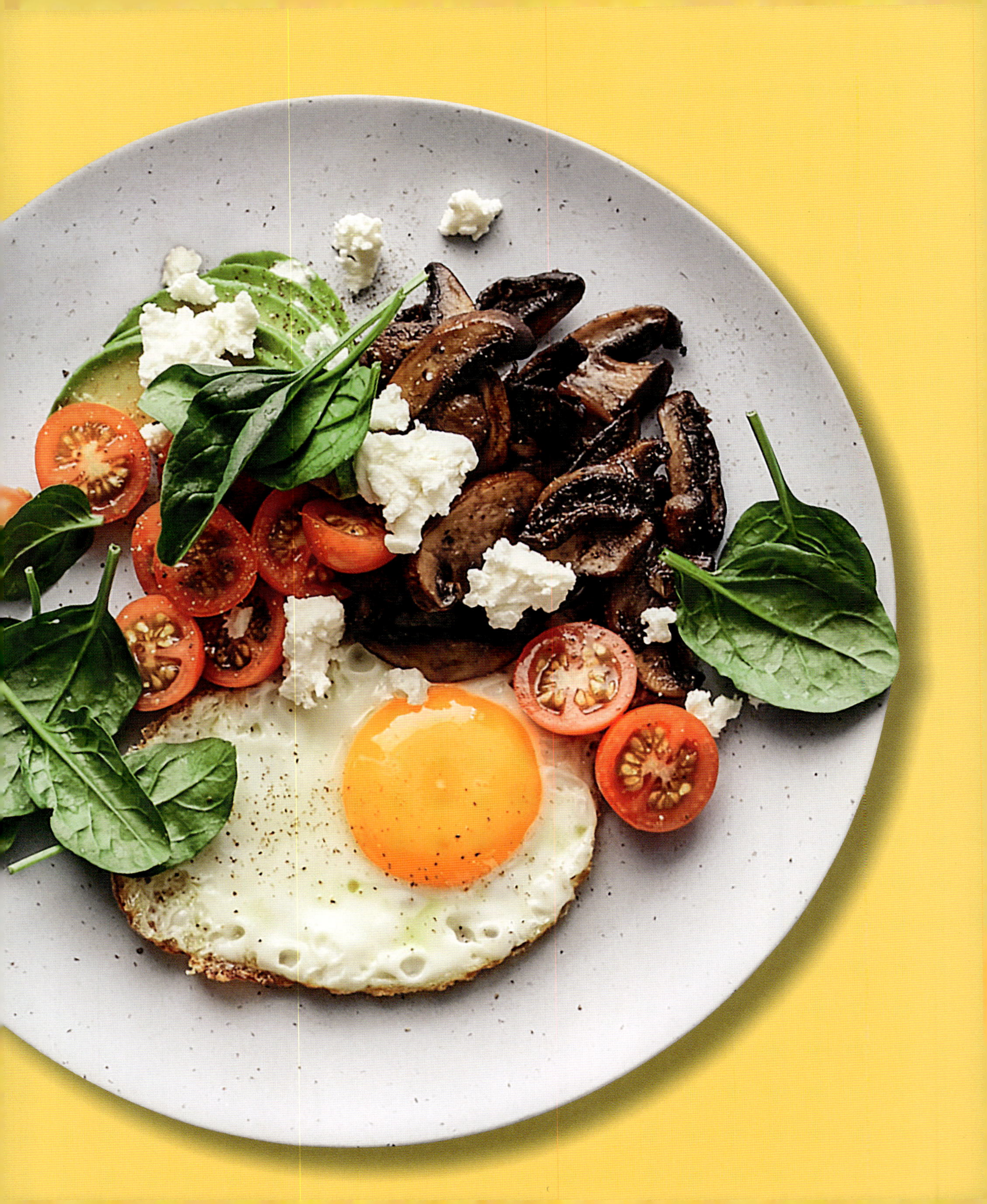

01.

Breakfast

UNITS PER SERVE:	
Breads, Cereals, Legumes, Starchy Veg	1
Dairy	0
Lean Meat, Fish, Poultry, Eggs, Tofu	0
Low–Moderate Carbohydrate Veg	0
Healthy Fats	3

Nutty Cinnamon and Vanilla Muesli

CARBS 13 g PER SERVE

SERVES: 6 | PREPARATION: 5 MINUTES | COOKING: 30 MINUTES

1½ cups (120 g) rolled oats
⅓ cup (35 g) walnuts
⅓ cup (35 g) raw unsalted almonds
1½ tablespoons pumpkin seeds (pepitas)
½ teaspoon ground cinnamon
1 tablespoon pure vanilla extract
3 teaspoons macadamia oil (or olive oil)

1. Preheat the oven to 180°C (160°C fan-forced) and line a large baking tray with baking paper.
2. Place all the ingredients in a large bowl and toss until well combined and coated in the oil. Transfer the muesli to the prepared baking tray and bake in the oven for 30 minutes, stirring occasionally, until toasted and golden.
3. Remove from the oven and set aside to cool before transferring to an airtight jar or container. The muesli will keep for 2 weeks. See note for serving suggestion pictured.

Note

Serving suggestion: Serve ⅓ cup (40 g) muesli with ¼ cup (65 g) low-fat natural yoghurt and ¼ cup berries. If you serve the muesli this way, you will need to add 0.5 units Dairy, 1 unit Low–Moderate Carbohydrate Vegetables and 8 g carbohydrates (taking a serve from 13 g carbs to 20 g).

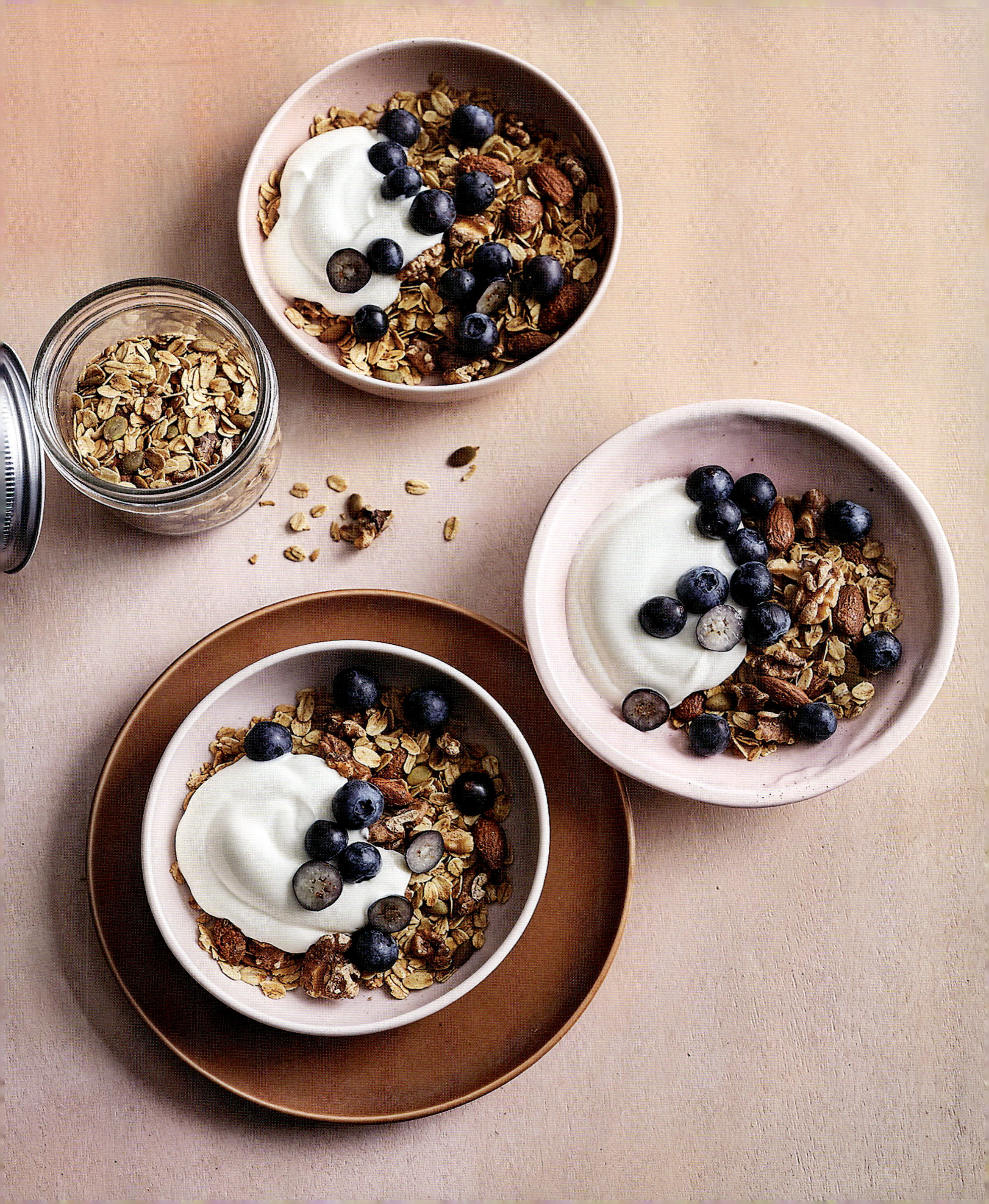

UNITS PER SERVE:	
Breads, Cereals, Legumes, Starchy Veg	1
Dairy	1
Lean Meat, Fish, Poultry, Eggs, Tofu	0
Low-Moderate Carbohydrate Veg	0
Healthy Fats	2

Lemony Avocado and Feta Vita-Weats

CARBS 11g PER SERVE

SERVES: 2 | PREPARATION: 5 MINUTES | COOKING: NIL

½ medium avocado, mashed
6 × 9-Grain Vita-Weats
40 g reduced-fat feta, crumbled
½ lemon, sliced into wedges
Pinch dried chilli flakes

Spread the avocado across the Vita-Weats. Top with the feta, a squeeze of lemon juice, the chilli flakes and ¼ teaspoon freshly ground black pepper. Divide the Vita-Weats between two plates and serve immediately.

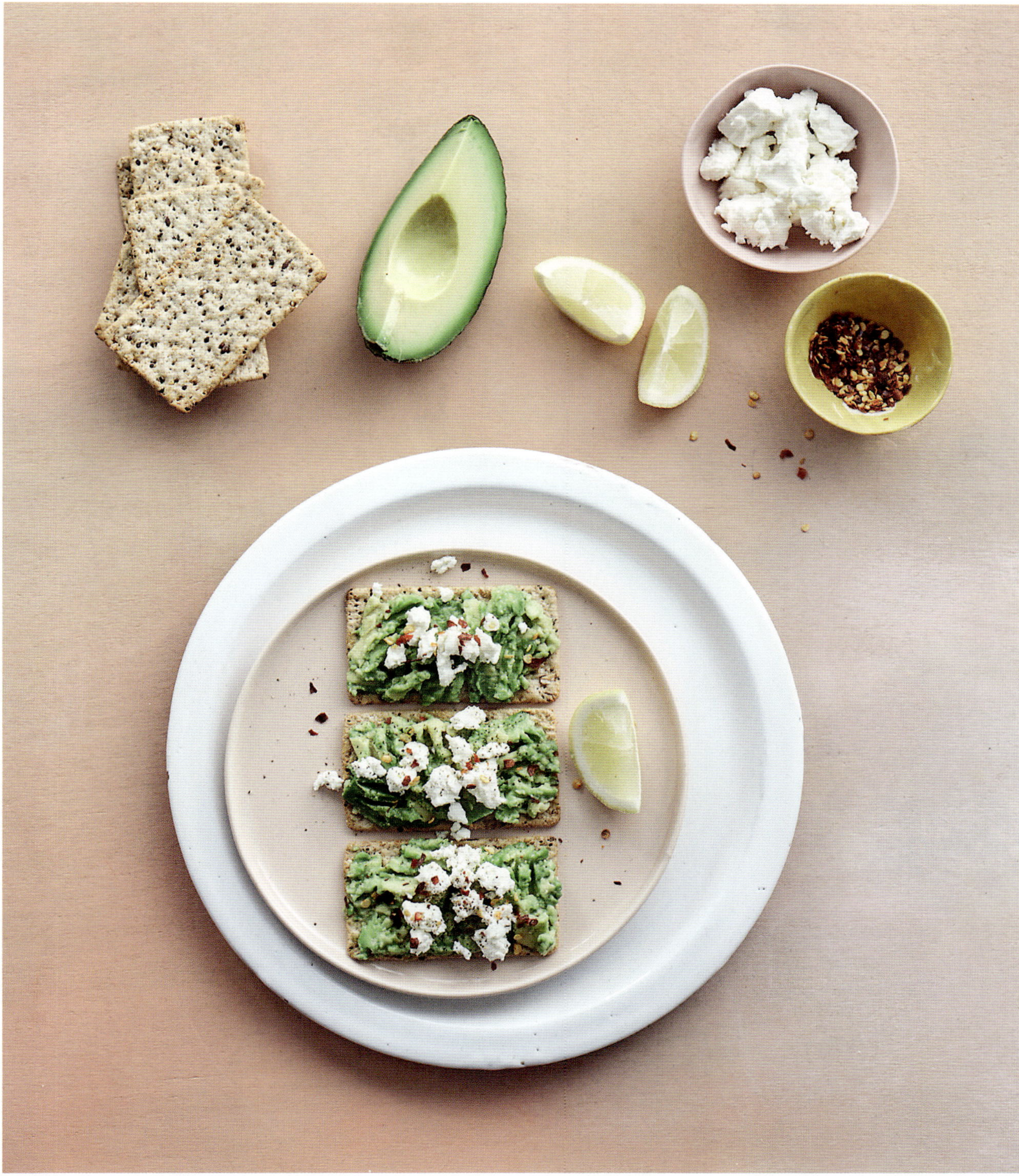

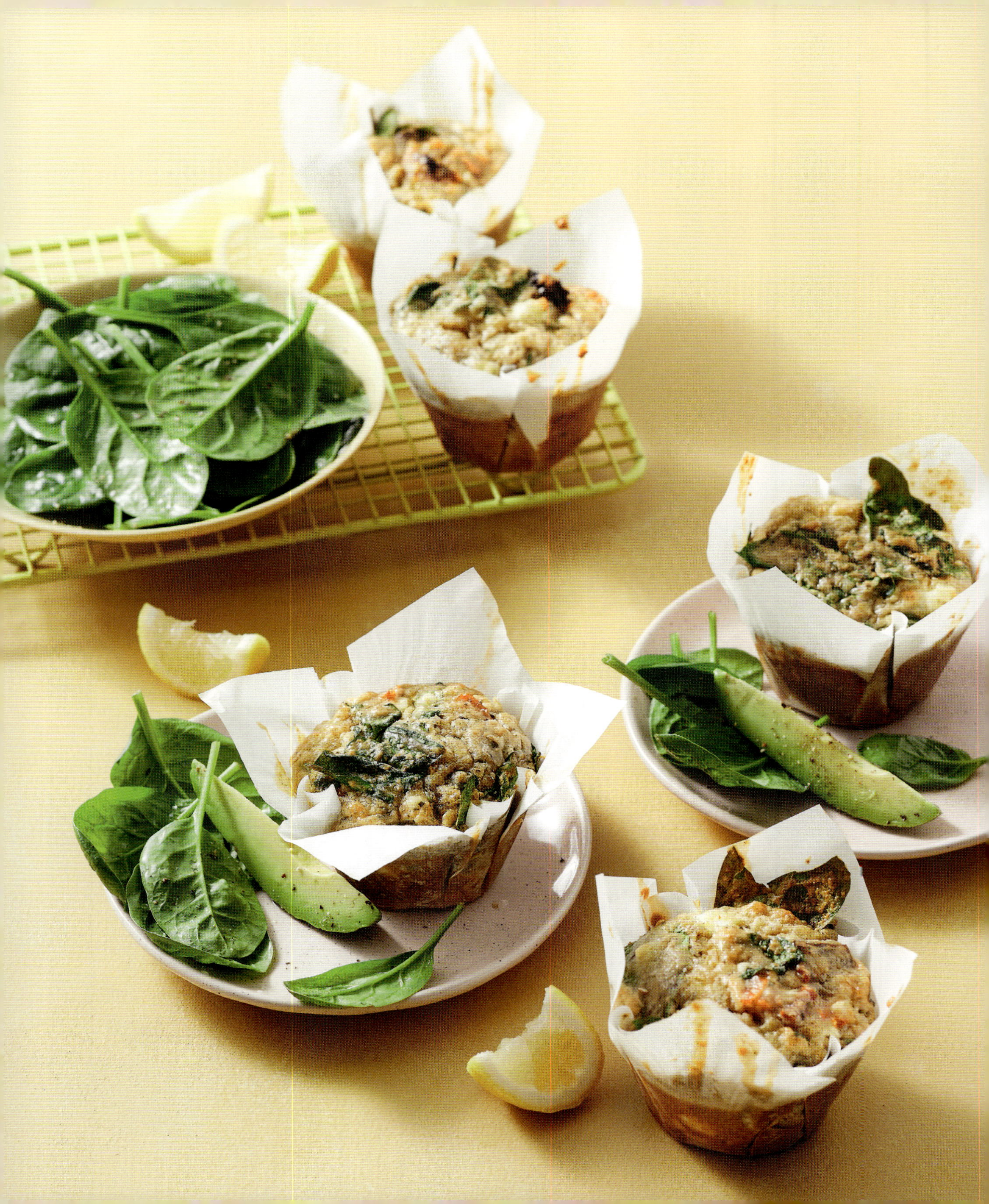

UNITS PER SERVE:	
Breads, Cereals, Legumes, Starchy Veg	0.5
Dairy	0.5
Lean Meat, Fish, Poultry, Eggs, Tofu	0.5
Low–Moderate Carbohydrate Veg	0.5
Healthy Fats	2

Feta, Spinach and Sundried Tomato Breakfast Muffins

CARBS 12g PER SERVE

SERVES: 6 | PREPARATION: 10 MINUTES | COOKING: 20 MINUTES

6 × 55 g free-range eggs
¼ cup (60 ml) full-fat milk
40 g reduced-fat firm feta
½ cup (70 g) sundried tomatoes, roughly chopped
1 tablespoon oil-free pesto
1 cup baby spinach leaves, roughly chopped
½ cup (60 g) wholemeal self-raising flour

TO SERVE

½ teaspoon Nuttelex or canola margarine
½ cup baby spinach leaves
1 × 20 g slice avocado
Lemon wedges

1. Preheat the oven to 200°C (180°C fan-forced) and line 6 holes of a muffin tin with patty pans.
2. In a large bowl, whisk the eggs and milk. Add the remaining ingredients and ¼ teaspoon freshly ground black pepper and mix until well combined.
3. Pour the batter into 6 holes of the muffin tin. Bake in the oven for 20 minutes until the egg has cooked through and the muffins are set.
4. Remove from the oven and allow to cool in the tin. Divide the muffins into ziplock bags or place in an airtight container to store.
5. To serve, warm one muffin, split it open and spread with Nuttelex or margarine. Serve with the baby spinach, avocado and a squeeze of lemon juice.

UNITS PER SERVE:	
Breads, Cereals, Legumes, Starchy Veg	1
Dairy	1
Lean Meat, Fish, Poultry, Eggs, Tofu	0.5
Low–Moderate Carbohydrate Veg	2
Healthy Fats	2

Vegetarian Big Breakfast

CARBS 16 g PER SERVE

SERVES: 2 | PREPARATION: 5 MINUTES | COOKING: 10 MINUTES

1½ teaspoons extra virgin olive oil
300 g sliced Swiss brown mushrooms
1 clove garlic, crushed
2 cups baby spinach leaves
2 × 55 g free-range eggs
150 g cherry tomatoes, halved
½ small avocado, sliced into wedges
2 thin slices multigrain bread, toasted
40 g reduced-fat feta, crumbled

1. Heat the olive oil in a large frying pan over medium heat and cook the mushrooms and garlic for 3 minutes until the mushrooms are browned. (Optional – if you'd like your spinach cooked, add it to the mushrooms and stir it through for 1 minute, or until wilted.)
2. Tip the mushrooms into a bowl and place the pan back on the heat. Crack in the eggs and allow to cook for 5 minutes or until the egg whites are set.
3. Divide the eggs, mushrooms, spinach, cherry tomatoes, avocado and toast between two plates. Sprinkle the crumbled feta over the top and season with freshly ground black pepper.

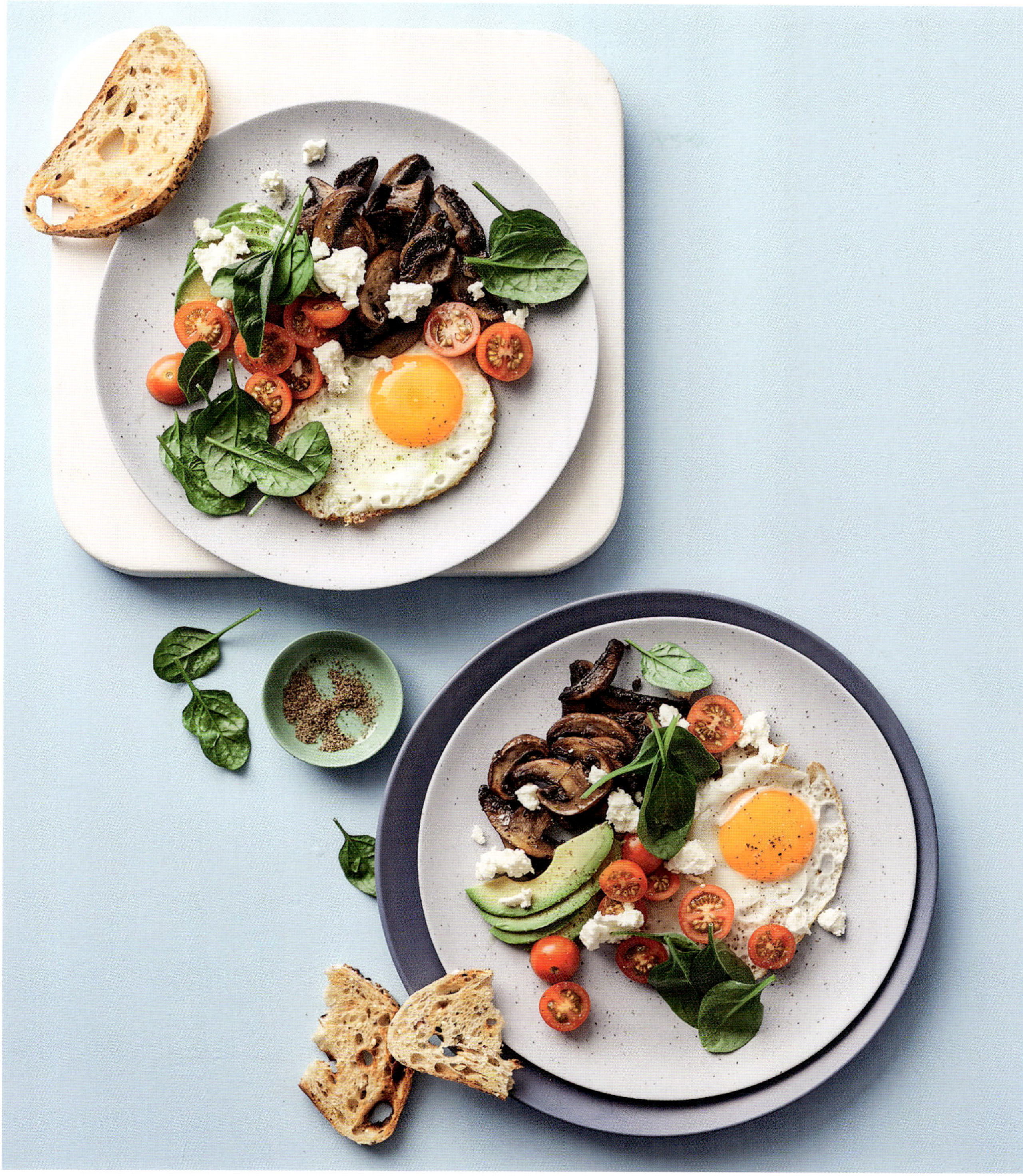

UNITS PER SERVE:	
Breads, Cereals, Legumes, Starchy Veg	1
Dairy	1
Lean Meat, Fish, Poultry, Eggs, Tofu	0.5
Low–Moderate Carbohydrate Veg	0
Healthy Fats	2

Scrambled Eggs with Goat's Cheese

CARBS 18 g PER SERVE

SERVES: 2 | PREPARATION: 2 MINUTES | COOKING: 4 MINUTES

2 × 55 g free-range eggs
2 tablespoons full-fat milk
2 teaspoons extra virgin olive oil
40 g soft goat's cheese
2 tablespoons finely chopped chives
2 slices multigrain bread, toasted
2 teaspoons Nuttelex

1. Whisk the eggs and milk together with a pinch of freshly ground black pepper.
2. Heat the olive oil in a non-stick frying pan over medium heat. Pour in the whisked egg and let it sit in the pan for 1 minute before adding the goat's cheese and sprinkling in half the chives. Use a spatula to push the egg around the pan gently for 30 seconds–1 minute, until mostly cooked through. Remove the pan from the heat.
3. Butter the toast with the Nuttelex, then divide between two plates. Serve with the scrambled egg sprinkled with the remaining chopped chives.

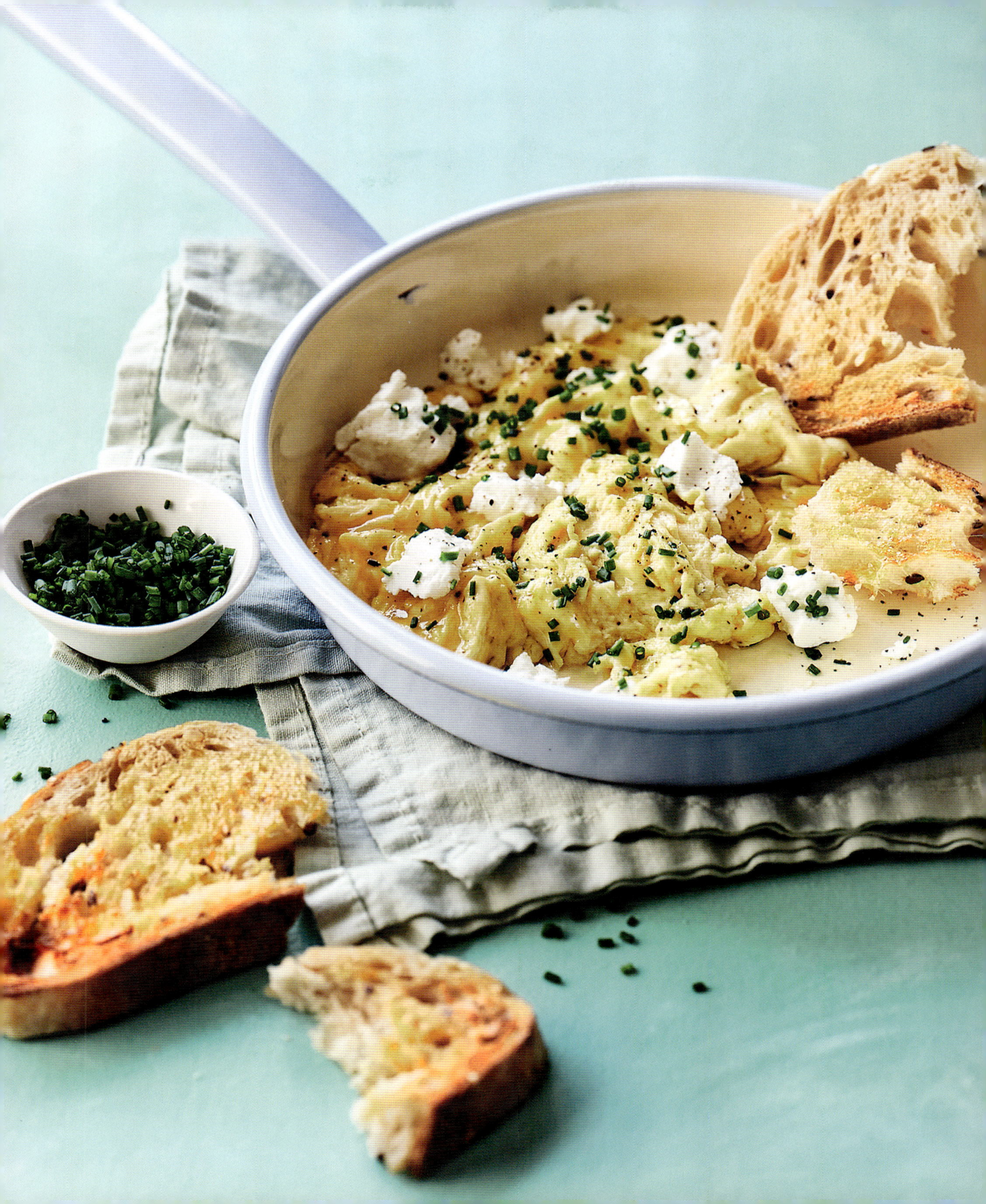

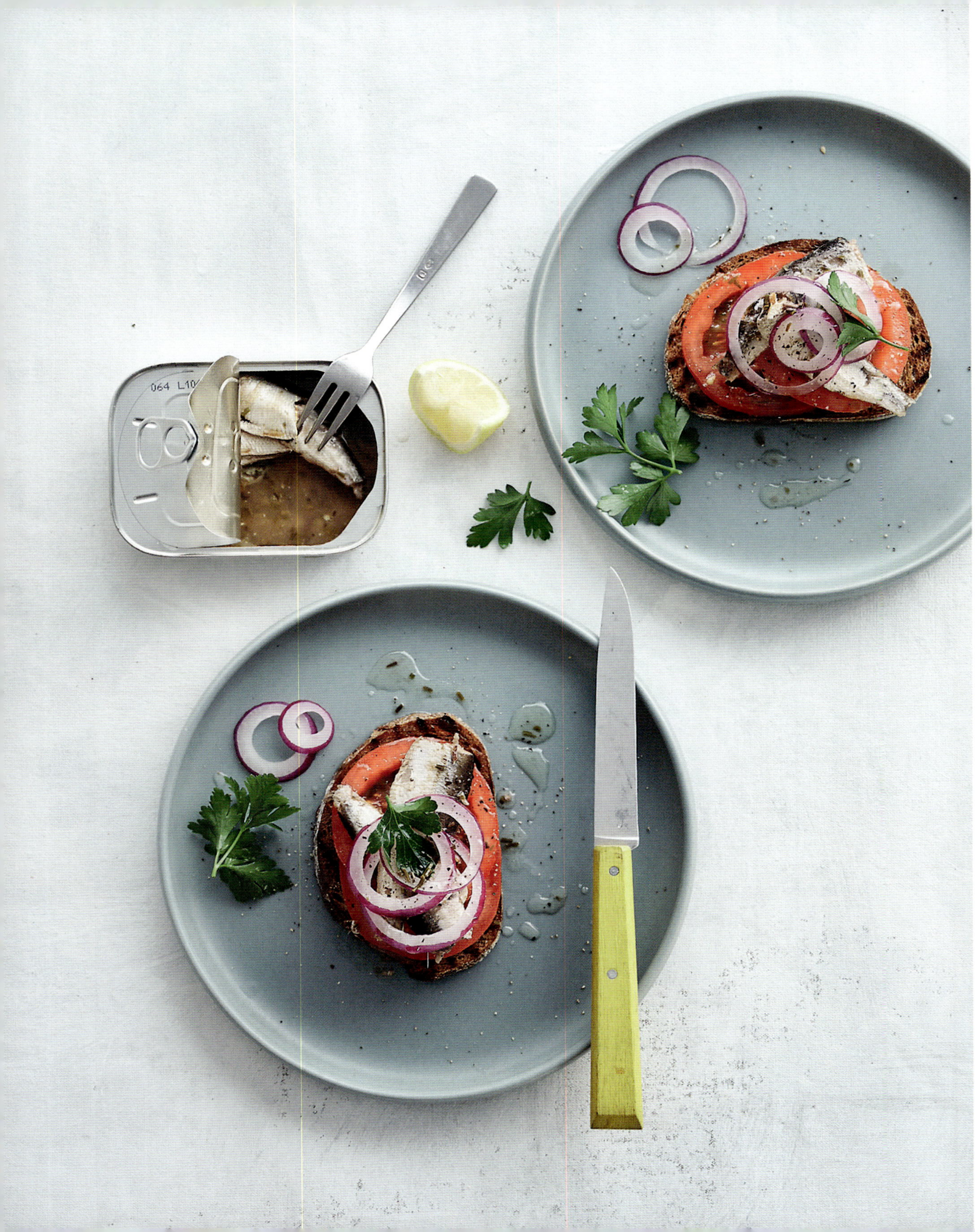

UNITS PER SERVE:	
Breads, Cereals, Legumes, Starchy Veg	1
Dairy	0
Lean Meat, Fish, Poultry, Eggs, Tofu	0.5
Low–Moderate Carbohydrate Veg	1
Healthy Fats	2

Tomato and Sardines on Rye

CARBS 19g PER SERVE

SERVES: 2 | PREPARATION: 2 MINUTES | COOKING: 2 MINUTES

1 tomato, sliced
90 g tinned sardines in extra virgin olive oil (undrained)
2 thin slices rye bread, toasted
¼ small red onion, thinly sliced
Parsley leaves, to serve
Lemon wedges, to serve (optional)

Divide the tomato and sardines between the two slices of toast – including 2 teaspoons of the olive oil from the tin per slice of bread. Top with the red onion, season with ¼ teaspoon freshly ground black pepper, divide between two plates and serve sprinkled with the parsley, with lemon wedges on the side (if using).

UNITS PER SERVE:	
Breads, Cereals, Legumes, Starchy Veg	1
Dairy	0.5
Lean Meat, Fish, Poultry, Eggs, Tofu	0.5
Low–Moderate Carbohydrate Veg	1
Healthy Fats	2

Chilli Egg and Mushroom Savoury Porridge

CARBS 19 g PER SERVE

SERVES: 2 | PREPARATION: 3 MINUTES | COOKING: 13 MINUTES

2 teaspoons extra virgin olive oil
300 g Swiss brown mushrooms, halved or quartered
3 sprigs thyme, leaves picked
1 clove garlic, thinly sliced
2 × 55 g free-range eggs
2 teaspoons chilli oil
½ heaped cup (55 g) rolled oats
1½ cups (375 ml) salt-reduced chicken stock (see note)
1 cup baby spinach leaves
20 g parmesan, shaved

1. Place the olive oil, mushrooms, thyme and garlic in a frying pan over medium–high heat. Cook for 3 minutes until the mushrooms are brown and tender, then transfer to a bowl and set aside.
2. Place the frying pan back on the heat and crack in the eggs. Spoon the chilli oil around the edges, then cook for 5 minutes until the whites are set. Remove the pan from the heat.
3. Place the oats, stock and ¼ teaspoon freshly ground black pepper in a small saucepan over low–medium heat. Cook, stirring, for 5–6 minutes until the oats are tender and have taken on most of the stock to create a porridge consistency.
4. Divide the porridge between two bowls. Top with the mushrooms, egg, spinach and parmesan, season with more pepper and serve.

Note

Commercial chicken stock is usually very high in sodium. We recommend shopping for 'chicken broth', which is a similar product you can find in the refrigerator section of supermarkets and grocers. Broth is sold in small batches and contains less sodium. Check the label to ensure your stock contains less than 50 mg sodium per 100 g. Alternatively, if you'd like to make your own homemade stock, see the recipe on page 131.

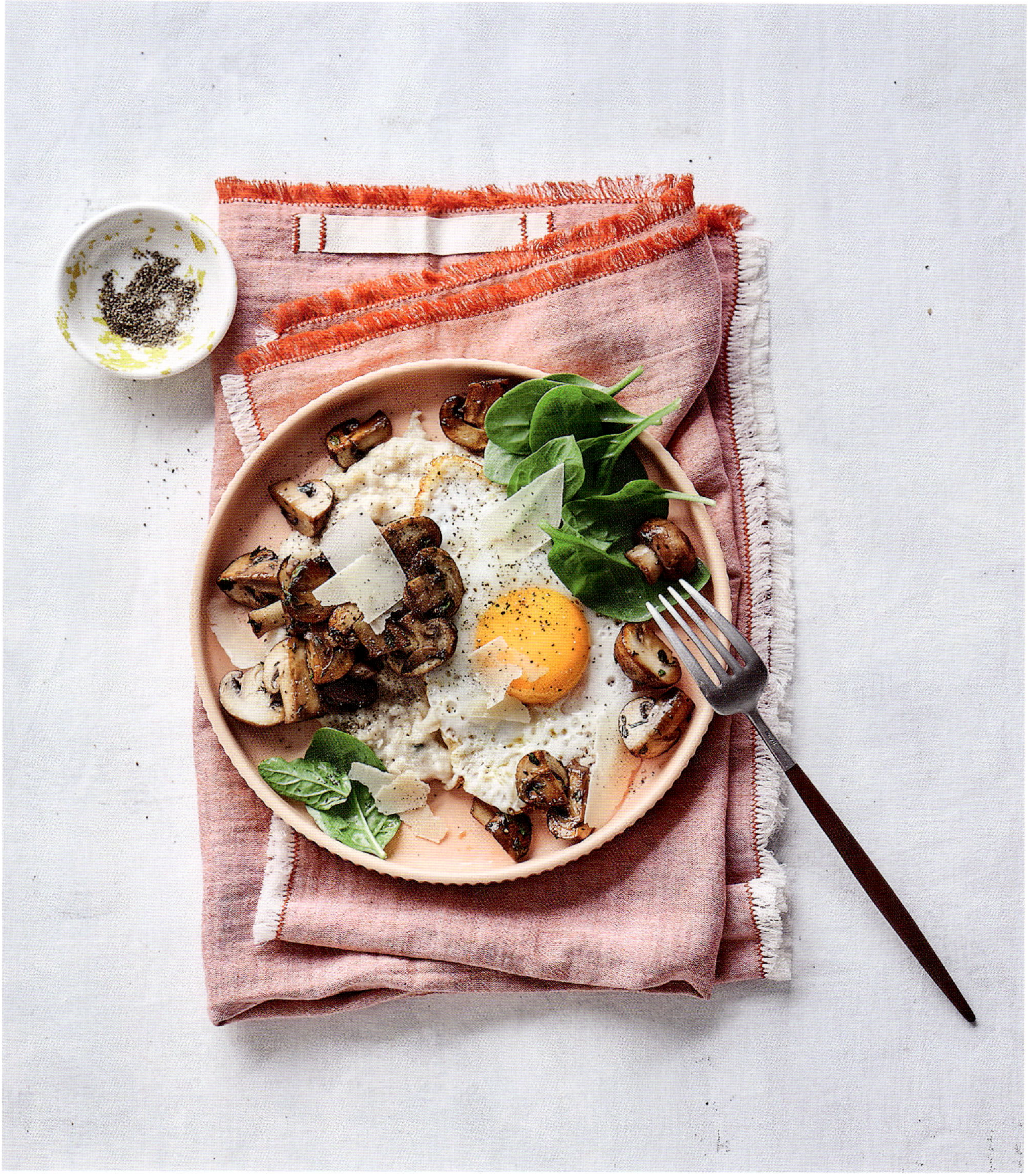

UNITS PER SERVE:	
Breads, Cereals, Legumes, Starchy Veg	1
Dairy	1
Lean Meat, Fish, Poultry, Eggs, Tofu	0.5
Low–Moderate Carbohydrate Veg	0
Healthy Fats	1.5

Egg and Goat's Cheese on Cruskits

CARBS 20g PER SERVE

SERVES: 2 | PREPARATION: 2 MINUTES | COOKING: 12 MINUTES

2 × 55 g free-range eggs
40 g soft goat's cheese
8 rye Cruskits
¼ cup (55 g) hummus
2 teaspoons finely chopped chives
Pinch paprika, to serve

1. Bring a saucepan of water to the boil, then add the eggs and cook, undisturbed, for 8 minutes. Remove the eggs using a slotted spoon and run them under water until they are cool to the touch. Peel and chop into pieces.
2. Spread the goat's cheese thinly on four of the Cruskits and spread the hummus on the other four. Top with the egg and chives and season with freshly ground black pepper. Divide the Cruskits between two plates, sprinkle with paprika and serve.

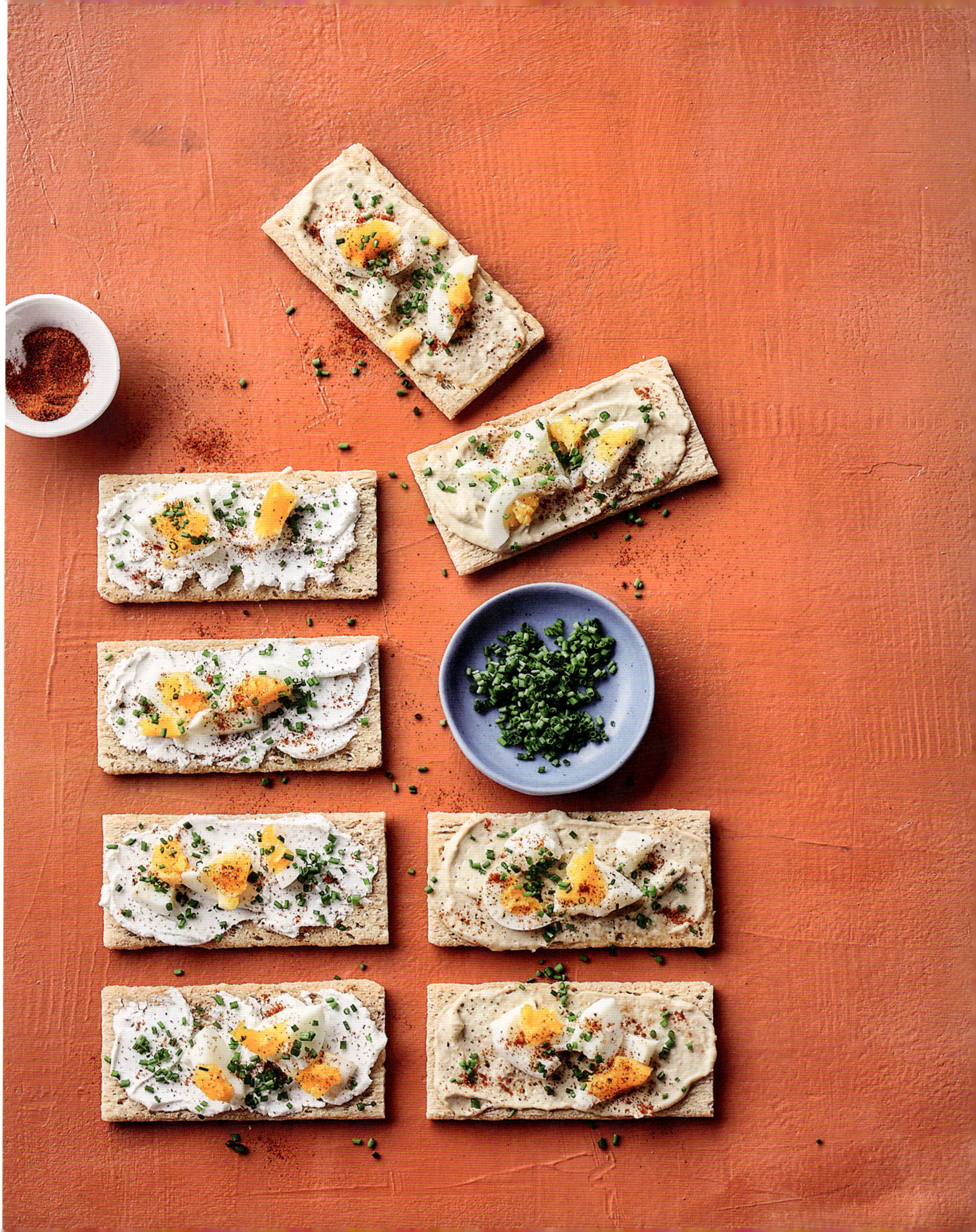

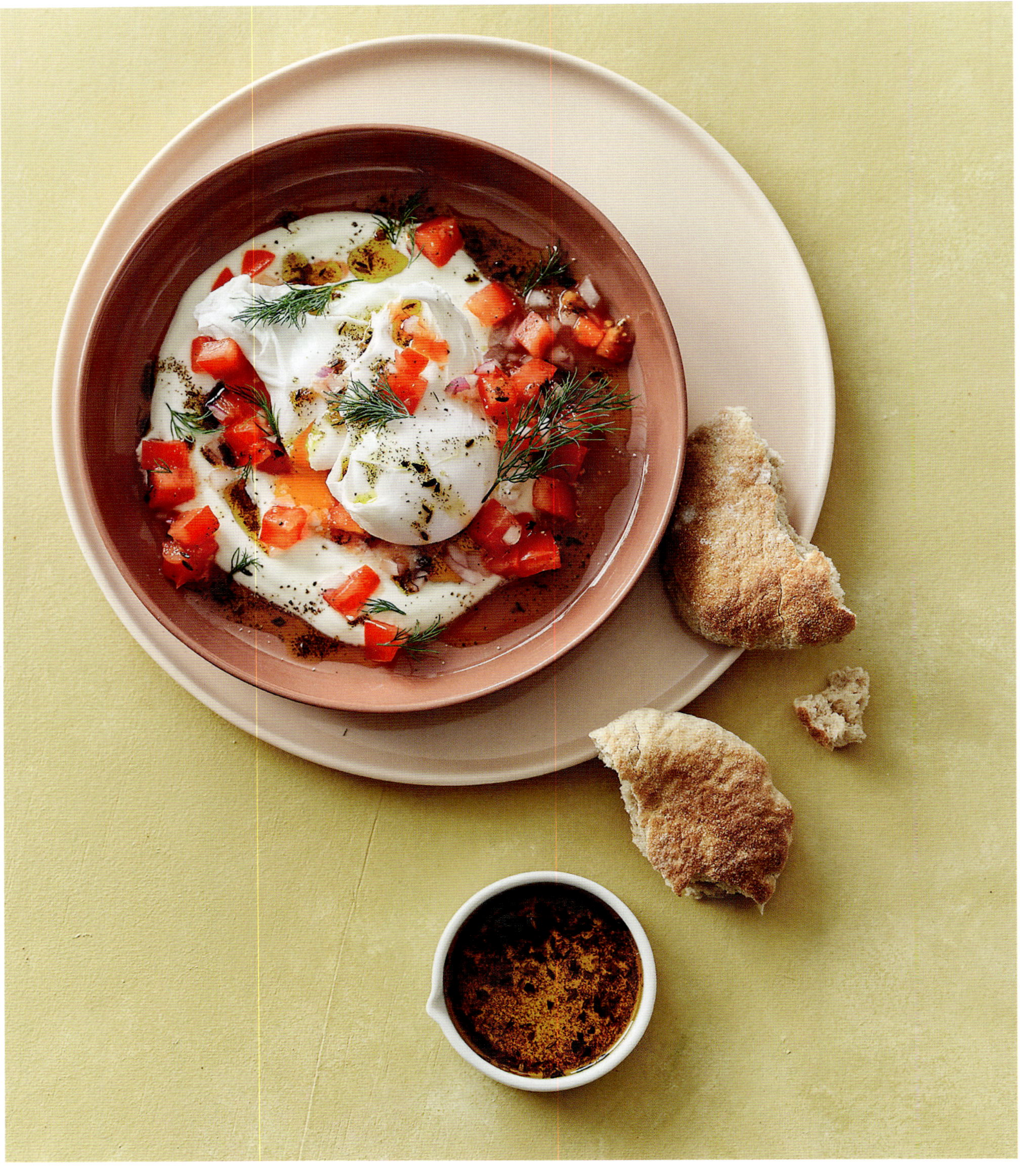

UNITS PER SERVE:	
Breads, Cereals, Legumes, Starchy Veg	1
Dairy	1
Lean Meat, Fish, Poultry, Eggs, Tofu	1
Low–Moderate Carbohydrate Veg	1
Healthy Fats	2

Turkish Poached Eggs with Chilli Oil

CARBS 15g PER SERVE

SERVES: 2 | PREPARATION: 3 MINUTES | COOKING: 12 MINUTES

1 tablespoon extra virgin olive oil
½ teaspoon cumin seeds
½ teaspoon smoked paprika
Pinch dried chilli flakes
1 tomato, diced
¼ small red onion, finely diced
1 teaspoon white vinegar
4 × 55 g free-range eggs
½ cup (130 g) natural yoghurt
1 tablespoon dill leaves
1 small wholemeal pita bread, sliced into quarters, warmed in the microwave

1. Heat the olive oil in a small non-stick frying pan over medium heat. Add the cumin seeds, paprika and chilli flakes and toast for 1 minute until fragrant. Set aside.
2. Place the tomato and red onion in a bowl and toss to combine.
3. To poach the eggs, bring a wide saucepan of water to the boil. Reduce the heat to a simmer and add the vinegar. Crack an egg into a mug, then slide it into the simmering water. Repeat with the other eggs and poach for 4 minutes. Remove the eggs from the pan using a slotted spoon and transfer to a paper towel–lined plate.
4. Spread the yoghurt across the bottom of two small shallow bowls, then add the eggs. Top with the tomato and red onion, and drizzle the chilli oil over. Garnish with the dill leaves, then season with ¼ teaspoon freshly ground black pepper and serve with the pita bread.

UNITS PER SERVE:	
Breads, Cereals, Legumes, Starchy Veg	1
Dairy	1
Lean Meat, Fish, Poultry, Eggs, Tofu	0
Low-Moderate Carbohydrate Veg	0.5
Healthy Fats	1

Strawberry Cashew Yoghurt Bowl

CARBS 20g PER SERVE

SERVES: 2 | PREPARATION: 5 MINUTES | COOKING: NIL

¾ cup (200 g) reduced-fat natural yoghurt
1 teaspoon pure vanilla extract
6 medium strawberries, hulled and sliced
2 teaspoons cashew butter (see notes)
50 g untoasted natural muesli (see notes)
2 teaspoons shredded coconut

Divide the yoghurt between two bowls, then stir ½ teaspoon vanilla extract through each serving. Top each bowl with the strawberries, cashew butter, muesli and shredded coconut, then serve.

Notes

When purchasing nut butters, it is important to look at the food label. Make sure your nut butter has no added sugar or salt.

Ensure your purchased muesli is fruit and sugar free. There are a lot of great options on the market that are a mix of oats and nuts.

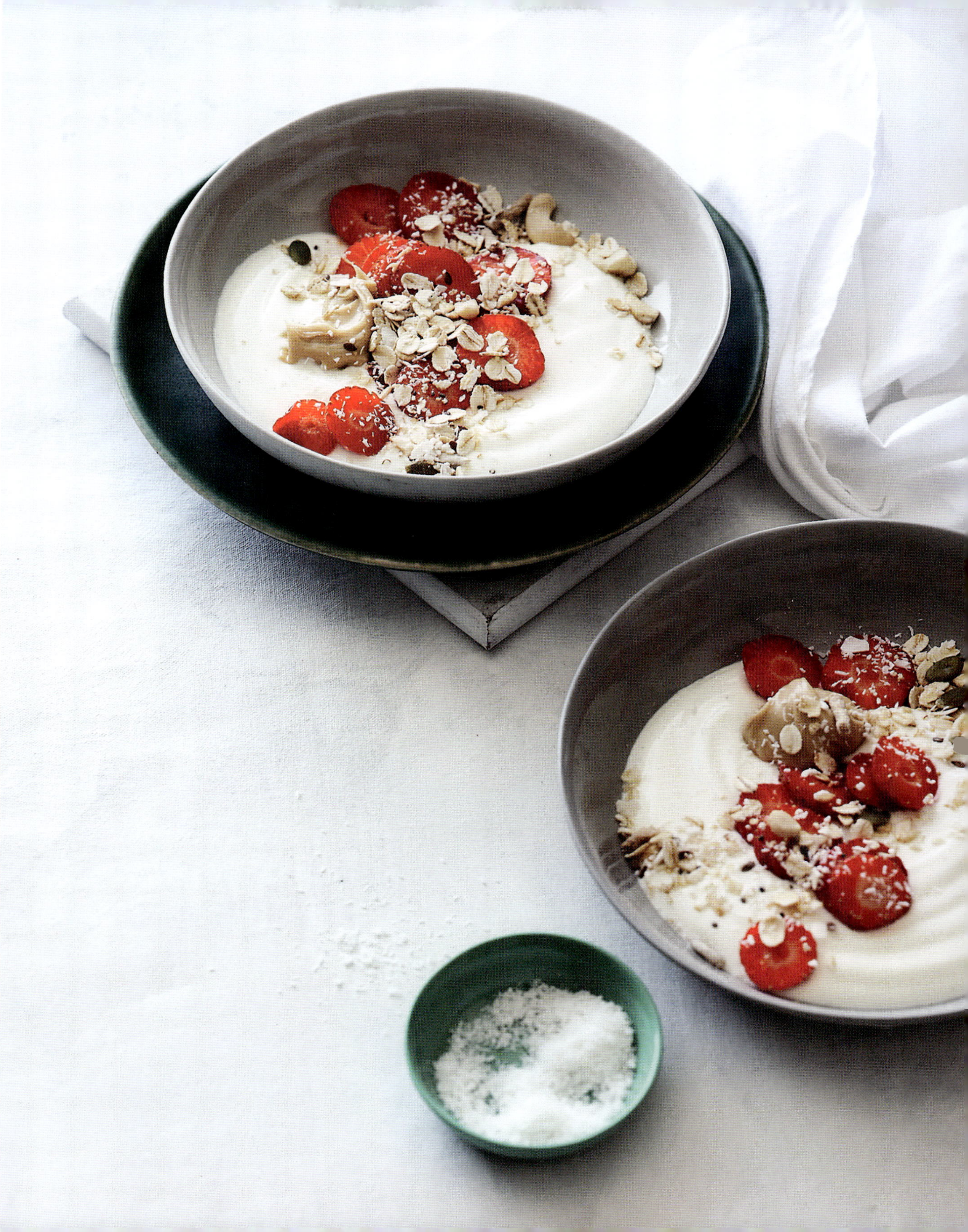

UNITS PER SERVE:	
Breads, Cereals, Legumes, Starchy Veg	0.5
Dairy	0
Lean Meat, Fish, Poultry, Eggs, Tofu	1
Low–Moderate Carbohydrate Veg	4
Healthy Fats	2

Smoky Shakshuka

CARBS 19g PER SERVE

SERVES: 4 | PREPARATION: 5 MINUTES | COOKING: 12 MINUTES

2 tablespoons extra virgin olive oil
1 onion, diced
1 red capsicum, seeded and sliced into 1 cm strips
1 zucchini, finely diced
4 cloves garlic, sliced
2 teaspoons smoked paprika
1 teaspoon ground cumin
Pinch cayenne pepper
400 g tinned whole peeled tomatoes
8 × 55 g free-range eggs
2 slices multigrain bread, toasted and sliced in half
4 cups baby spinach leaves
1 cup chopped flat-leaf parsley leaves

1. Heat the olive oil in a large frying pan over medium heat. Add the onion, capsicum and zucchini and cook for 5 minutes until tender. Add the garlic, paprika, cumin and cayenne pepper and stir through for 1 minute or until fragrant.
2. Pour in the tinned tomatoes, using a wooden spoon to break them up, then bring to a simmer. Make an indentation in the sauce with the spoon, then crack an egg into the hole. Repeat with the other eggs. Cover the pan with a lid and cook for 5 minutes, undisturbed, until the egg whites have set.
3. Remove the pan from the heat and divide the shakshuka between four plates. Serve with the toast and spinach, garnished with the parsley.

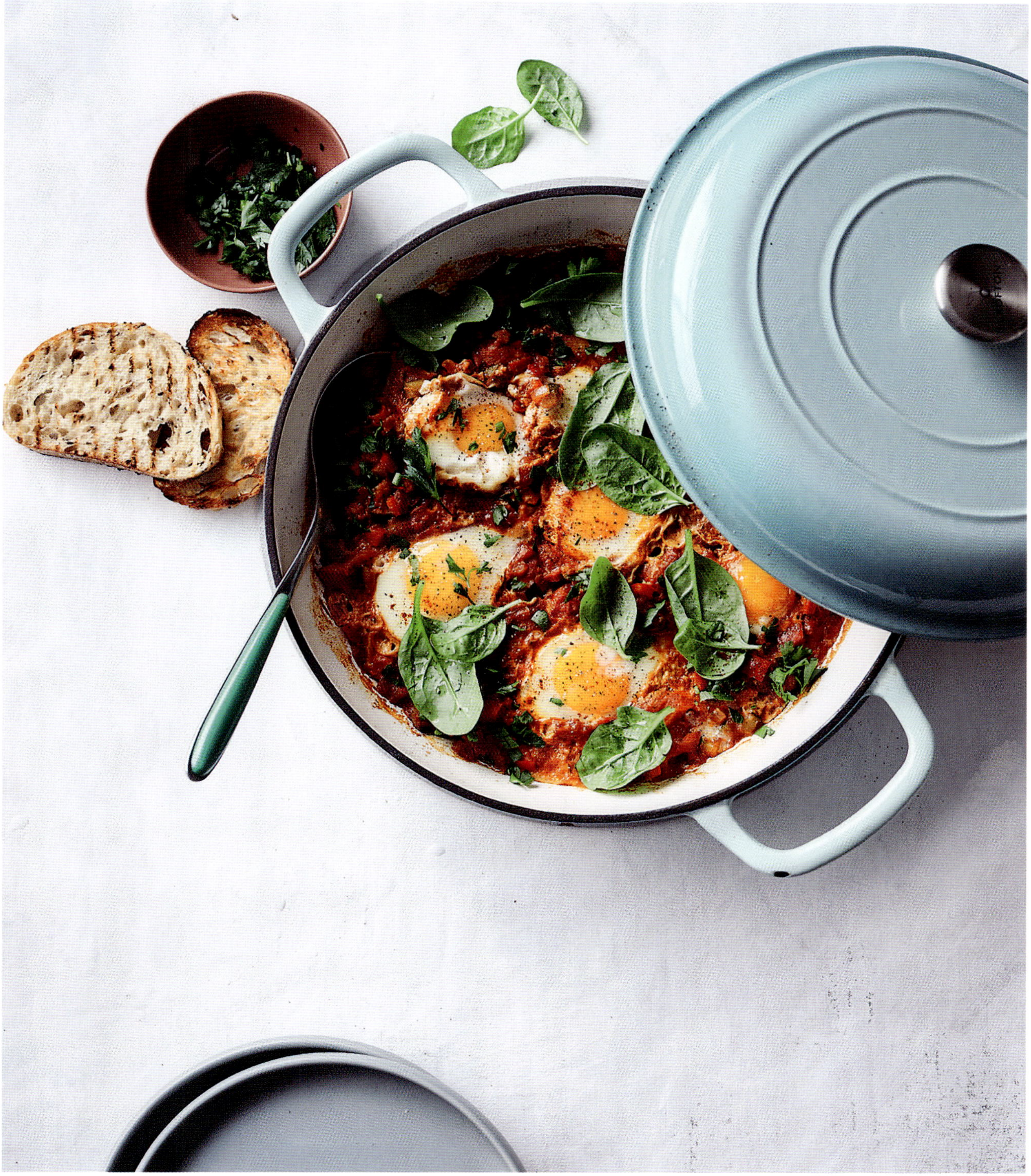

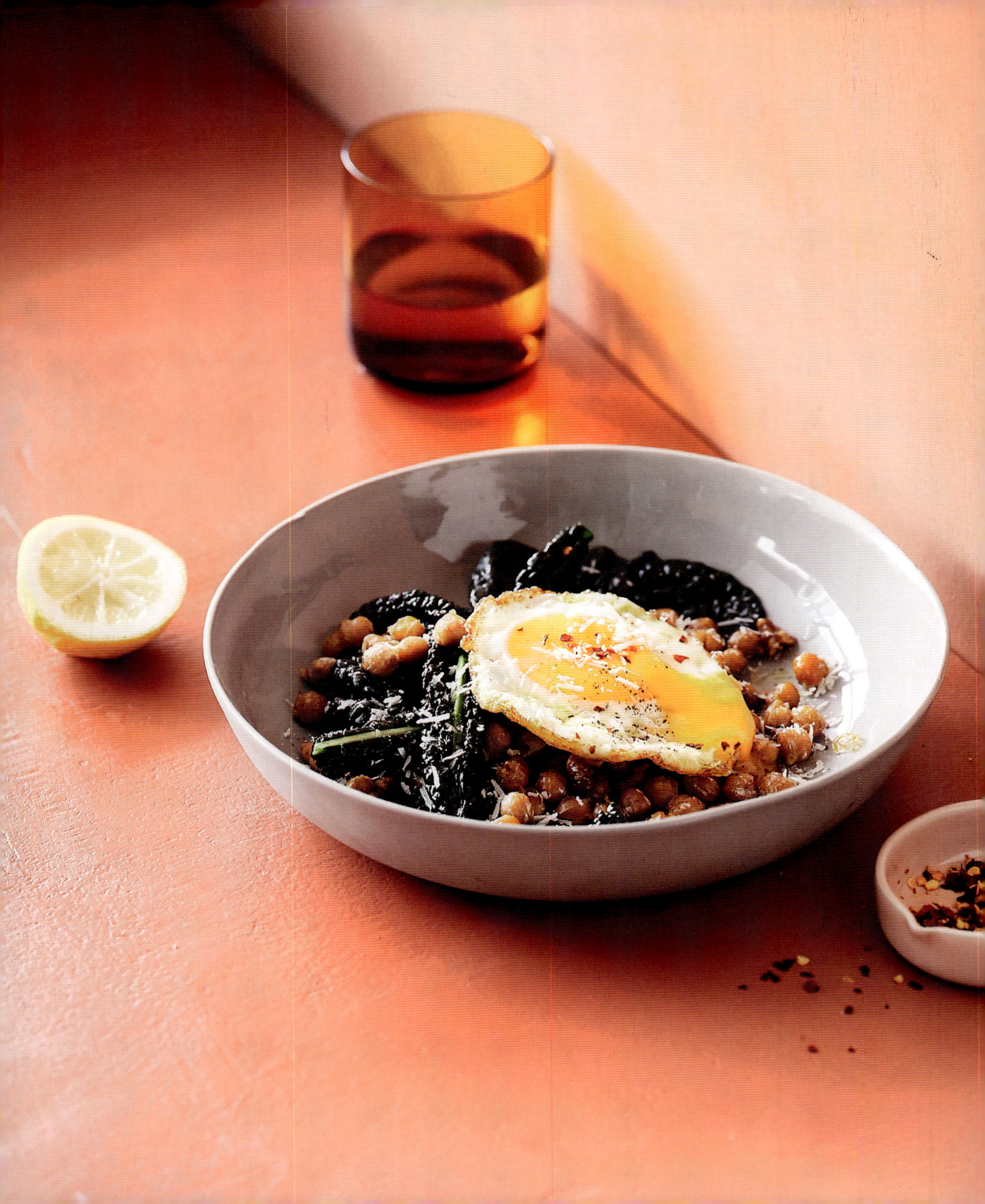

UNITS PER SERVE:	
Breads, Cereals, Legumes, Starchy Veg	1
Dairy	1
Lean Meat, Fish, Poultry, Eggs, Tofu	0.5
Low–Moderate Carbohydrate Veg	1
Healthy Fats	2

Chickpeas and Kale with Chilli Eggs

CARBS 16 g PER SERVE

SERVES: 2 | PREPARATION: 2 MINUTES | COOKING: 10 MINUTES

- 6 leaves kale (curly or Tuscan kale), stalks removed, leaves torn
- Juice of ½ lemon
- 2 teaspoons extra virgin olive oil
- 1 cup tinned salt-reduced chickpeas, drained and rinsed
- 2 tablespoons crumbled walnuts
- 2 × 55 g free-range eggs
- Pinch dried chilli flakes
- 40 g parmesan, grated

1. Place the kale in a large bowl, then add the lemon juice and massage it into the kale leaves for about 30 seconds until the kale softens. Set aside.
2. Heat half the olive oil in a frying pan over medium–high heat. Add the chickpeas and walnuts and cook for 4–5 minutes, tossing occasionally, until the chickpeas are golden around the edges. Transfer the mixture to a bowl and set aside.
3. Place the remaining olive oil in the pan. Once hot, crack in the eggs and sprinkle the chilli flakes around the edges. Cook for 4 minutes until the egg whites have set.
4. Divide the kale between two plates, top with the chickpeas, walnuts and chilli egg, sprinkle with parmesan and serve.

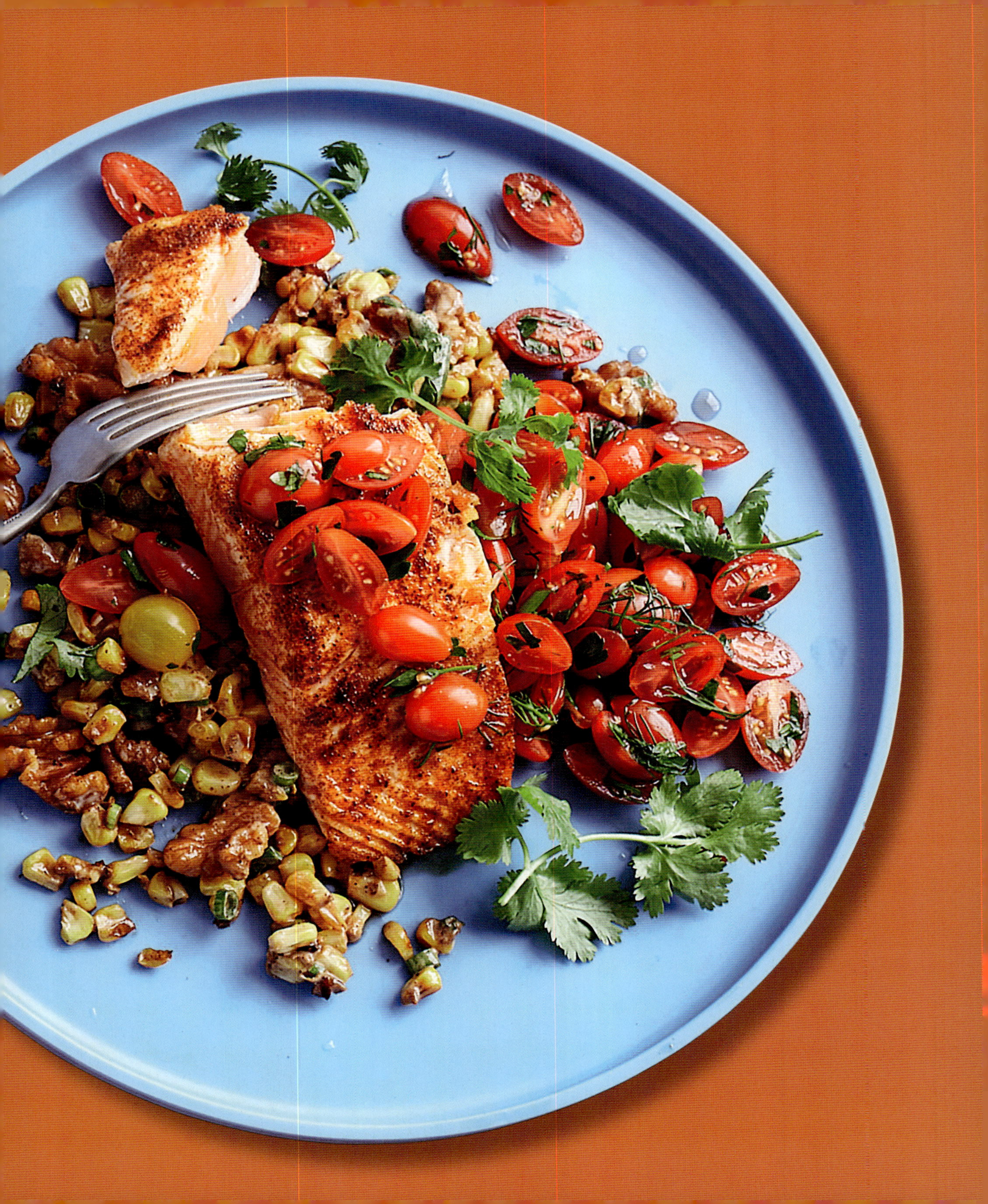

02.

Lunch

UNITS PER SERVE:	
Breads, Cereals, Legumes, Starchy Veg	1
Dairy	0
Lean Meat, Fish, Poultry, Eggs, Tofu	1
Low–Moderate Carbohydrate Veg	2
Healthy Fats	2.5

Spiced Beef Pita Pockets with Tomato Salad

CARBS 14g PER SERVE

SERVES: 4 | PREPARATION: 15 MINUTES | COOKING: 15 MINUTES

2 teaspoons extra virgin olive oil
1 onion, finely diced
500 g lean beef mince
3 cloves garlic, crushed
1 tablespoon Moroccan spice blend
2 tablespoons finely chopped flat-leaf parsley
2 small wholemeal pita breads, sliced in half, warmed in the microwave

TOMATO SALAD

250 g cherry tomatoes, sliced
½ small red onion, thinly sliced
½ cup chopped coriander
½ cup chopped flat-leaf parsley
1 Lebanese cucumber, diced
2 tablespoons red wine vinegar

TAHINI DRESSING

2 tablespoons tahini
½ small clove garlic, crushed
Juice of ½ lemon

1. To make the tomato salad, place all the ingredients in a bowl and toss to combine. Set aside to marinate.
2. Heat the olive oil in a large frying pan over medium–high heat. Add the onion and cook, tossing occasionally, for 3–4 minutes until golden. Add the beef mince and cook, breaking it up with a wooden spoon, for 5 minutes or until brown and cooked through. Add the garlic and Moroccan spice blend and stir for 1 minute until fragrant. Remove the pan from the heat and stir the parsley through.
3. In a small bowl, mix together the ingredients for the tahini dressing. Add 1–2 tablespoons of warm water and stir it through to thin out the sauce to a drizzling consistency.
4. Divide the spiced beef, tomato salad and warmed pita bread between four plates. Drizzle over the tahini dressing and serve.

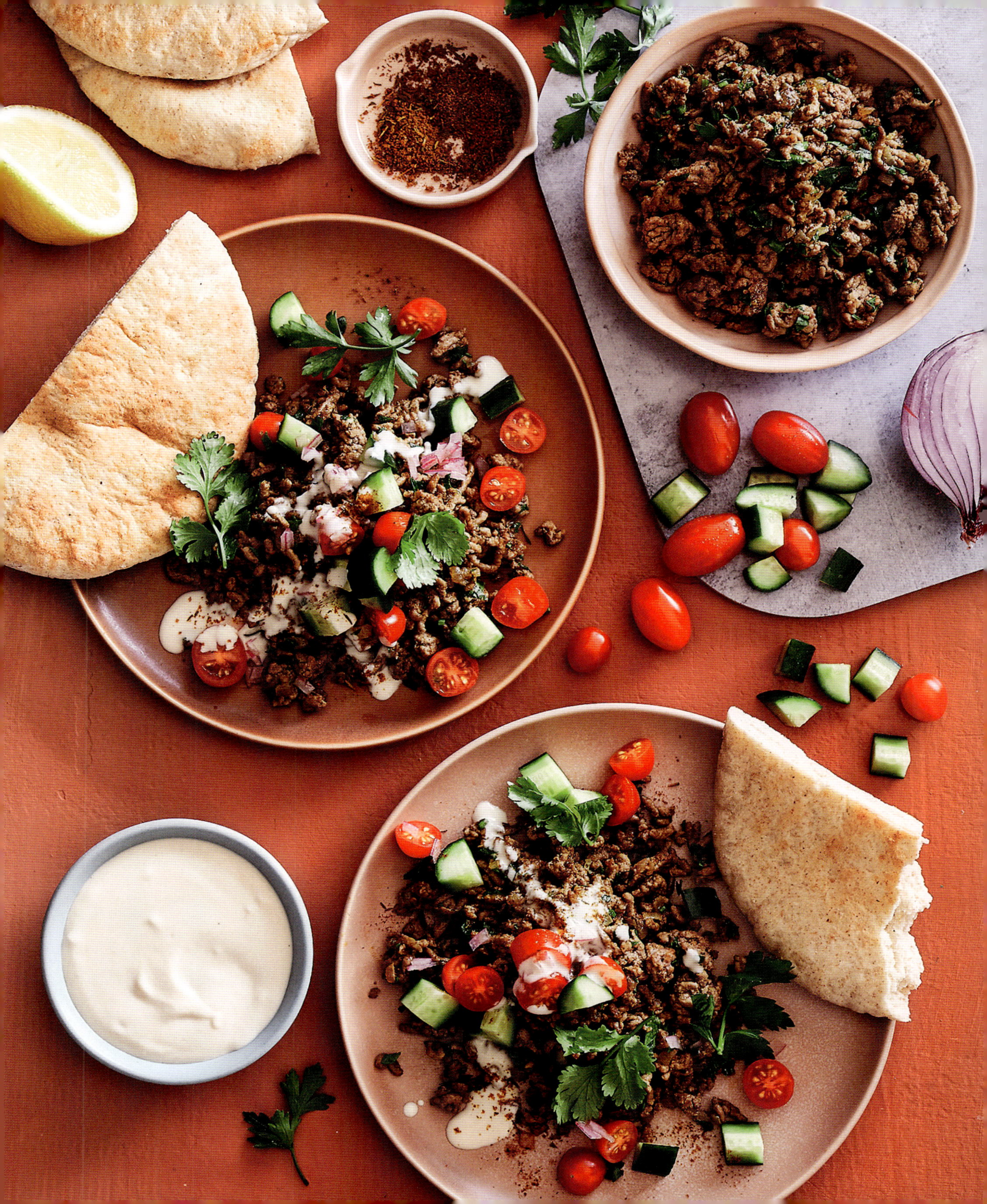

UNITS PER SERVE:	
Breads, Cereals, Legumes, Starchy Veg	1
Dairy	1
Lean Meat, Fish, Poultry, Eggs, Tofu	1
Low–Moderate Carbohydrate Veg	3
Healthy Fats	2

Open Chicken Sandwich Bento Box

CARBS 19g PER SERVE

SERVES: 1 | PREPARATION: 5 MINUTES | COOKING: NIL

- 100 g roast chicken, skin removed (see notes)
- 20 g slice cheddar
- 1 small Lebanese cucumber, thinly sliced
- 1 thin slice multigrain bread
- 2 teaspoons oil-based pesto (see notes)
- 1 cup lettuce leaves (cos, butter or iceberg)

Assemble all the ingredients in an airtight container or a stainless-steel bento box and serve.

Notes

If you are not cooking your own, you can use a purchased pre-roasted chicken or chicken breast. You can find these in the refrigerator section of the supermarket.

If you are using an oil-free pesto, you are able to remove the healthy fat unit count from your daily unit tally.

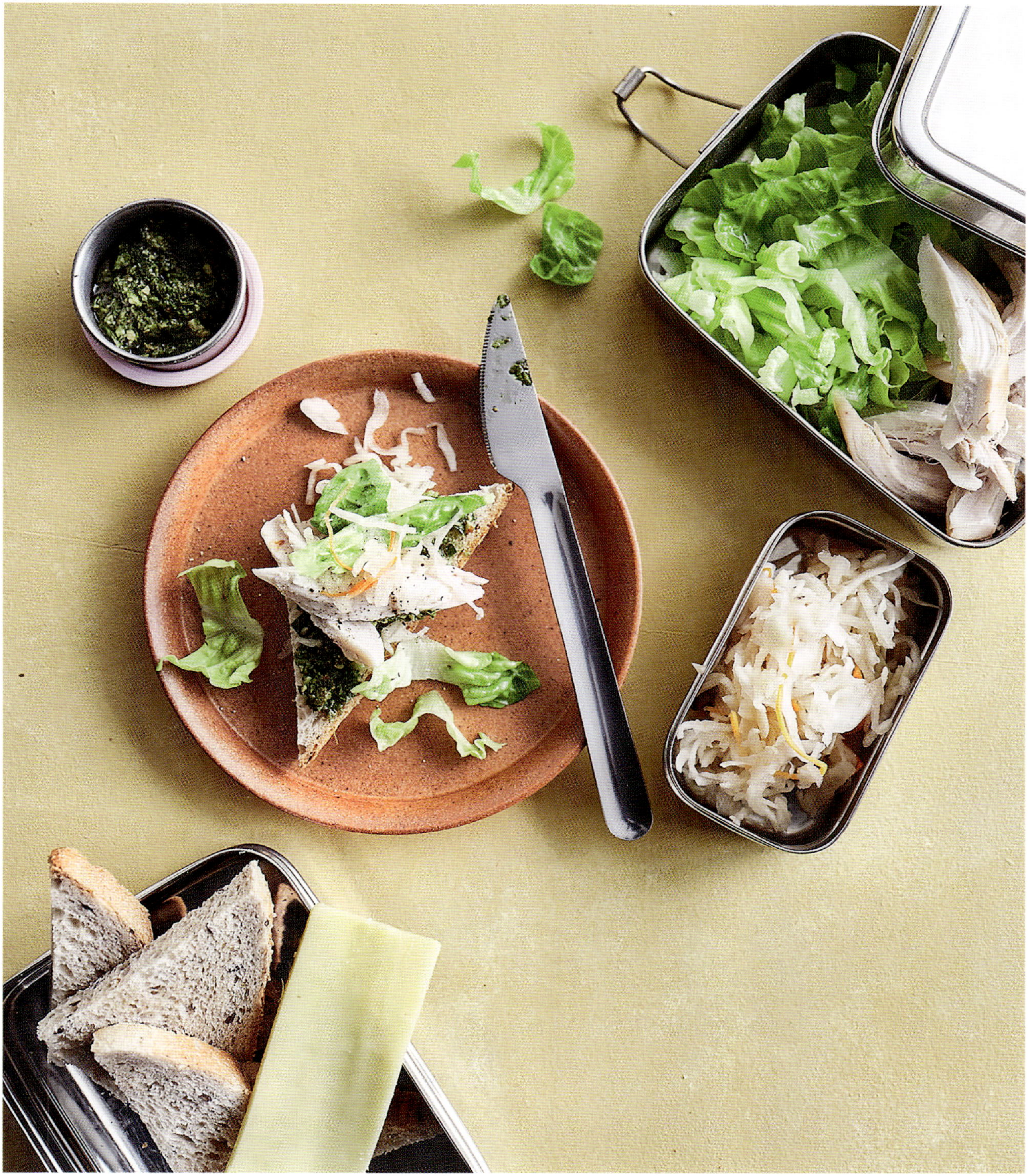

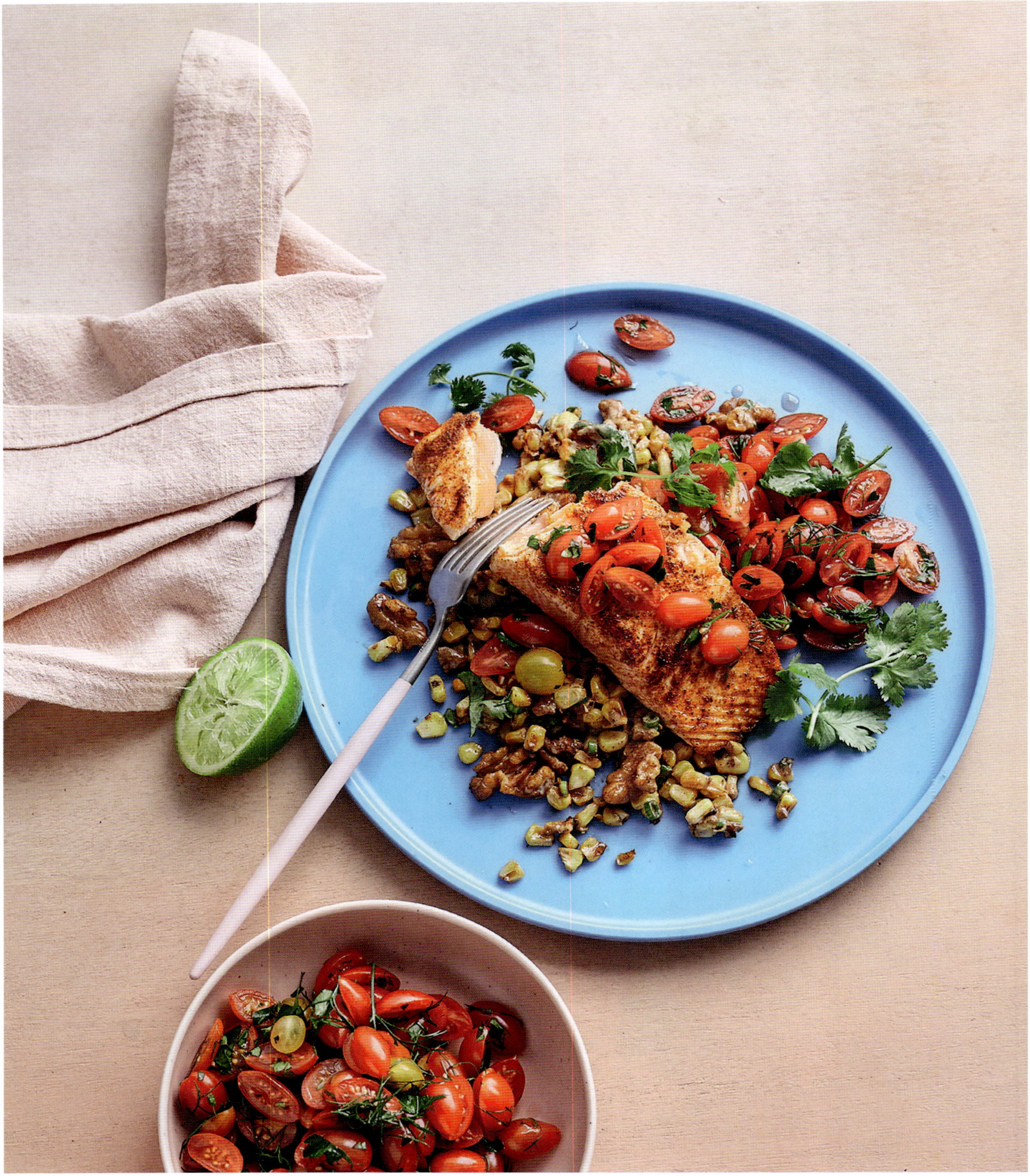

UNITS PER SERVE:	
Breads, Cereals, Legumes, Starchy Veg	1
Dairy	0
Lean Meat, Fish, Poultry, Eggs, Tofu	1.5
Low–Moderate Carbohydrate Veg	2
Healthy Fats	2.5

Seared Salmon with Corn Salad and Herby Tomatoes

CARBS 16 g PER SERVE

SERVES: 4 | PREPARATION: 10 MINUTES | COOKING: 15 MINUTES

1 teaspoon extra virgin olive oil
4 × 150 g boneless, skinless salmon fillets
1 tablespoon smoked paprika

HERBY TOMATOES

500 g cherry tomatoes, halved
2 tablespoons red wine vinegar
½ cup roughly chopped flat-leaf parsley
¼ cup dill leaves, roughly chopped

CORN SALAD

2½ corn cobs, husks and silks removed, kernels sliced off (200 g kernels)
¼ cup (35 g) walnuts, roughly chopped
¼ teaspoon smoked paprika
1 cup coriander leaves, roughly chopped
4 spring onions, finely chopped
Juice of ½ lime
1½ tablespoons whole-egg mayonnaise

1. To make the herby tomatoes, place all the ingredients in a large bowl and toss to combine. Set aside to marinate.
2. Heat the olive oil in a large frying pan over medium–high heat. Add the salmon, sprinkle with the paprika and cook for 4 minutes. Flip, then cook for another 3 minutes, or until the salmon is cooked to your liking. Transfer the salmon to a plate and loosely cover with foil.
3. To make the corn salad, drain out most of the salmon fat from the frying pan, leaving a few teaspoons. Add the corn kernels, walnuts and paprika and cook, tossing occasionally, for 3–4 minutes until the corn is tender and the walnuts are lightly toasted. Remove from the heat and place in a bowl. Allow to cool for a minute, then add the coriander, spring onion, lime juice, mayonnaise, ¼ teaspoon freshly ground black pepper and toss to combine.
4. Divide the salmon between four plates and serve with the herby tomatoes and corn salad.

UNITS PER SERVE:	
Breads, Cereals, Legumes, Starchy Veg	1
Dairy	1.5
Lean Meat, Fish, Poultry, Eggs, Tofu	0.5
Low–Moderate Carbohydrate Veg	2
Healthy Fats	2.5

Zucchini Pancakes with Crispy Chickpeas

CARBS 17 g PER SERVE

SERVES: 4 | PREPARATION: 15 MINUTES | COOKING: 30 MINUTES

750 g zucchini (about 4 medium zucchini)
4 × 55 g free-range eggs
⅓ cup flat-leaf parsley, finely chopped
⅓ cup (30 g) chickpea flour (besan)
2½ tablespoons extra virgin olive oil

YOGHURT DRESSING

½ cup (130 g) natural yoghurt
¼ teaspoon freshly ground black pepper
Juice of ½ lemon
40 g Danish feta

GREEN SALAD

1 cup baby spinach leaves
1 cup micro green sprouts
Juice of ½ lemon

CRISPY CHICKPEAS

2 teaspoons extra virgin olive oil
1 × 400 g tin salt-reduced chickpeas, drained, rinsed and patted dry
½ teaspoon ground turmeric

1. To make the pancakes, finely grate the zucchini on the small holes of a box grater. Use your hands to squeeze out the excess water from the zucchini over the sink, then place in a large bowl. Add the eggs and parsley and whisk to combine. Stir in the chickpea flour until well combined. Set aside for 10 minutes before cooking.
2. To make the yoghurt dressing, combine all the ingredients in a small bowl, mashing the feta in with a fork. Set aside.
3. To make the green salad, place the spinach and sprouts in a bowl, squeeze the lemon juice over and toss to coat. Set aside.
4. Heat a dash of the olive oil in a large frying pan over medium–high heat. Scoop up ¼ cup amounts of the zucchini batter and place in the frying pan – you should be able to cook three pancakes at once. Cook the pancakes for 3 minutes on each side until golden brown. Set aside and repeat with the remaining olive oil and batter. Transfer the pancakes to a plate and keep warm.
5. To make the crispy chickpeas, heat the olive oil in the same pan, add the chickpeas and cook, tossing occasionally, for 4–5 minutes, until the chickpeas are crisp on the edges. Sprinkle in the turmeric and toss again for 1 minute until fragrant.
6. Spread the yoghurt dressing across four plates, top with the pancakes, the green salad and crispy chickpeas and serve.

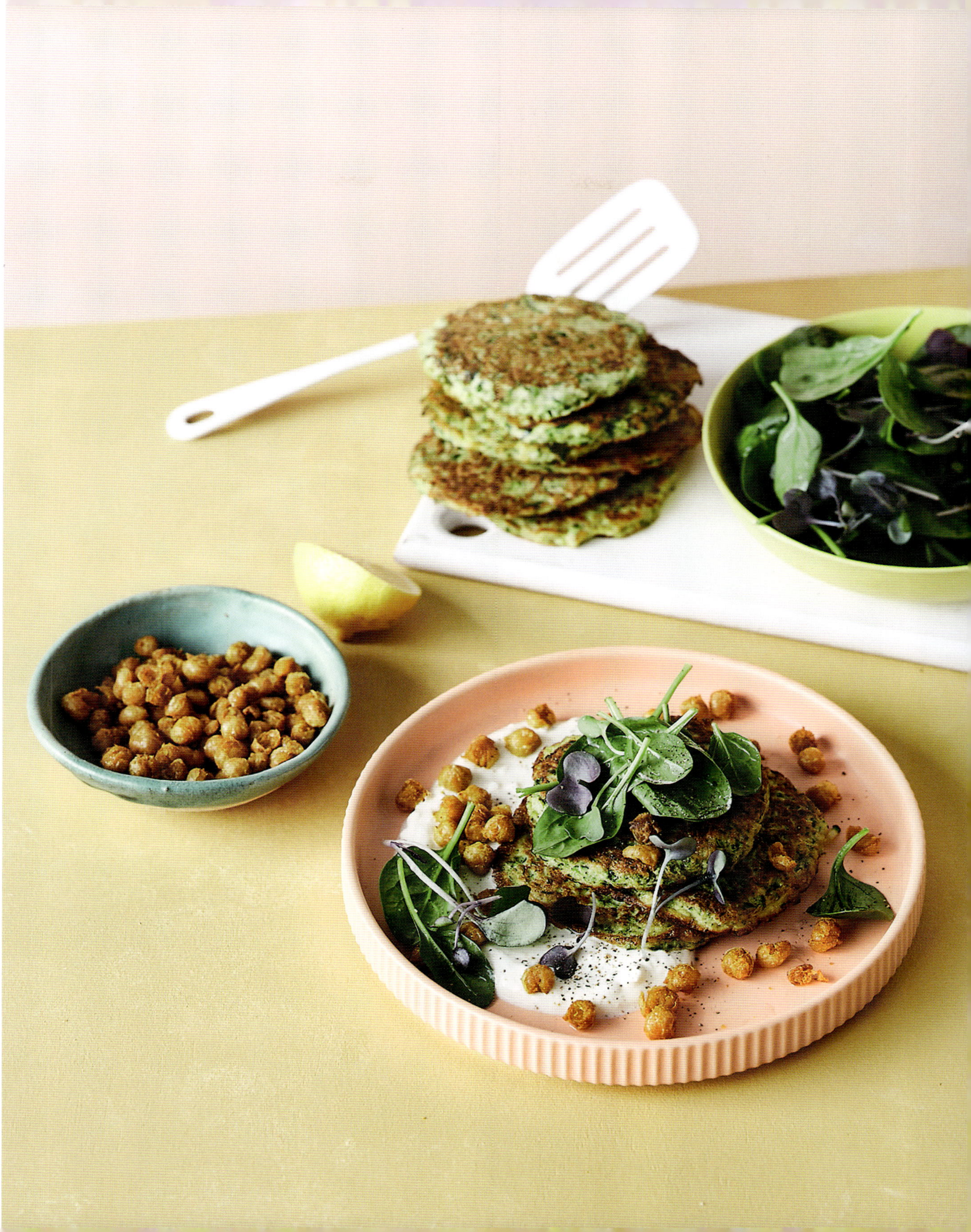

UNITS PER SERVE:	
Breads, Cereals, Legumes, Starchy Veg	1
Dairy	1.5
Lean Meat, Fish, Poultry, Eggs, Tofu	1
Low–Moderate Carbohydrate Veg	2.5
Healthy Fats	2

Spring Quinoa Pilaf with Asparagus and Salmon

CARBS 20g PER SERVE

SERVES: 4 | PREPARATION: 15 MINUTES | COOKING: 25 MINUTES

80 g (½ cup) white quinoa, rinsed well and drained
1 teaspoon extra virgin olive oil
2 × 200 g salmon fillets, skin on
Pinch of paprika
2 bunches asparagus, woody ends trimmed, stalks cut into 4 cm pieces diagonally
1 cup (100 g) sugar snap peas, ends trimmed and thinly sliced
3 cups baby spinach leaves
1 cup mint leaves
1 cup roughly chopped coriander
¼ cup finely chopped dill
3 tablespoons unsalted almonds, roughly chopped
3 tablespoons unsalted pistachios, roughly chopped
2 tablespoons pumpkin seeds (pepitas)

YOGHURT DRESSING

½ cup (130 g) natural yoghurt
¼ teaspoon freshly ground black pepper
Juice of 1 lemon
40 g soft goat's cheese

1. Place the quinoa in a sieve and rinse under cold tap water for 1 minute. Place in a saucepan with 1 cup (250 ml) water over high heat and bring to the boil. Reduce to a simmer, cover and cook for 10 minutes. Remove the pan from the heat and stand, covered, for 10 minutes. Remove the lid, fluff the quinoa with a fork and allow to cool to room temperature. (You can put it in the refrigerator to speed this up.)
2. To make the yoghurt dressing, place all the ingredients in a small bowl and mix to combine, mashing the goat's cheese in well with a fork.
3. Heat the olive oil in a large frying pan over medium–high heat. Add the salmon, skin side down, sprinkle with the paprika and cook for 4 minutes. Flip, then cook for another 3 minutes, or until the salmon is cooked to your liking. Transfer the salmon to a plate and loosely cover with foil.
4. Place the cooled quinoa, asparagus, sugar snap peas, spinach, mint, coriander, dill, almonds, pistachios and pumpkin seeds in a bowl and toss to combine.
5. Divide the pilaf between four shallow bowls. Flake the salmon and place it on top of the pilaf, drizzle generously with the yoghurt dressing and serve.

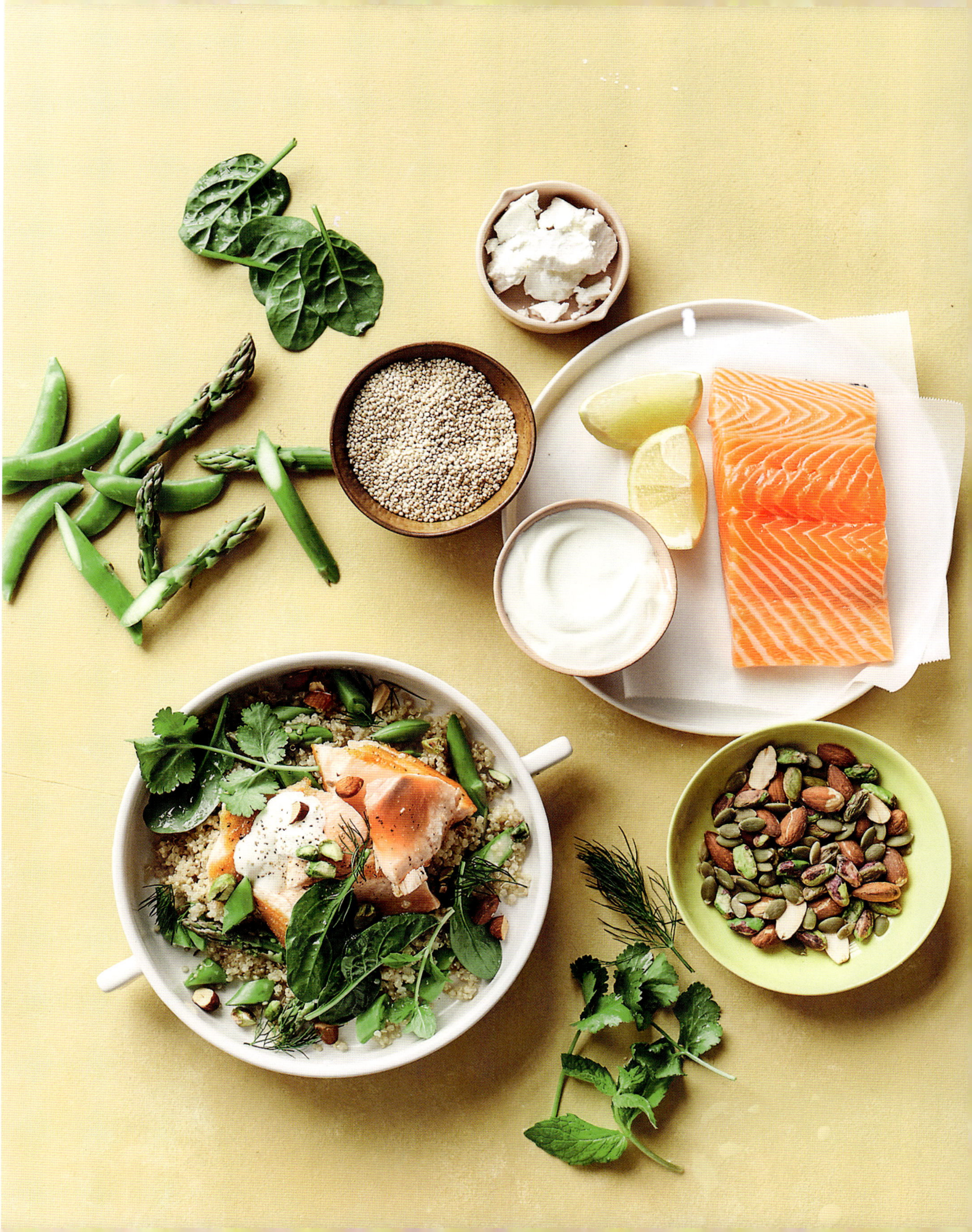

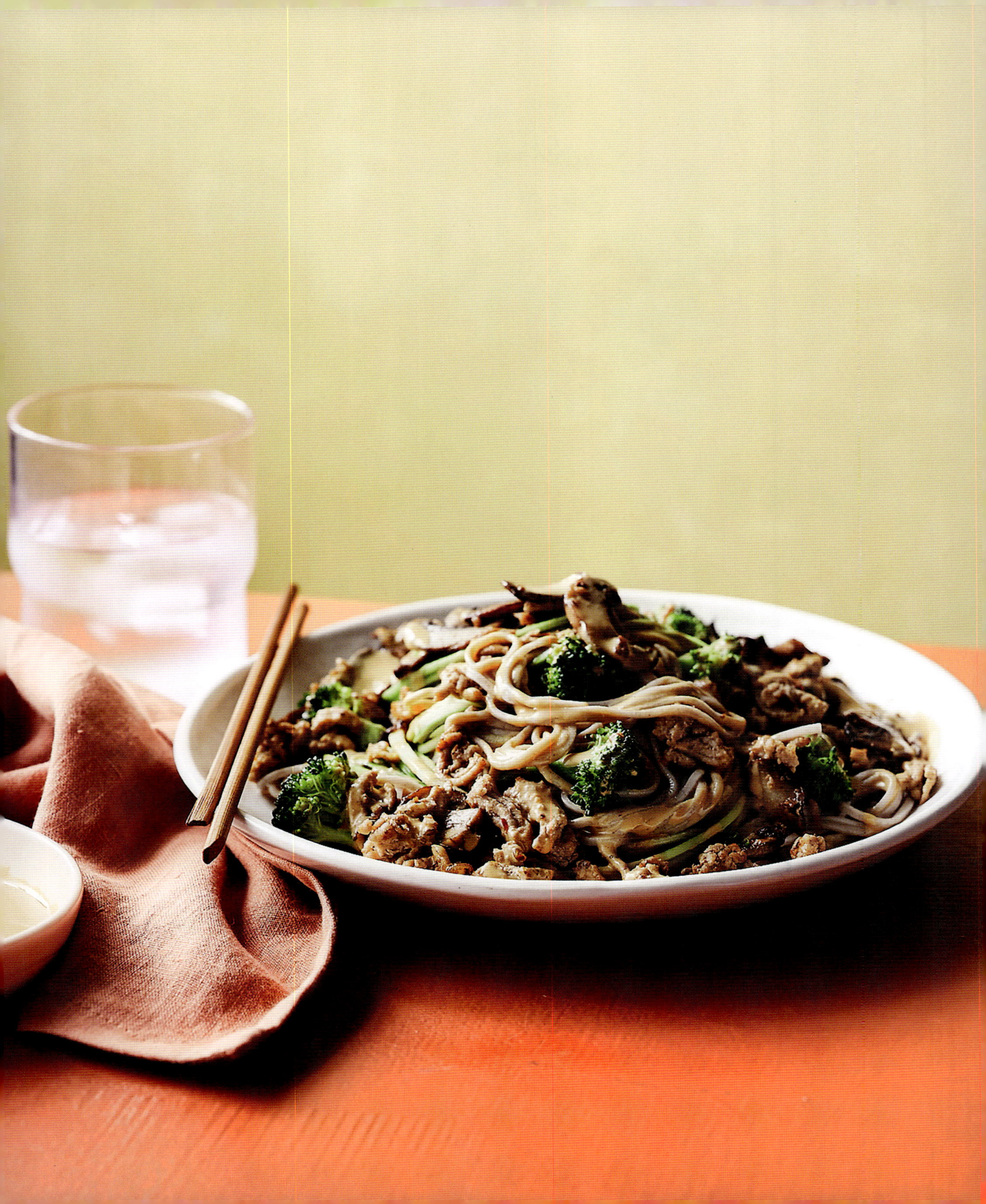

UNITS PER SERVE:	
Breads, Cereals, Legumes, Starchy Veg	0.5
Dairy	0
Lean Meat, Fish, Poultry, Eggs, Tofu	1
Low–Moderate Carbohydrate Veg	2.5
Healthy Fats	3

Garlicky Pork Soba Noodle Salad

CARBS 15g PER SERVE

SERVES: 4 | PREPARATION: 10 MINUTES | COOKING: 25 MINUTES

1 teaspoon extra virgin olive oil
2 golden shallots, thinly sliced
400 g lean pork mince
300 g sliced Swiss brown mushrooms
1 head broccoli (275 g), florets and stem chopped into 1–2 cm pieces
4 cloves garlic, thinly sliced
½ teaspoon dried chilli flakes
60 g soba noodles
5 cups (730 g) purchased zucchini noodles (see notes)

TAHINI DRESSING

2 tablespoons tahini
3 teaspoons salt-reduced tamari (see notes)
2 tablespoons rice wine vinegar
3 teaspoons sesame oil

1. Heat the olive oil in a large frying pan over medium–high heat, add the shallot and cook for 3–4 minutes until golden and tender. Add the pork mince and cook, breaking it up with a wooden spoon, for 3–4 minutes or until brown and cooked through. Add the mushrooms, broccoli, garlic and dried chilli flakes and cook for 2–3 minutes until the mushrooms are browned and any excess liquid has evaporated.
2. Place a medium saucepan of water over high heat.
3. To make the tahini dressing, combine all the ingredients in a small bowl. Add 1–2 tablespoons of warm water and stir it through to thin out the sauce to a drizzling consistency.
4. Place the soba noodles in the pan of boiling water and cook according to the packet instructions. Remove the pan from the heat and add the zucchini noodles. Leave for 30 seconds to blanch, then drain all the noodles and rinse under cool water.
5. Transfer the noodles to the frying pan with the pork mince mixture and mix to combine. Add the tahini dressing and toss well to coat.
6. Divide the saucy noodles between four wide bowls to serve.

Notes

You'll find zucchini noodles in the fresh produce section at the supermarket. If unavailable, you can simply cut 4 zucchini into thin matchsticks and use as directed in the recipe.

Tamari is a higher-salt product, so ideally use low-salt or no-added-salt alternatives. If you are following a low-sodium diet, omit this ingredient.

UNITS PER SERVE:	
Breads, Cereals, Legumes, Starchy Veg	0.5
Dairy	0.5
Lean Meat, Fish, Poultry, Eggs, Tofu	1.5
Low–Moderate Carbohydrate Veg	2
Healthy Fats	3

BBQ Jerk Chicken and Marinated Tomatoes

CARBS 19g PER SERVE

SERVES: 4 | PREPARATION: 15 MINUTES | COOKING: 30 MINUTES

1½ tablespoons dried thyme
1 teaspoon ground allspice
1 teaspoon ground cinnamon
¼ teaspoon cayenne pepper
4 cloves garlic, crushed
Juice of 1 lime
1 × 1.5 kg chicken, butterflied, skin removed (150 g shredded meat per serve once cooked) (see note)
1 teaspoon olive oil

MARINATED TOMATOES

500 g truss tomatoes, chopped
1 tablespoon extra virgin olive oil
2 tablespoons finely chopped flat-leaf parsley
1 clove garlic, crushed
Pinch dried chilli flakes

CORN AND AVOCADO SALAD

2 corn cobs, husks and silks removed
1 small avocado, sliced
4 cups cos lettuce leaves
¼ cup roughly chopped mint leaves
¼ cup roughly chopped basil leaves
2 teaspoons extra virgin olive oil
1 tablespoon red wine vinegar
¼ cup (65 g) reduced-fat natural yoghurt

1. Preheat a barbecue grill plate to high, or preheat the oven to 220°C (200°C fan-forced).
2. Place the thyme, allspice, cinnamon, cayenne pepper, garlic, lime juice and 1 teaspoon freshly ground black pepper in a small bowl and mix until combined into a thick paste.
3. Massage the paste into the butterflied chicken, then drizzle with the olive oil.
4. For the marinated tomatoes, place all the ingredients in a bowl and toss to combine.
5. Place the chicken on the barbecue grill, or in the oven, with the tomatoes and one of the corn cobs. Cook the chicken for 15 minutes on each side and the corn for 6 minutes, turning the chicken once and the corn regularly. Once cooked, set the chicken and tomatoes aside to rest.
6. Once cool enough to handle, slice the kernels off the grilled corn cob using a sharp knife, and also off the uncooked corn cob (the raw corn adds a great texture and freshness to the salad).
7. To make the corn and avocado salad, place the corn kernels in a large bowl with the avocado, lettuce, mint and basil. To make a dressing, combine the olive oil, vinegar and yoghurt in a small bowl and mix well. Drizzle the dressing over the salad.
8. Carve the chicken into pieces and serve with the marinated tomatoes and corn and avocado salad.

Note

You can buy your chicken already butterflied from your butcher, and also from many supermarkets (but buy it without any added flavouring).

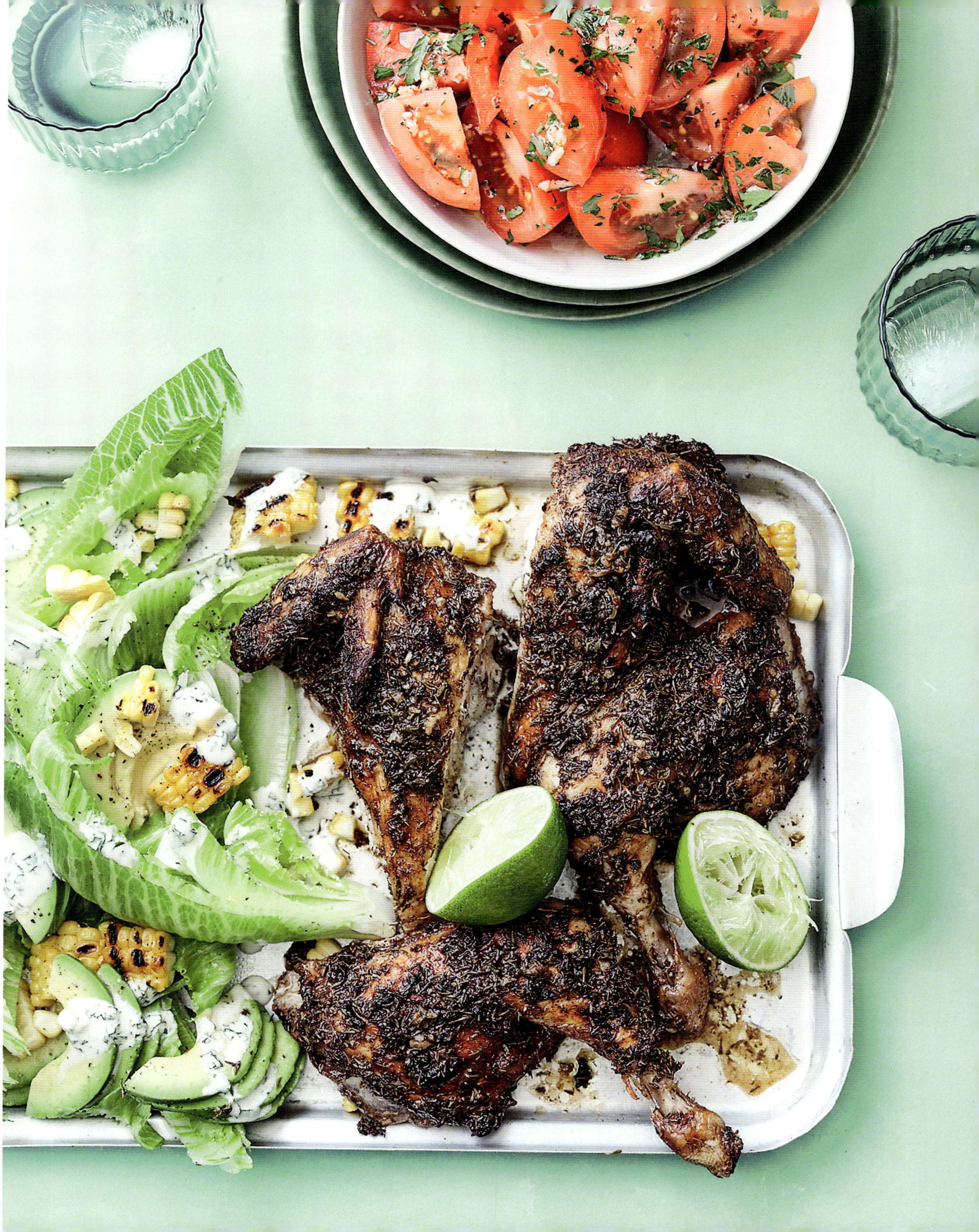

UNITS PER SERVE:	
Breads, Cereals, Legumes, Starchy Veg	1
Dairy	0
Lean Meat, Fish, Poultry, Eggs, Tofu	1
Low–Moderate Carbohydrate Veg	2
Healthy Fats	3

Egg Bento Box with Hummus, Olives and Spinach

CARBS 11g PER SERVE

SERVES: 1 | PREPARATION: 5 MINUTES | COOKING: 12 MINUTES

2 × 55 g free-range eggs
100 g cherry tomatoes, halved
1 tablespoon hummus
3 pitted kalamata olives
1 cup baby spinach leaves
½ wholemeal mountain bread wrap

1. Place a saucepan of water over high heat. Once boiling, add the eggs and cook, undisturbed, for 8 minutes. Remove the eggs from the pan using a slotted spoon and run them under water until cool to the touch.
2. Peel the eggs and slice in half, then transfer to an airtight container or a stainless steel bento box, along with the cherry tomatoes, hummus, olives and spinach. Add the mountain bread to wrap the ingredients in when you are ready to eat.

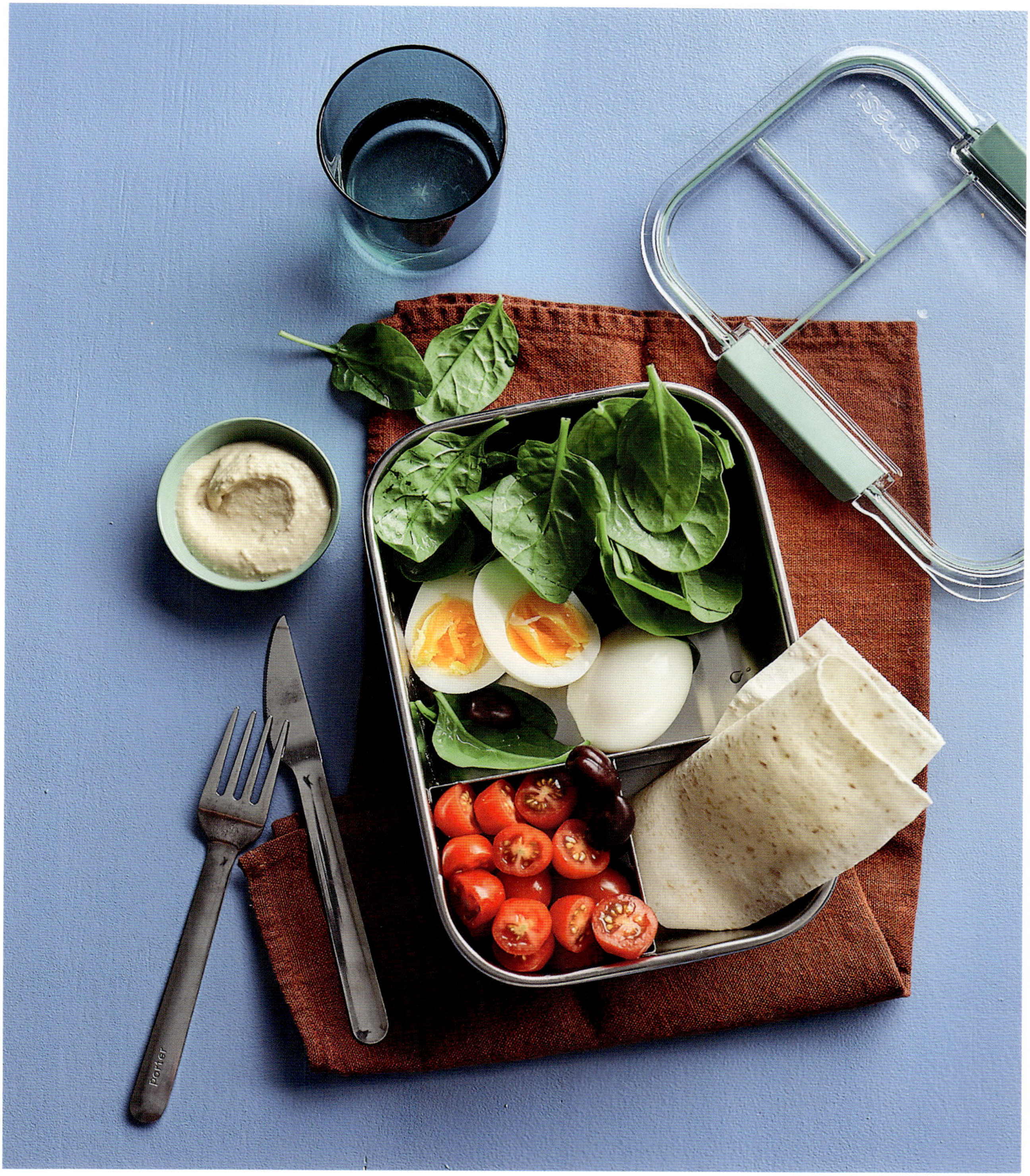

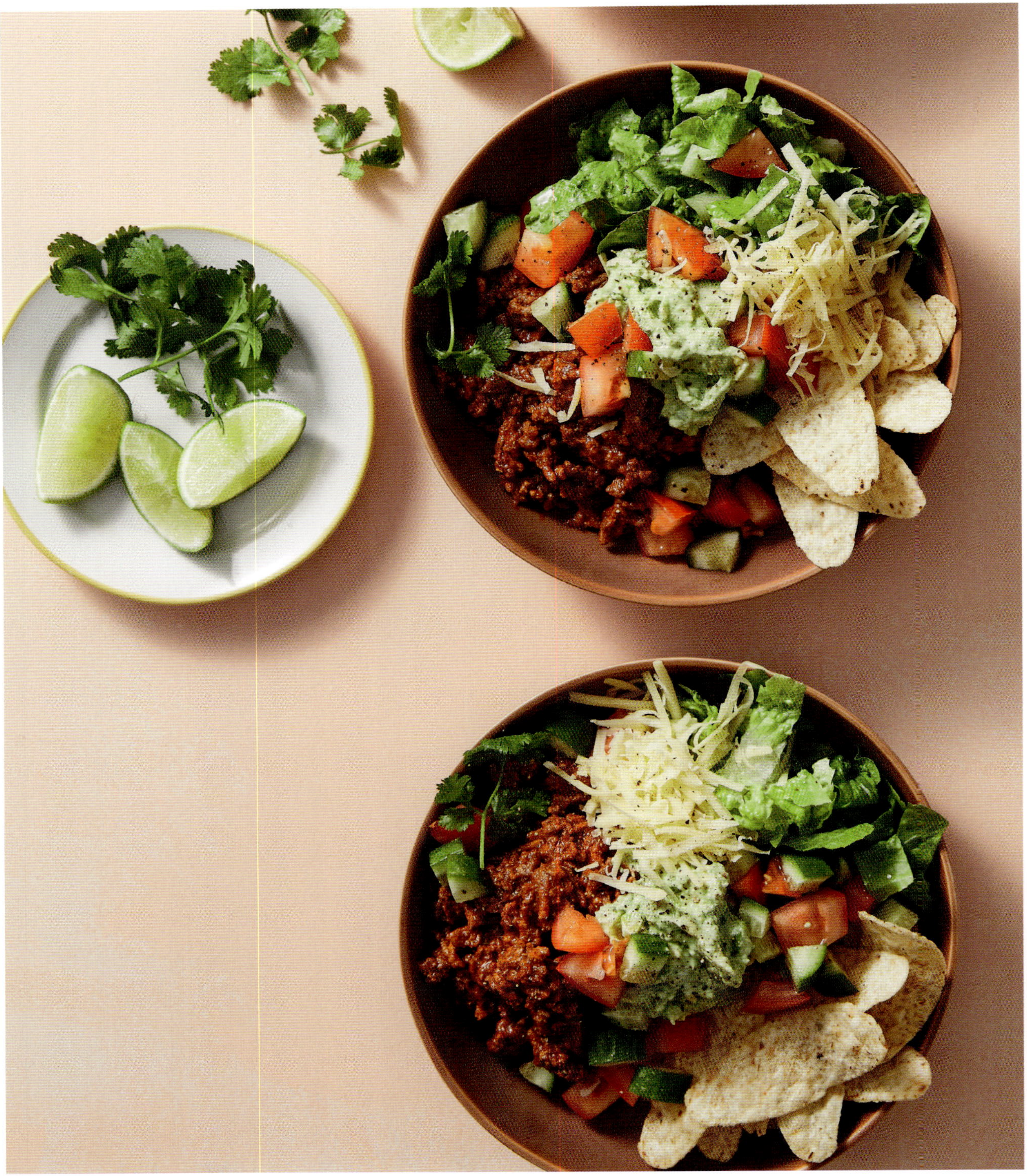

UNITS PER SERVE:	
Breads, Cereals, Legumes, Starchy Veg	1
Dairy	1
Lean Meat, Fish, Poultry, Eggs, Tofu	1.5
Low–Moderate Carbohydrate Veg	2
Healthy Fats	2.5

Beef Nachos Bowl with Quick Guac

CARBS 20g PER SERVE

SERVES: 4 | PREPARATION: 10 MINUTES | COOKING: 10 MINUTES

2 teaspoons extra virgin olive oil
600 g lean beef mince
1 tablespoon smoked paprika
2 teaspoons ground cumin
2 teaspoons ground coriander
3 cloves garlic, crushed
1 tablespoon tomato paste (no added sugar or salt)

QUICK GUAC

1 avocado
1 tablespoon low-fat natural yoghurt
Juice of 1 lime
½ cup coriander leaves, finely chopped

TO SERVE

2 tomatoes, diced
2 baby cos lettuces, shredded
1 Lebanese cucumber, diced
100 g unsalted corn chips
80 g grated cheddar
Coriander sprigs

1. Heat the olive oil in a large frying pan over medium–high heat. Add the beef mince and cook, breaking it up with a wooden spoon, for 4–5 minutes or until brown and cooked through. Add the paprika, cumin, ground coriander and garlic and stir through for 1 minute or until fragrant. Add the tomato paste and ⅓ cup (80 ml) water and stir for 1–2 minutes until well combined. Set aside.
2. To make the quick guac, mash the avocado in a bowl with a fork. Add the yoghurt, lime juice and chopped coriander and stir until combined.
3. Divide the beef between four bowls and serve with the tomato, lettuce, cucumber, corn chips, cheese, corainder sprigs and a dollop of guac.

UNITS PER SERVE:	
Breads, Cereals, Legumes, Starchy Veg	1
Dairy	0.5
Lean Meat, Fish, Poultry, Eggs, Tofu	1
Low–Moderate Carbohydrate Veg	2.5
Healthy Fats	1

Creamy Chicken and Celery Wraps

CARBS 14g PER SERVE

SERVES: 4 | PREPARATION: 10 MINUTES | COOKING: NIL

400 g shredded roast chicken, skin removed (see note)
2 sticks celery, finely chopped
¾ cup chopped kale, stalks removed
1 Lebanese cucumber, diced
¼ cup (35 g) walnuts, toasted
1 tablespoon finely chopped dill
3 spring onions, finely chopped
4 cups roughly chopped cos lettuce
2 wholemeal mountain bread wraps, sliced in half

DRESSING

Juice of ½ lemon
2 teaspoons Dijon mustard
½ cup (130 g) low-fat natural yoghurt
¼ teaspoon freshly ground black pepper

1. To make the dressing, place the ingredients in a large bowl and mix to combine. Add the chicken, celery, kale, cucumber, walnuts, dill and spring onion and mix well to coat in the dressing.
2. Place one-quarter of the cos lettuce and one-quarter of the chicken mixture on each mountain bread half and roll up. Serve immediately.

Note

If you are not cooking your own, you can use a purchased pre-roasted chicken or chicken breast. You can find these in the refrigerator section of the supermarket.

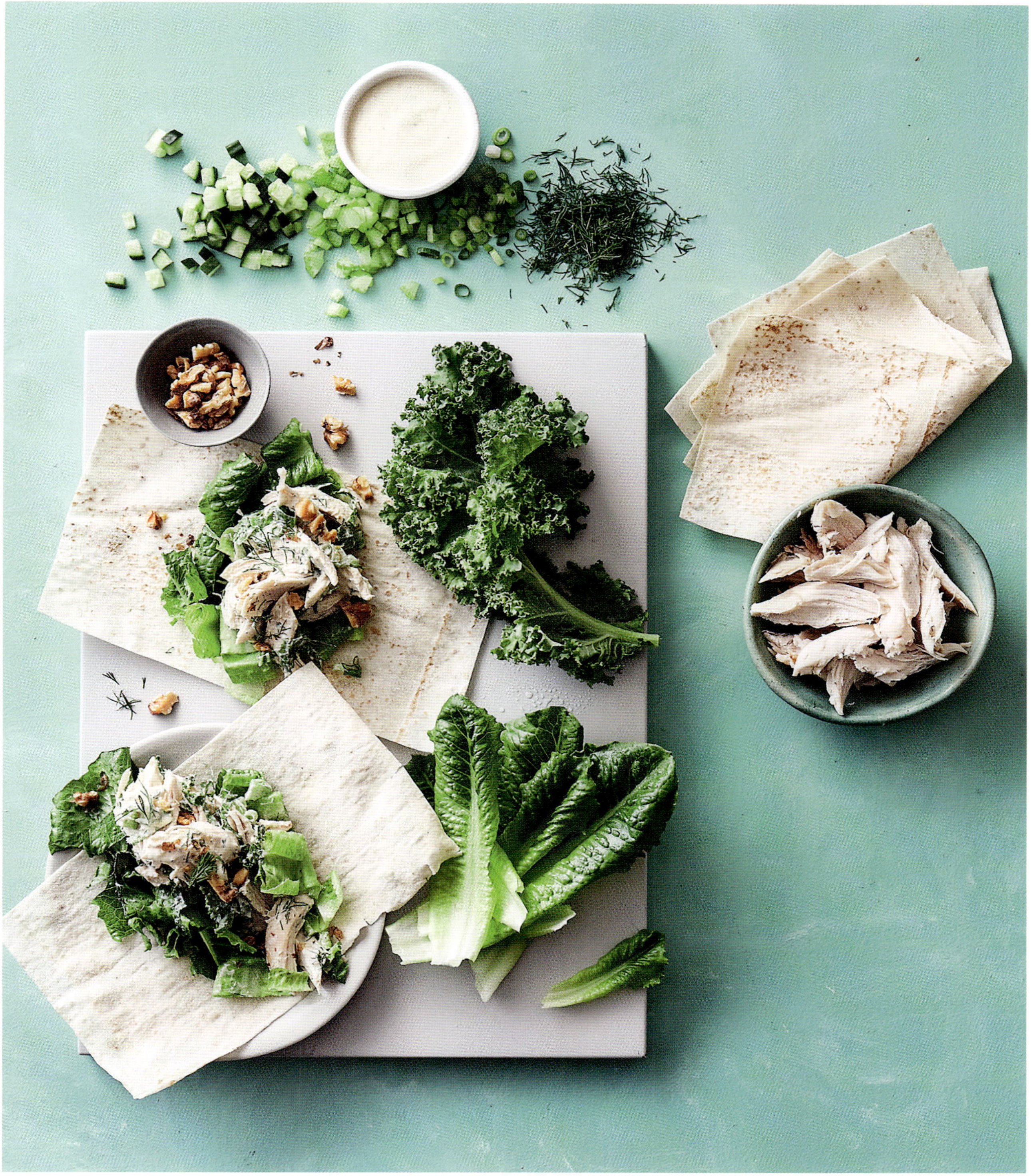

UNITS PER SERVE:	
Breads, Cereals, Legumes, Starchy Veg	1
Dairy	0
Lean Meat, Fish, Poultry, Eggs, Tofu	1.5
Low–Moderate Carbohydrate Veg	3
Healthy Fats	3

Salmon Nori Rolls

CARBS 20g PER SERVE

SERVES: 4 | PREPARATION: 20 MINUTES | COOKING: NIL

6 sheets nori
3 Lebanese cucumbers, very thinly sliced (use a mandoline if you have one), patted dry with paper towel
6 cups rocket leaves, baby spinach leaves or shredded kale, stalks removed
¾ cup (140 g) cooked basmati rice

SALMON FILLING

600 g tinned salmon in spring water (no added salt), drained well
2 teaspoons salt-reduced tamari (see note)
2 teaspoons rice vinegar
2 teaspoons sesame oil
2½ tablespoons whole-egg mayonnaise
1 tablespoon sriracha or other hot chilli sauce
4 spring onions, thinly sliced

1. To make the salmon filling, place all the ingredients in a bowl and mash well with a fork to combine.
2. Place a nori sheet flat on a workbench and top it with one-quarter of the cucumber, rocket, spinach or kale and rice, smoothing over the surface.
3. Add one-quarter of the salmon filling, roll up the nori sheet tightly, running water along the far edge to seal. Slice in half, then set aside and repeat with the remaining nori rolls and filling.

Note

Tamari is a higher-salt product, so ideally use low-salt or no-added-salt alternatives. If you are following a low-sodium diet, omit this ingredient.

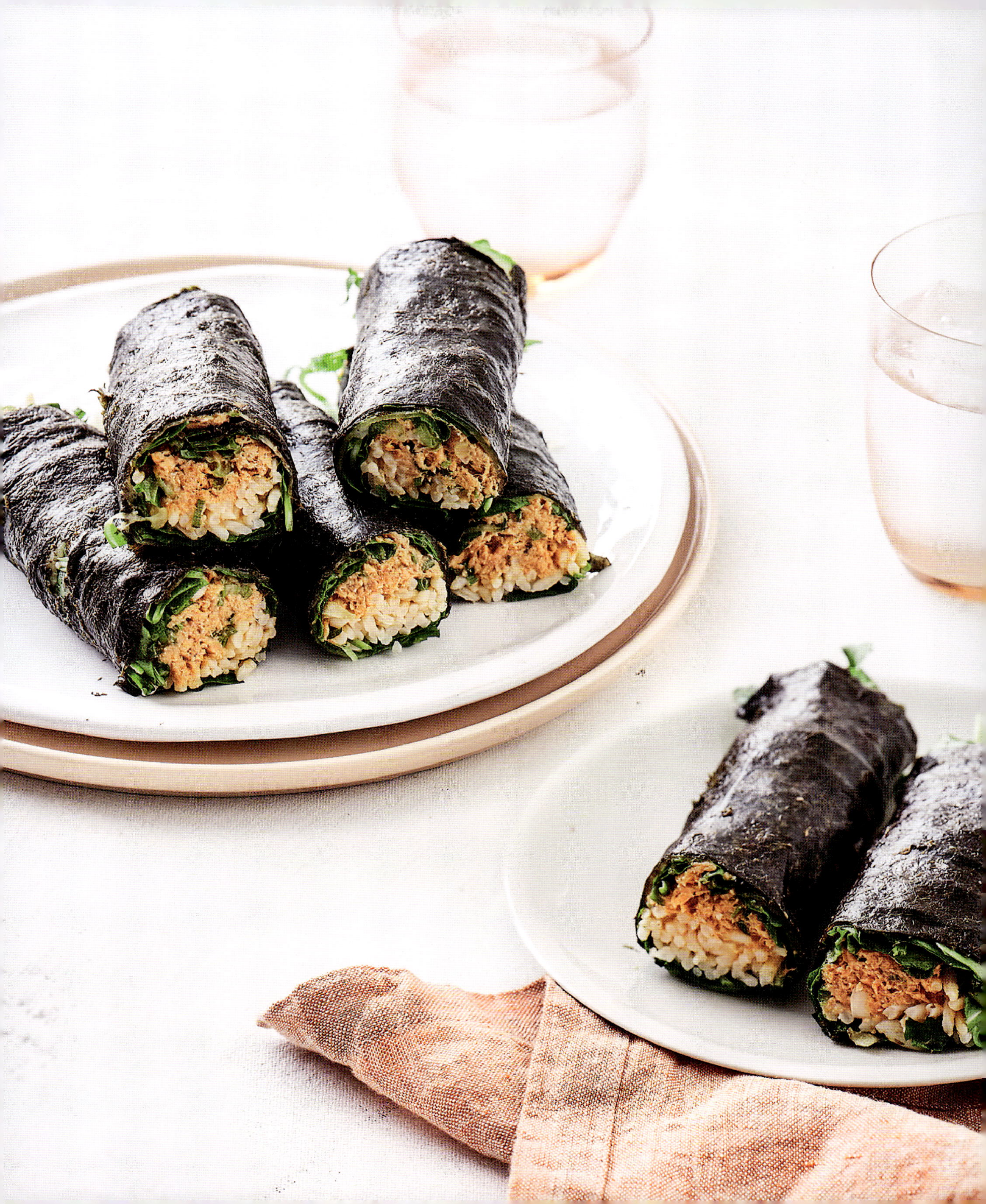

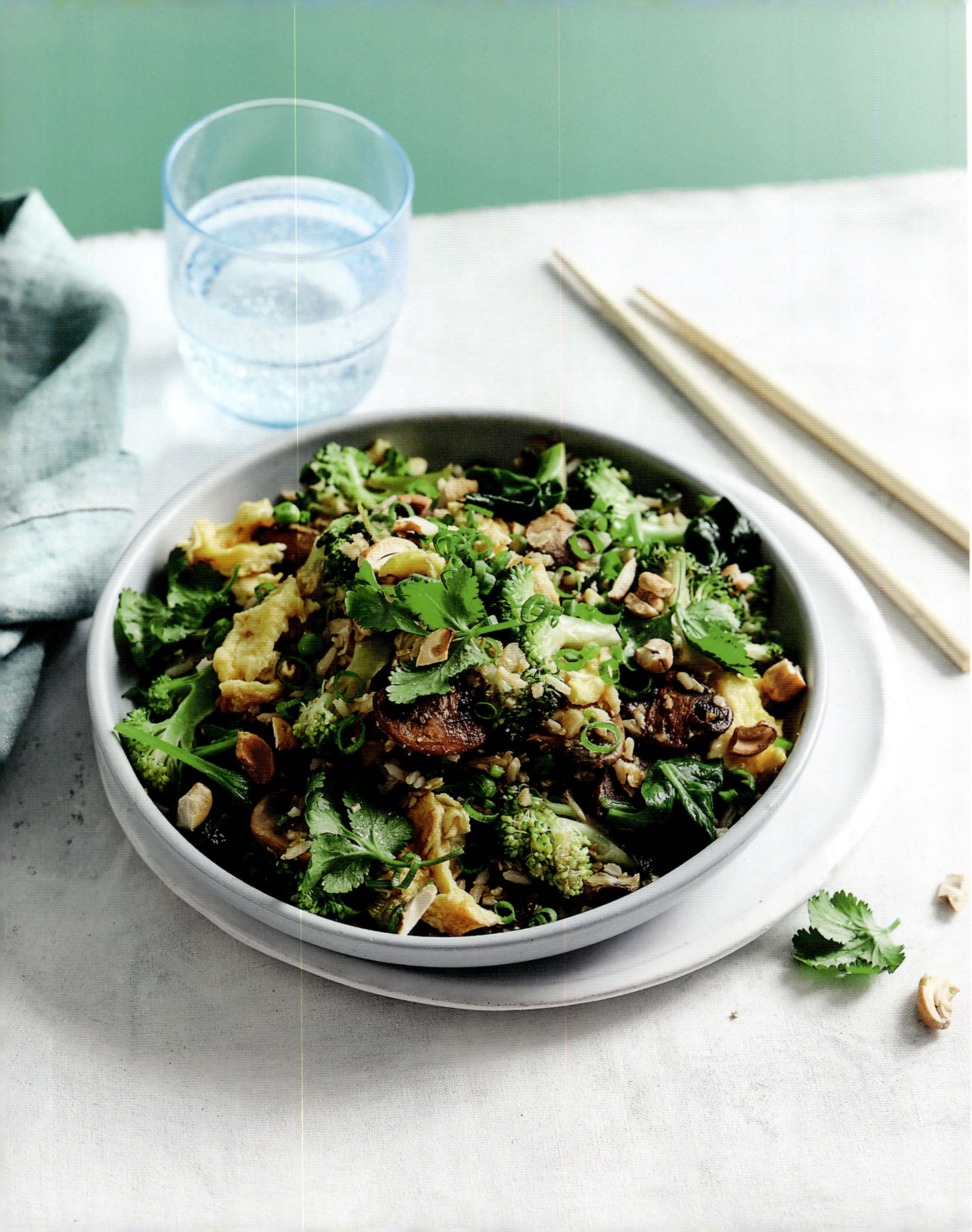

UNITS PER SERVE:	
Breads, Cereals, Legumes, Starchy Veg	1
Dairy	0
Lean Meat, Fish, Poultry, Eggs, Tofu	0.5
Low–Moderate Carbohydrate Veg	3
Healthy Fats	2

Mushroom and Egg Fried Rice with Chilli Oil

CARBS 18 g PER SERVE

SERVES: 4 | PREPARATION: 10 MINUTES | COOKING: 40 MINUTES

60 g (⅓ cup) basmati rice
1 tablespoon sesame oil
1 zucchini, diced
1 large head broccoli, stem sliced and florets chopped into 2 cm pieces
1 bunch coriander, leaves and stems finely chopped
450 g Swiss brown mushrooms, sliced
2 cloves garlic, crushed
¼ cup (35 g) frozen green peas
3 cups baby spinach leaves
2 cups (200 g) cauliflower rice (see notes)
1 tablespoon salt-reduced tamari (see notes)
4 × 55 g free-range eggs

TO SERVE

2 tablespoons unsalted roasted cashews, roughly chopped
4 spring onions, finely chopped
2 teaspoons chilli oil

1. Place the rice and ⅔ cup (170 ml) water in a saucepan over medium–high heat and bring to the boil. Reduce to a simmer and allow to cook for 10 minutes, undisturbed. Remove the pan from the heat and allow the rice to sit, covered, for 10–15 minutes. Remove the lid and fluff the rice with a fork.
2. Meanwhile, heat the sesame oil in a large non-stick frying pan over medium–high heat. Add the zucchini, broccoli stems and coriander stems and cook for 5 minutes, tossing occasionally, until softened. Add the mushrooms, broccoli florets and garlic, toss together, then place a lid on the pan. Cook, undisturbed, for 5 minutes to allow the mushrooms to reduce. Remove the lid and cook, stirring occasionally, for 2 minutes until the excess liquid evaporates. Add the peas, spinach, cauliflower rice, the cooked basmati rice and tamari and stir until warmed through. Push the rice to one side of the pan, then crack in the eggs. Softly scramble the eggs for 30 seconds, then mix with the rice.
3. Remove the pan from the heat and stir the coriander leaves through. Divide the fried rice between four bowls, top with the cashews and spring onion, drizzle the chilli oil over and serve.

Notes

You can find cauliflower rice in the fresh produce section at your local supermarket. If unavailable, use the frozen variety instead.

Tamari is a higher-salt product, so ideally use low-salt or no-added-salt alternatives. If you are following a low-sodium diet, omit this ingredient.

To freeze, place cooked and cooled individual portions of this meal in freezer-safe containers and freeze for up to 2 months. The day before serving, transfer to the refrigerator and thaw overnight. Reheat in the microwave, or heat through in a frying pan for a few minutes.

UNITS PER SERVE:	
Breads, Cereals, Legumes, Starchy Veg	1
Dairy	0
Lean Meat, Fish, Poultry, Eggs, Tofu	1
Low–Moderate Carbohydrate Veg	2.5
Healthy Fats	1

Sushi Bento Box with Salmon, Avocado and Spinach

CARBS 20g PER SERVE

SERVES: 1 | PREPARATION: 10 MINUTES | COOKING: NIL

¼ cup (45 g) cooked basmati rice
1 small Lebanese cucumber, thinly sliced
100 g smoked salmon fillet
¼ small avocado
1 cup baby spinach leaves
2 sheets nori

Assemble the ingredients in an airtight container or a stainless steel bento box. Use the nori sheets to wrap the ingredients to eat.

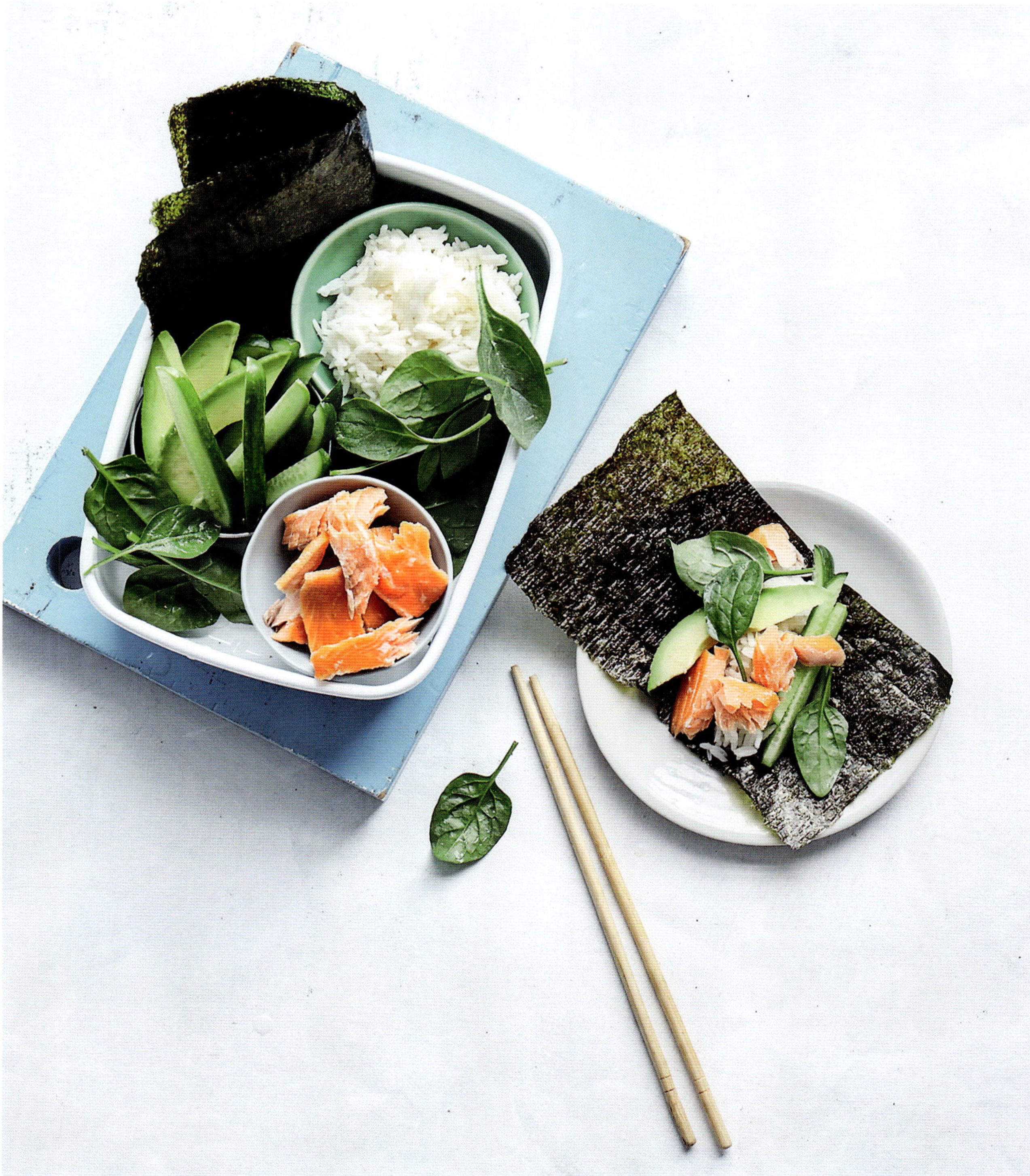

UNITS PER SERVE:	
Breads, Cereals, Legumes, Starchy Veg	1
Dairy	1
Lean Meat, Fish, Poultry, Eggs, Tofu	1
Low–Moderate Carbohydrate Veg	2.5
Healthy Fats	2

Chicken Lentil Salad with Dijon Mustard Dressing

CARBS 15g PER SERVE

SERVES: 4 | PREPARATION: 15 MINUTES | COOKING: NIL

⅓ cup (50 g) frozen green peas
400 g shredded purchased roast or poached chicken, skin removed (see note)
240 g cooked brown lentils, drained and rinsed
6 cups baby spinach leaves
2 zucchini, shredded
2 spring onions, thinly sliced
¼ cup flat-leaf parsley, roughly chopped
¼ cup (35 g) pumpkin seeds (pepitas)
60 g Danish feta, crumbled

DRESSING

2 teaspoons Dijon mustard
1 tablespoon extra virgin olive oil
Juice of ½ lemon

1. Place the frozen peas in a sieve and run under water until thawed. Add to a large bowl with the remaining ingredients and toss to combine.
2. Shake the dressing ingredients in a jar until combined, then pour over the salad and toss to coat. Divide between four bowls to serve.

Note

If you are not cooking your own, you can use a purchased pre-roasted chicken or chicken breast. You can find these in the refrigerator section of the supermarket.

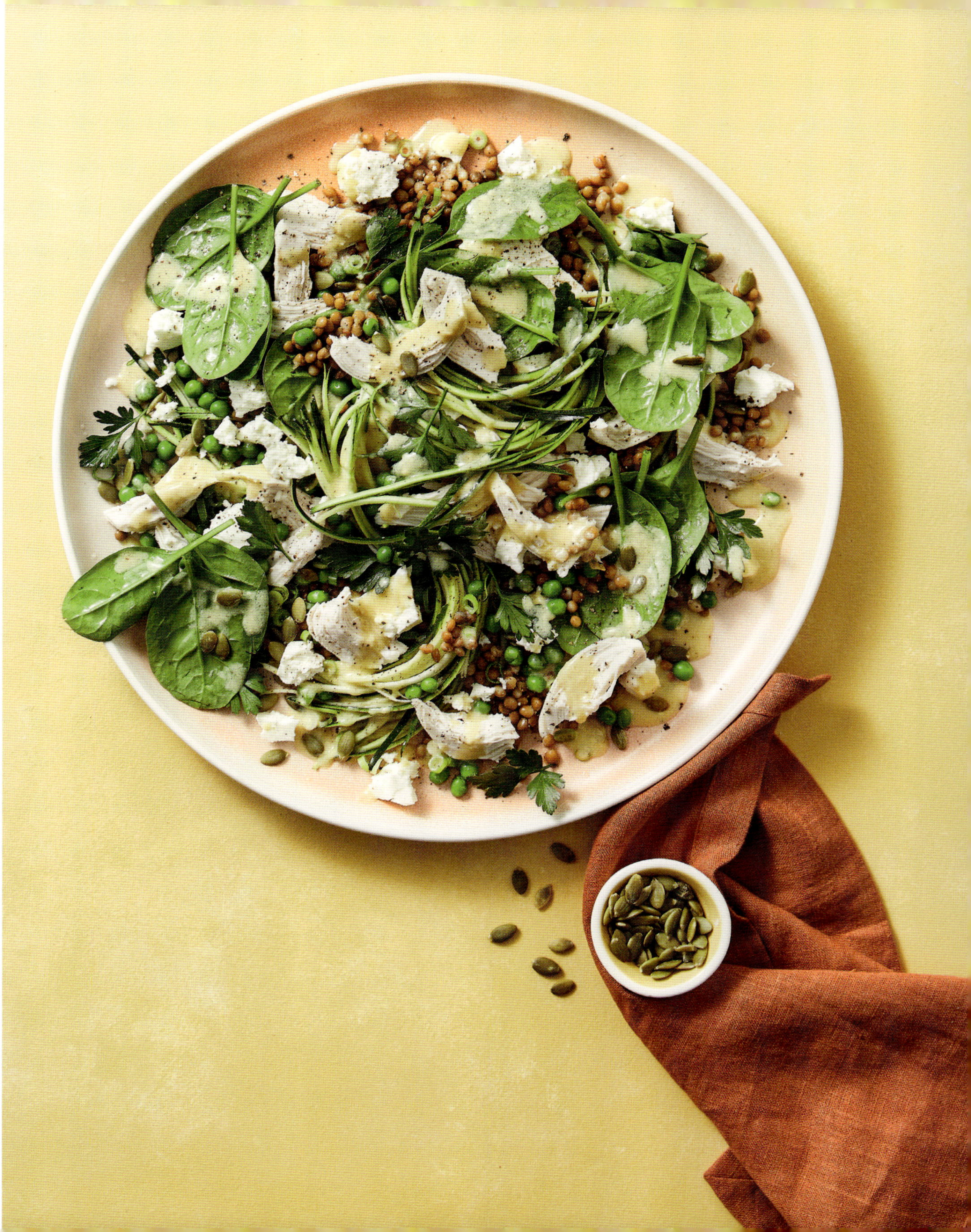

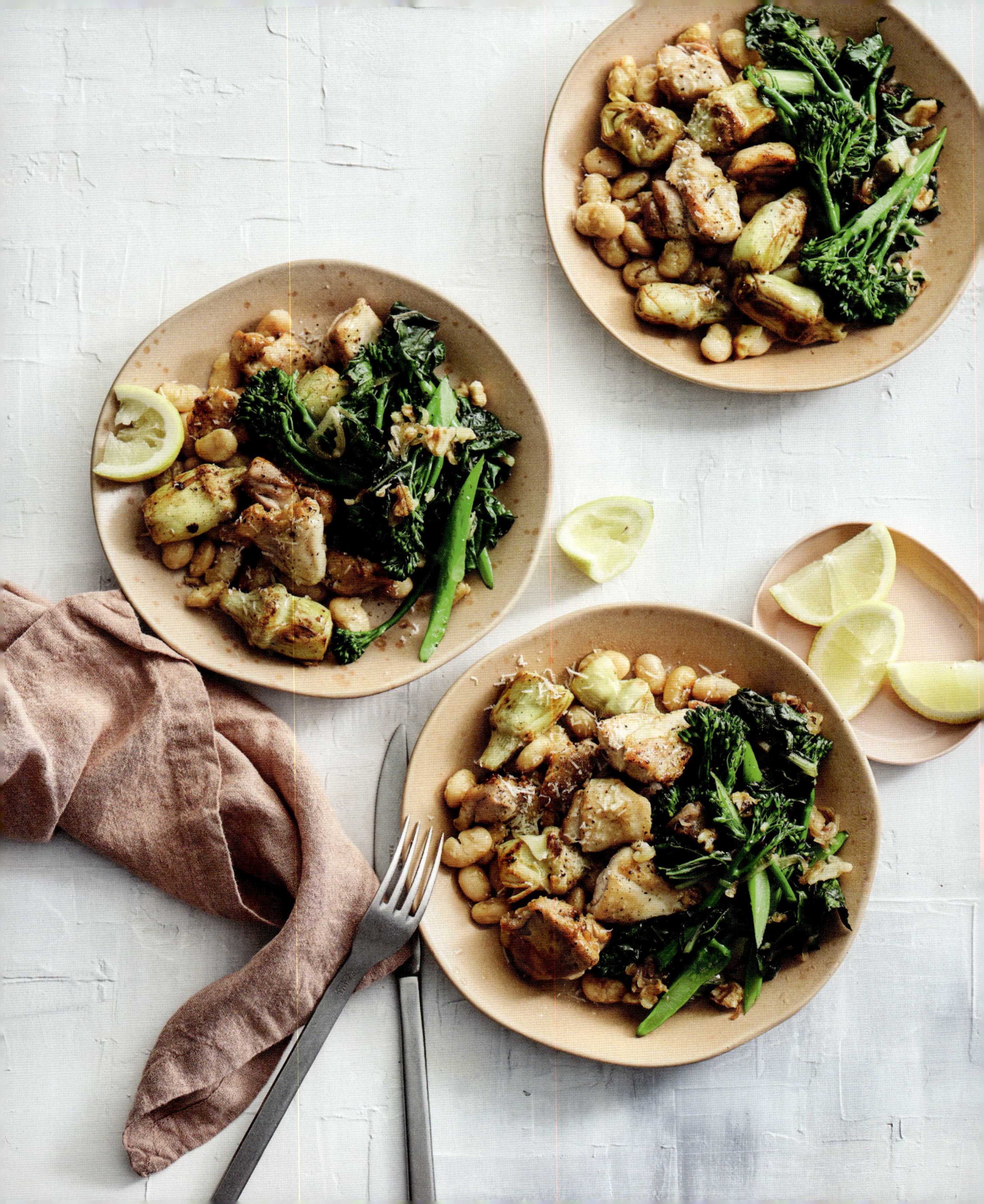

UNITS PER SERVE:	
Breads, Cereals, Legumes, Starchy Veg	1
Dairy	0.5
Lean Meat, Fish, Poultry, Eggs, Tofu	1
Low–Moderate Carbohydrate Veg	3
Healthy Fats	3

Chicken with Lemony Butter Beans and Garlicky Greens

CARBS 20g PER SERVE

SERVES: 4 | PREPARATION: 15 MINUTES | COOKING: 15 MINUTES

2 tablespoons extra virgin olive oil
400 g chicken thigh fillets, visible fat removed, chopped into 1 cm pieces
200 g tinned butter beans, drained and rinsed
300 g tinned artichoke hearts, drained and rinsed
Juice of 1 lemon
40 g parmesan, shaved

GARLICKY GREENS

2 teaspoons extra virgin olive oil
4 golden shallots, thinly sliced
2 cloves garlic, thinly sliced
2 tablespoons crumbled walnuts
1 bunch broccolini, stems sliced in half lengthways
½ cup (125 ml) salt-reduced chicken stock (see note)
600 g kale or silverbeet, stalks removed and leaves roughly chopped

1. Heat 1 teaspoon of the olive oil in a large frying pan over medium–high heat. Add the chicken and cook for 4 minutes – not tossing, but leaving the chicken to brown on the bottom of the pan – then flip and cook for another 3 minutes, until browned and cooked through. Add the butter beans, artichoke, remaining olive oil and lemon juice and toss just until warmed through. Transfer everything to a plate and sprinkle with the parmesan and a pinch of freshly ground black pepper.
2. To make the garlicky greens, add the olive oil to the same frying pan over medium–high heat. Add the shallots and garlic and cook for 3 minutes until golden. Add the walnuts and continue cooking for 2–3 minutes until nicely browned and crisp. Transfer to a bowl and set aside.
3. Place the broccolini and stock in the same frying pan, cover and cook for 3–4 minutes until the broccolini is almost tender. Add the kale or silverbeet and cook, tossing everything together, for 2 minutes until very wilted. Transfer to a bowl and top with the crispy shallot, garlic and walnut mixture.
4. Divide the chicken, butter beans, artichoke and garlicky greens between four bowls and serve.

Note

Commercial chicken stock is usually very high in sodium. We recommend shopping for 'chicken broth', which is a similar product you can find in the refrigerator section of supermarkets and grocers. Broth is sold in small batches and contains less sodium. Check the label to ensure your stock contains less than 50 mg sodium per 100 g. Alternatively, if you'd like to make your own homemade stock, see the recipe on page 131.

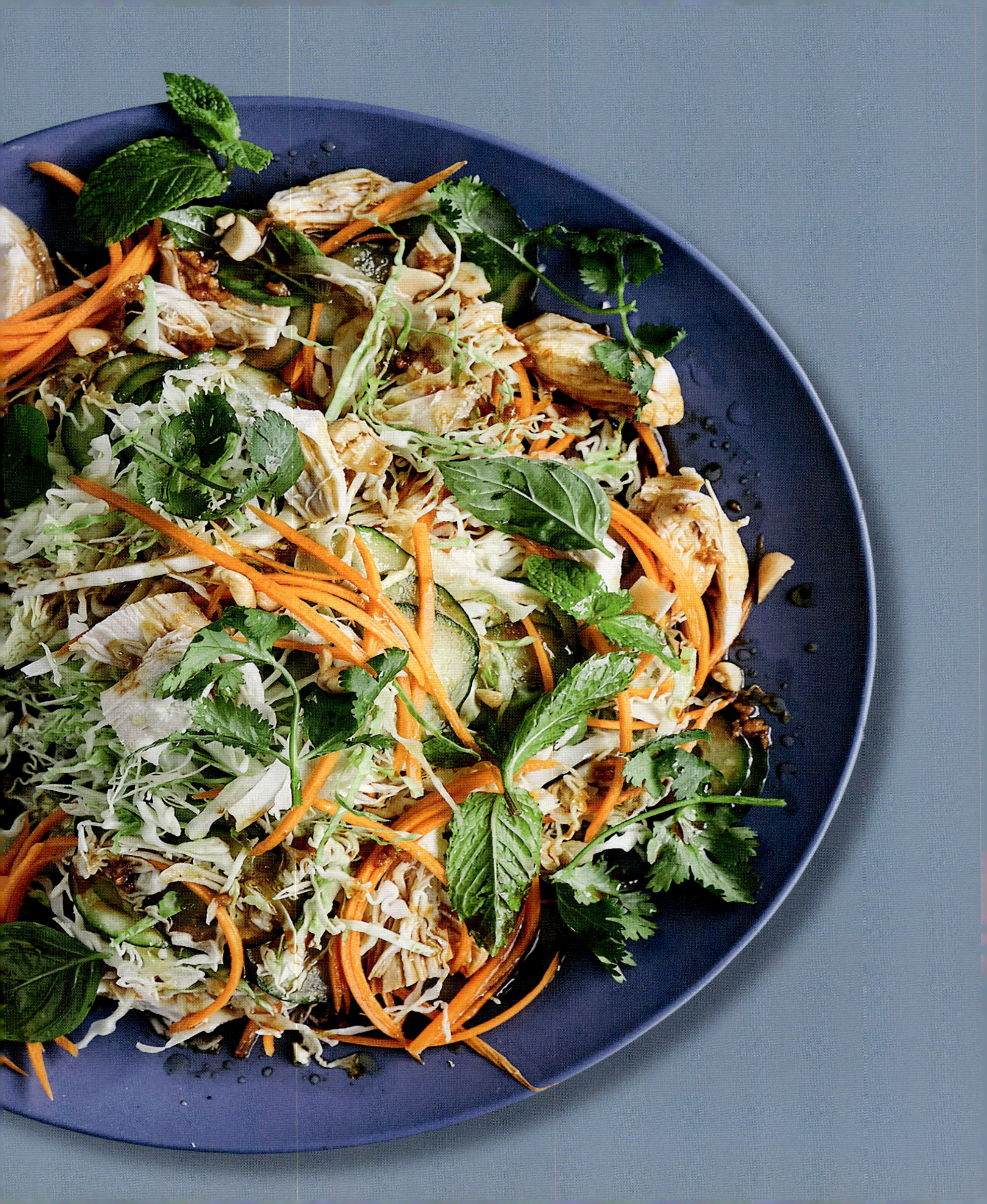

03.

For One or Two

UNITS PER SERVE:	
Breads, Cereals, Legumes, Starchy Veg	0
Dairy	1
Lean Meat, Fish, Poultry, Eggs, Tofu	1.5
Low–Moderate Carbohydrate Veg	3
Healthy Fats	3

Harissa Tofu Salad

CARBS **8g** PER SERVE

SERVES: 2 | PREPARATION: 10 MINUTES | COOKING: 8 MINUTES

3 teaspoons extra virgin olive oil
300 g firm tofu, crumbled
1 tablespoon harissa paste
1 small carrot, finely shredded
250 g cherry tomatoes, halved
1 baby cos lettuce, roughly chopped
40 g Danish feta, crumbled

HARISSA TAHINI DRESSING

3 teaspoons tahini
1 tablespoon room temperature water
2 teaspoons harissa paste
Juice of ½ lemon

1. To make the harissa tahini dressing, place all the ingredients in a bowl and mix to combine.
2. Heat the olive oil in a large frying pan over medium–high heat. Add the tofu and cook, tossing occasionally, for 5 minutes until the tofu is crisp and golden on the edges. Add the harissa paste and toss through for 1 minute.
3. Divide the harissa tofu, carrot, cherry tomatoes and lettuce between two bowls – or one bowl for dinner and a container for lunch the next day. Top with the feta and drizzle over the harissa tahini dressing. (Keep the dressing in a small jar or airtight container if serving for lunch the next day and drizzle over when ready to eat.)

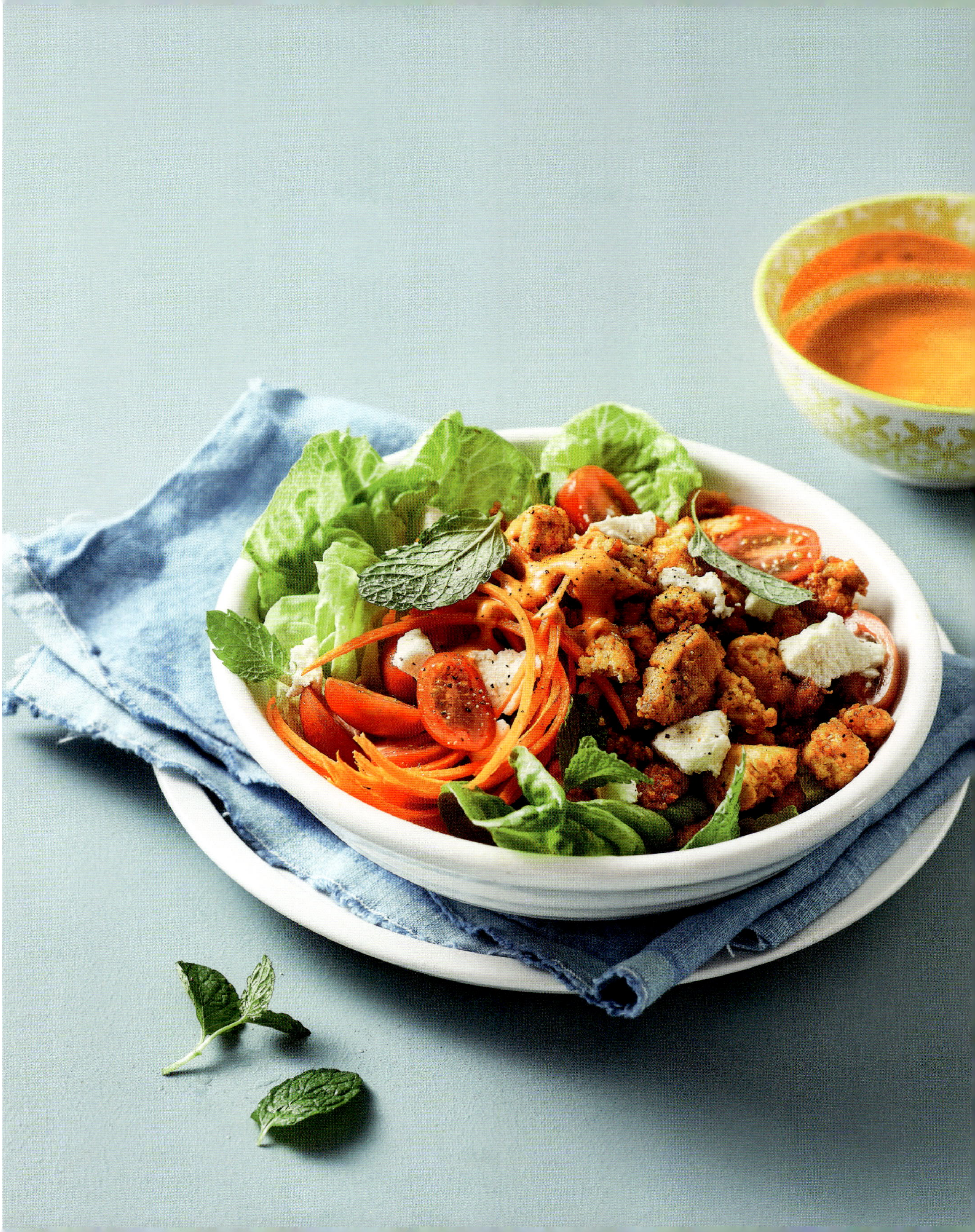

UNITS PER SERVE:	
Breads, Cereals, Legumes, Starchy Veg	0
Dairy	0
Lean Meat, Fish, Poultry, Eggs, Tofu	1.5
Low–Moderate Carbohydrate Veg	3
Healthy Fats	3

Herby Vietnamese Chicken Salad

CARBS 8 g PER SERVE

SERVES: 2 | PREPARATION: 15 MINUTES | COOKING: NIL

1 small carrot, julienned
1 small Lebanese cucumber, thinly sliced
2 cups tightly packed shredded savoy cabbage
2 cups baby spinach leaves
1 cup coriander, leaves picked
½ cup mint leaves
½ cup Thai basil leaves (or regular basil)
250 g shredded roast or poached chicken, skin removed (see notes)
2 tablespoons unsalted roasted peanuts, finely chopped

DRESSING

2 teaspoons salt-reduced tamari (see notes)
1 tablespoon extra virgin olive oil
Juice of 1 lime
½ clove garlic, crushed (about ¼ teaspoon)

1. To make the dressing, place all the ingredients in a small bowl and mix to combine.
2. Place all the salad ingredients in a bowl, drizzle the dressing over, then use your hands to toss everything together. Divide between two bowls to serve.

Notes

If you are not cooking your own, you can use a purchased pre-roasted chicken or chicken breast. You can find these in the refrigerator section of the supermarket.

Tamari is a higher-salt product, so ideally use low-salt or no-added-salt alternatives. If you are following a low-sodium diet, omit this ingredient.

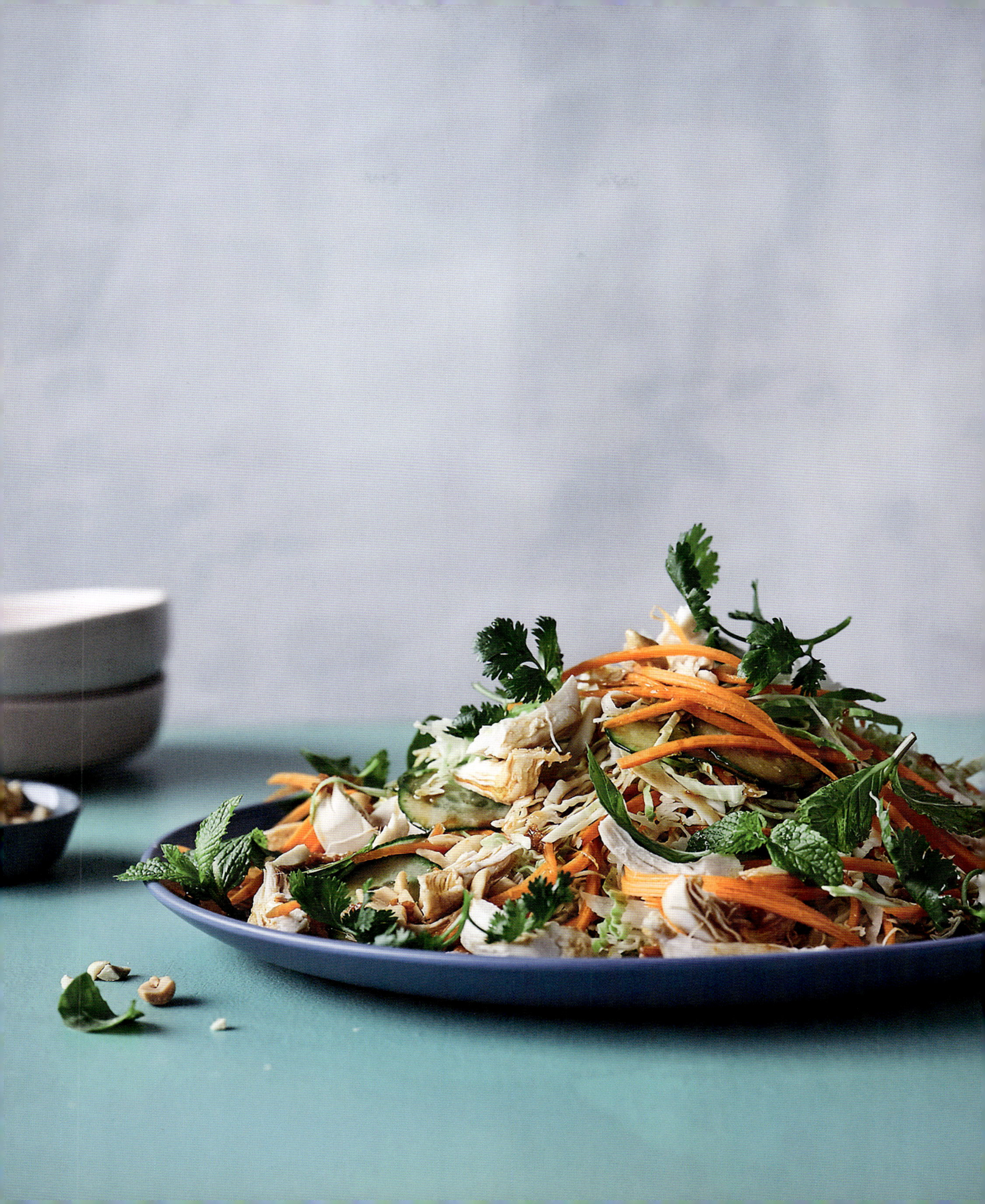

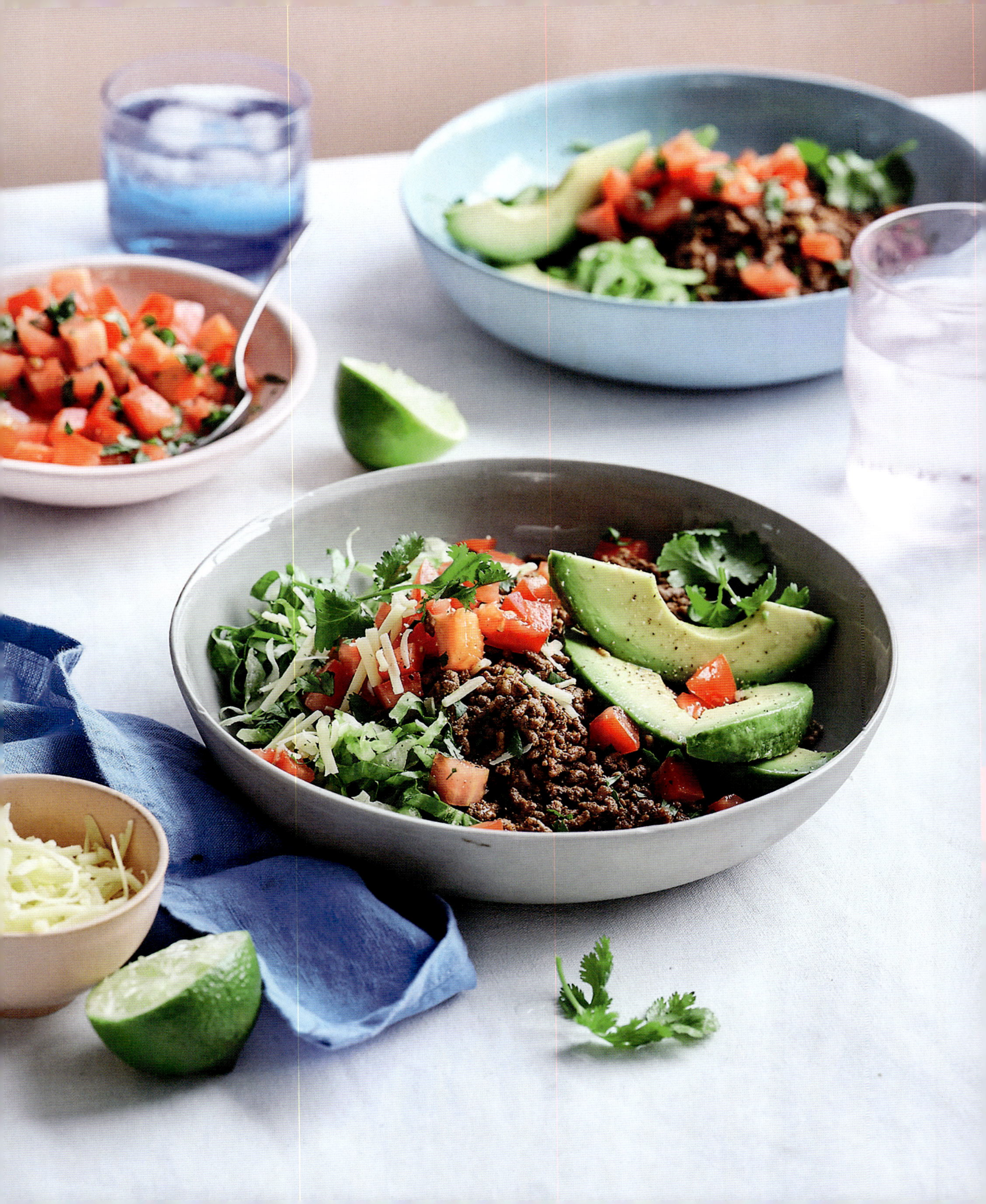

UNITS PER SERVE:	
Breads, Cereals, Legumes, Starchy Veg	0
Dairy	1
Lean Meat, Fish, Poultry, Eggs, Tofu	1.5
Low–Moderate Carbohydrate Veg	3
Healthy Fats	2.5

Mexican Beef Bowl with Pico de Gallo

CARBS 7g PER SERVE

SERVES: 2 | PREPARATION: 10 MINUTES | COOKING: 6 MINUTES

2 teaspoons extra virgin olive oil
300 g lean beef mince
1 tablespoon purchased Mexican spice blend (no added sugar or salt)
2 cups finely shredded lettuce
½ small avocado, sliced into wedges
40 g grated cheddar

PICO DE GALLO

½ cup coriander, roughly chopped
1 clove garlic, crushed
2 tomatoes, diced
Juice of 1 lime
¼ teaspoon freshly ground black pepper

1. To make the pico de gallo, place all the ingredients in a bowl and toss to combine. Set aside.
2. Heat the olive oil in a large frying pan over medium–high heat. Add the beef mince and cook, breaking it up with a wooden spoon, for 4 minutes or until brown and cooked through. Add the Mexican spice blend and stir it through for 1 minute until fragrant.
3. Divide the beef, lettuce, avocado, cheese and pico de gallo between two bowls – or a bowl for dinner and two airtight containers for lunch the next day (one for the beef mince so you can reheat it easily in the microwave, and another container for the salad ingredients).

UNITS PER SERVE:	
Breads, Cereals, Legumes, Starchy Veg	0
Dairy	0
Lean Meat, Fish, Poultry, Eggs, Tofu	1.5
Low–Moderate Carbohydrate Veg	3
Healthy Fats	2.5

Salmon Cobb Salad with Lemon Mustard Dressing

CARBS 6g PER SERVE

SERVES: 2 | PREPARATION: 5 MINUTES | COOKING: 15 MINUTES

2 × 55 g free-range eggs
½ teaspoon extra virgin olive oil
2 × 150 g boneless, skinless salmon or ocean trout fillets
200 g cherry tomatoes, halved
1 cos lettuce, roughly chopped
1 small Lebanese cucumber, diced
¼ small red onion, thinly sliced
½ avocado, diced

DRESSING

2 teaspoons Dijon mustard
3 teaspoons extra virgin olive oil
Juice of ½ lemon
¼ teaspoon freshly ground black pepper

1. Place a small saucepan of water over high heat. Once boiling, add the eggs and cook, undisturbed, for 8 minutes. Remove the eggs with a slotted spoon and run them under water until they are cool to the touch. Peel and chop roughly.
2. Heat the oil in a frying pan over medium–high heat. Add the salmon and cook for 4 minutes. Flip, then cook for 3 minutes or until cooked to your liking.
3. Place all the dressing ingredients in a jar and shake to combine.
4. Divide the tomatoes, lettuce, cucumber, onion and avocado between two bowls (or a bowl for dinner and a container for lunch the next day). Divide the cooked salmon and egg between the bowls, drizzle over the dressing and serve.

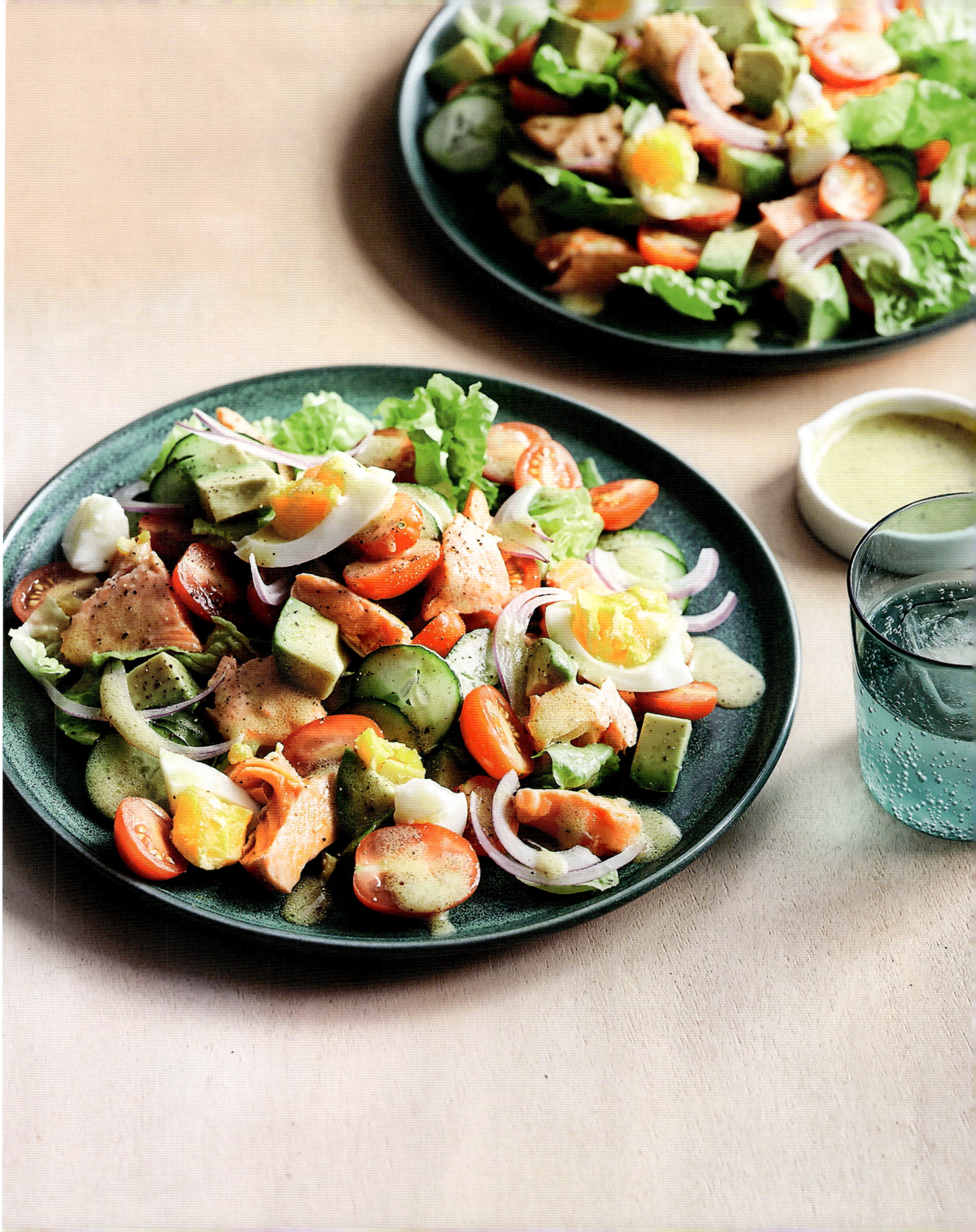

UNITS PER SERVE:	
Breads, Cereals, Legumes, Starchy Veg	0
Dairy	1
Lean Meat, Fish, Poultry, Eggs, Tofu	1.5
Low–Moderate Carbohydrate Veg	3
Healthy Fats	2.5

Steak Salad with Endive, Radish and Asparagus

CARBS 5g PER SERVE

SERVES: 2 | PREPARATION: 10 MINUTES | COOKING: 8 MINUTES + RESTING

300 g steak (flank, hanger, skirt, flat-iron, porterhouse or rib-eye), visible fat removed
2 teaspoons extra virgin olive oil
1 head curly endive, roughly torn
3 radishes, thinly sliced
½ small bulb fennel, trimmed and very thinly sliced
1 bunch thin asparagus spears, woody ends trimmed, cut in half
30 g parmesan, shaved

DRESSING

2 teaspoons Dijon mustard
2 tablespoons finely chopped chives
Juice of ½ lemon
3 teaspoons extra virgin olive oil

1. Season the steak on both sides with freshly ground black pepper. Heat the olive oil in a large frying pan over medium–high heat, add the steak and cook for 4 minutes on one side. Flip and cook for another 3 minutes, or until crisp and brown on the edges and pink in the centre, or cooked to your liking. Set the steak aside and allow it to rest for 10 minutes before slicing it into thin strips.
2. Place the dressing ingredients in a large bowl and whisk with a fork to combine. Add the endive, radish, fennel, asparagus and parmesan to the bowl and toss well to coat everything in the dressing.
3. Divide the salad between two plate – or a plate for dinner and a container for lunch the next day. Serve the salad with the steak. To reheat the next day, place the steak on a plate and microwave briefly for 45 seconds until warmed through. Toss the steak through the salad, add the parmesan and serve.

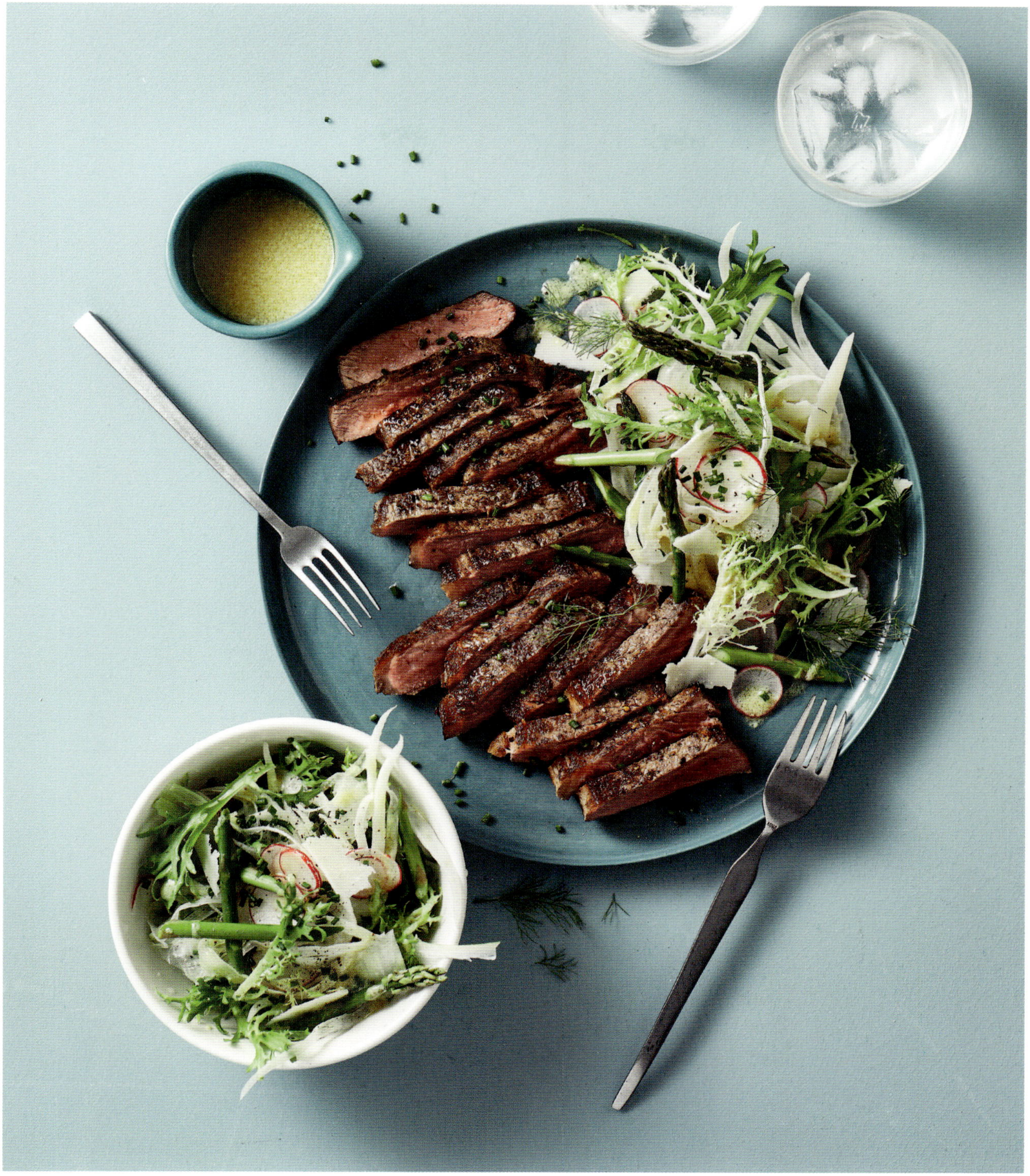

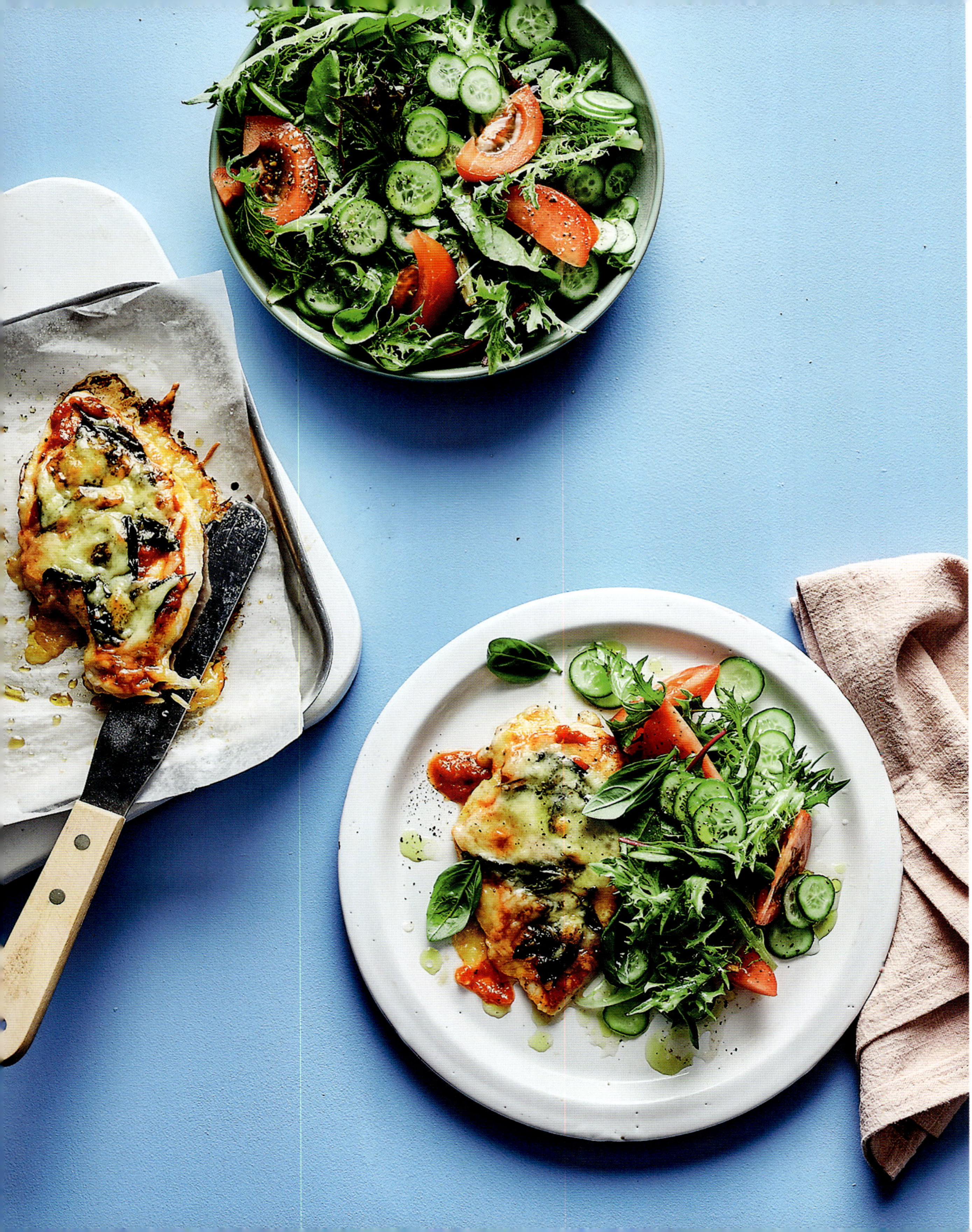

UNITS PER SERVE:	
Breads, Cereals, Legumes, Starchy Veg	0
Dairy	2
Lean Meat, Fish, Poultry, Eggs, Tofu	1.5
Low–Moderate Carbohydrate Veg	3
Healthy Fats	2

Cheat's Chicken Parmigiana

CARBS 7g PER SERVE

SERVES: 2 | PREPARATION: 5 MINUTES | COOKING: 13 MINUTES

1 × 300 g chicken breast fillet, sliced in half horizontally to make 2 thin steaks
¼ cup (60 ml) tomato passata (no added sugar or salt)
1 clove garlic, crushed
¼ cup basil leaves, plus extra for serving
80 g cheddar, grated

SALAD

4 cups mixed salad leaves
1 tomato, diced
1 small Lebanese cucumber, sliced
2 teaspoons white wine vinegar
1 tablespoon extra virgin olive oil

1. Preheat the oven to 200°C (180°C fan-forced) and line a baking tray with baking paper.
2. Place the chicken steaks on the baking tray. Top each piece with two large spoonfuls of the passata, then sprinkle with the crushed garlic. Top with the basil and grated cheese and season with freshly ground black pepper. Bake in the oven for 10 minutes until the cheese is melted and the chicken is cooked through. Move to the top shelf of the oven and turn on the grill. Grill for 3 minutes until the cheese is golden brown.
3. For the salad, place all the ingredients in a large bowl and toss to combine.
4. Divide the chicken parmigiana between two plates (be careful with the topping as it can slip off) and serve with the salad, garnished with the extra basil leaves. To reheat leftovers, place the chicken on a baking tray and cook in a preheated 200°C (180°C fan-forced) oven for 5 minutes until warmed through. Serve with the salad.

UNITS PER SERVE:	
Breads, Cereals, Legumes, Starchy Veg	0
Dairy	0
Lean Meat, Fish, Poultry, Eggs, Tofu	1.5
Low–Moderate Carbohydrate Veg	2
Healthy Fats	3

Creamy Prawn Lettuce Cups

CARBS 5g PER SERVE

SERVES: 2 | PREPARATION: 15 MINUTES | COOKING: NIL

1 teaspoon Dijon mustard
1½ tablespoons whole-egg mayonnaise
Juice of 1 lime
¼ cup dill leaves, finely chopped
300 g cooked, peeled and deveined prawns, roughly chopped (see note)
1 Lebanese cucumber, finely diced
1 baby cos lettuce, 8 leaves picked

1. Place the mustard, mayonnaise, lime juice, dill and ¼ teaspoon freshly ground black pepper in a large bowl and mix to combine. Add the prawns and cucumber and toss to coat.
2. Divide the lettuce leaves between two plates – or between a plate for dinner and a container for lunch the next day. Top with the creamy prawn mixture and serve.

Note

You can purchase raw frozen peeled prawns and thaw in the refrigerator. To cook, heat a non-stick frying pan over low–medium heat. Add the prawns, cover, and allow the prawns to steam softly in the pan for 3–5 minutes until pink. Allow to cool, then use as per recipe.

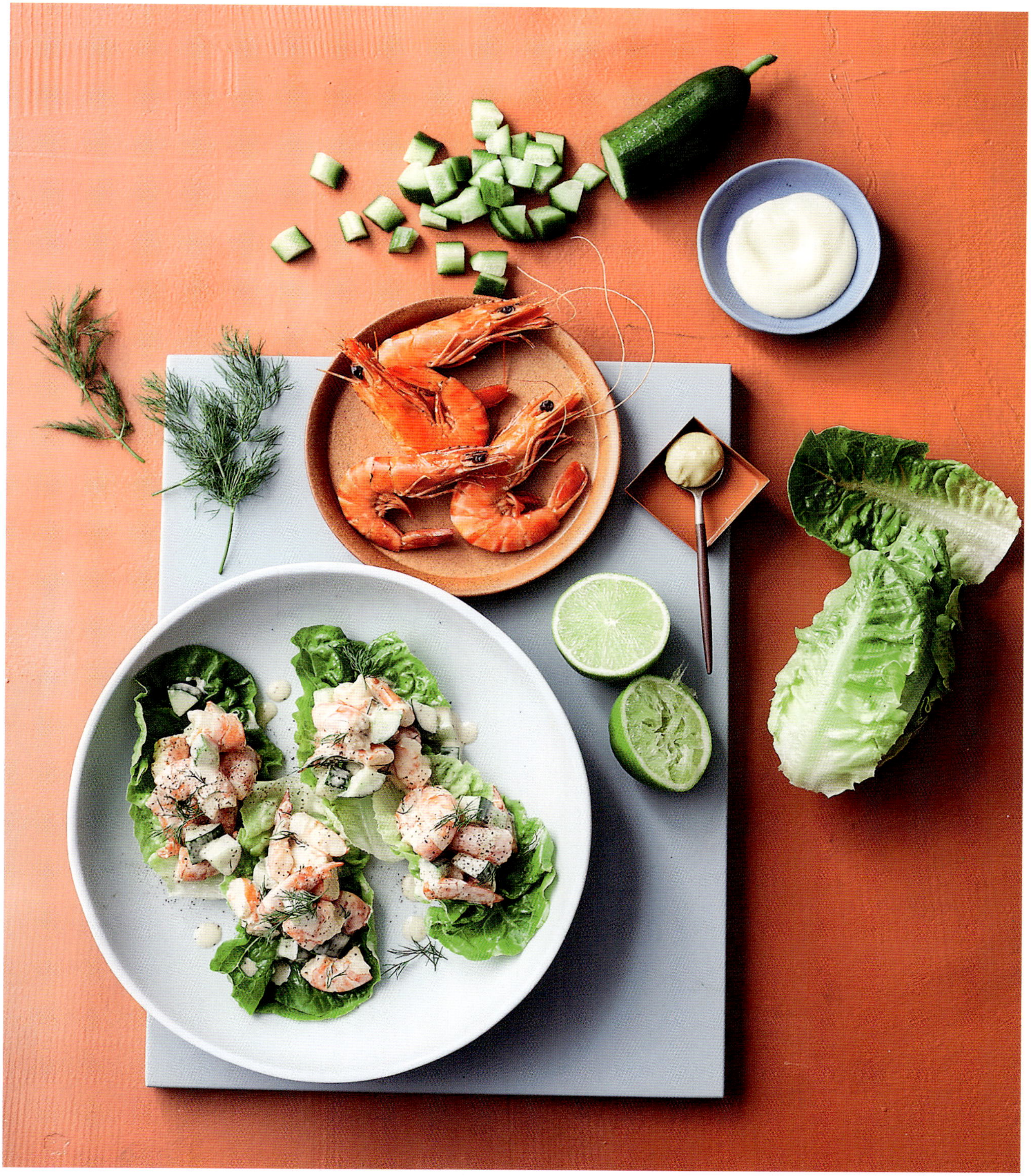

UNITS PER SERVE:	
Breads, Cereals, Legumes, Starchy Veg	0
Dairy	0.5
Lean Meat, Fish, Poultry, Eggs, Tofu	1.5
Low–Moderate Carbohydrate Veg	2.5
Healthy Fats	2.5

Lamb Cutlets with Spring Pea Salad

CARBS 7g PER SERVE

SERVES: 2 | PREPARATION: 20 MINUTES | COOKING: 6 MINUTES

6 × 100 g French-trimmed lamb cutlets (3 cutlets per serve; about 150 g meat)
1 tablespoon sumac
2 teaspoons extra virgin olive oil

SPRING PEA SALAD

¾ cup (110 g) frozen green peas
1 large zucchini, shredded
1 baby cos lettuce, roughly chopped
½ cup chopped flat-leaf parsley
½ cup chopped mint
¼ cup chopped dill
2 tablespoons roasted unsalted almonds, roughly chopped
2 teaspoons extra virgin olive oil
Juice of ½ lemon
40 g reduced-fat feta, crumbled

1. Preheat a barbecue chargrill plate to high, or place a chargrill pan on your stovetop over high heat.
2. Place the lamb cutlets, sumac and olive oil in a bowl and toss with your hands to combine well.
3. Once the barbecue or chargrill pan is hot, add the lamb and cook for 3 minutes on each side until browned. Transfer to a plate and set aside to rest.
4. To make the spring pea salad, place the frozen peas in a sieve and run under tap water to thaw. Place them in a large bowl with the zucchini, lettuce, parsley, mint, dill, almonds, olive oil and lemon juice, then toss gently. Add the feta and toss again gently to combine.
5. Divide the lamb cutlets and spring pea salad between two plates – or a plate for dinner and a container for lunch the next day. To reheat, cook the lamb cutlets in a frying pan over medium heat for 3–4 minutes until warmed through. Or place on a microwave-safe plate and heat for 45 seconds until warmed through.

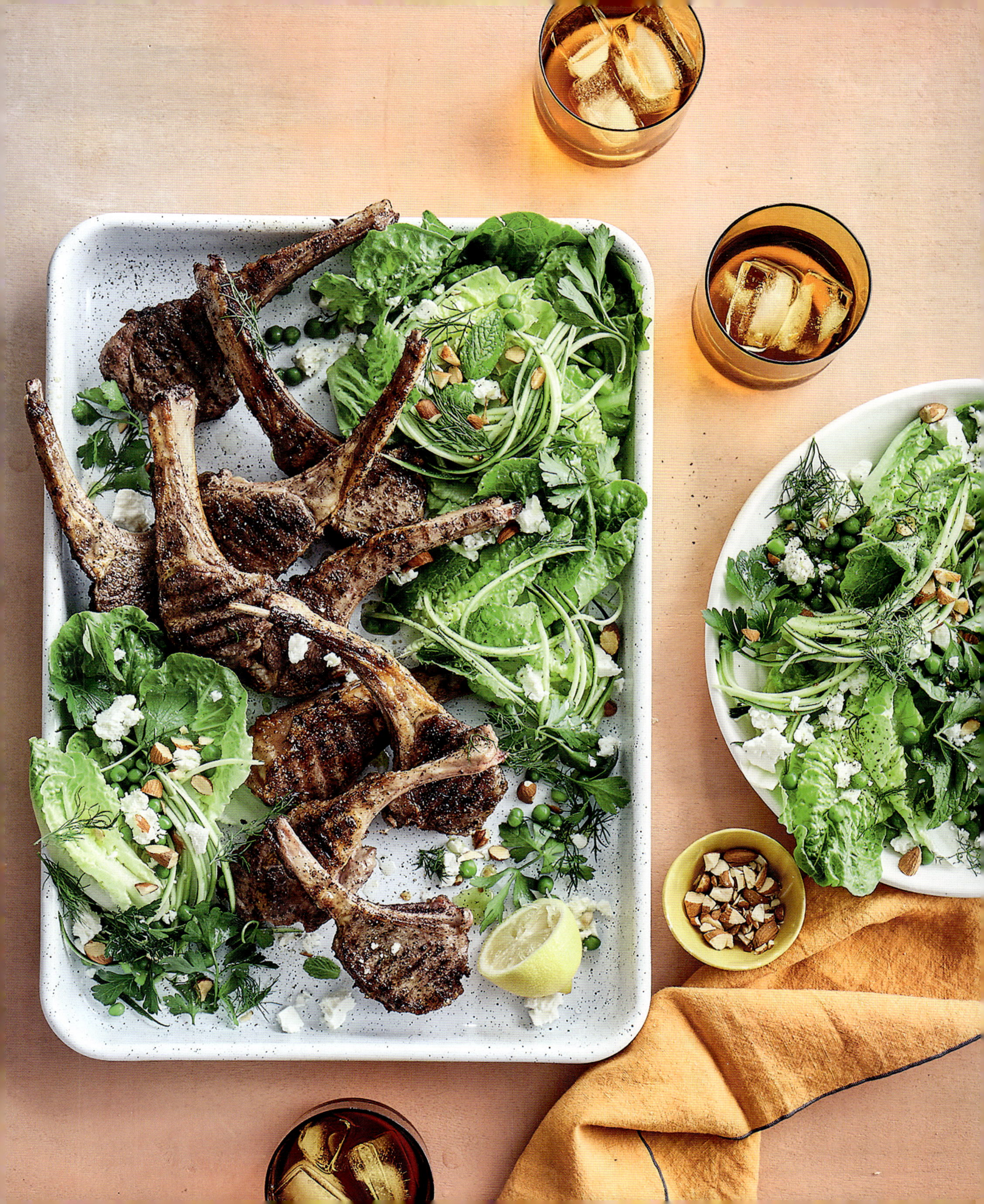

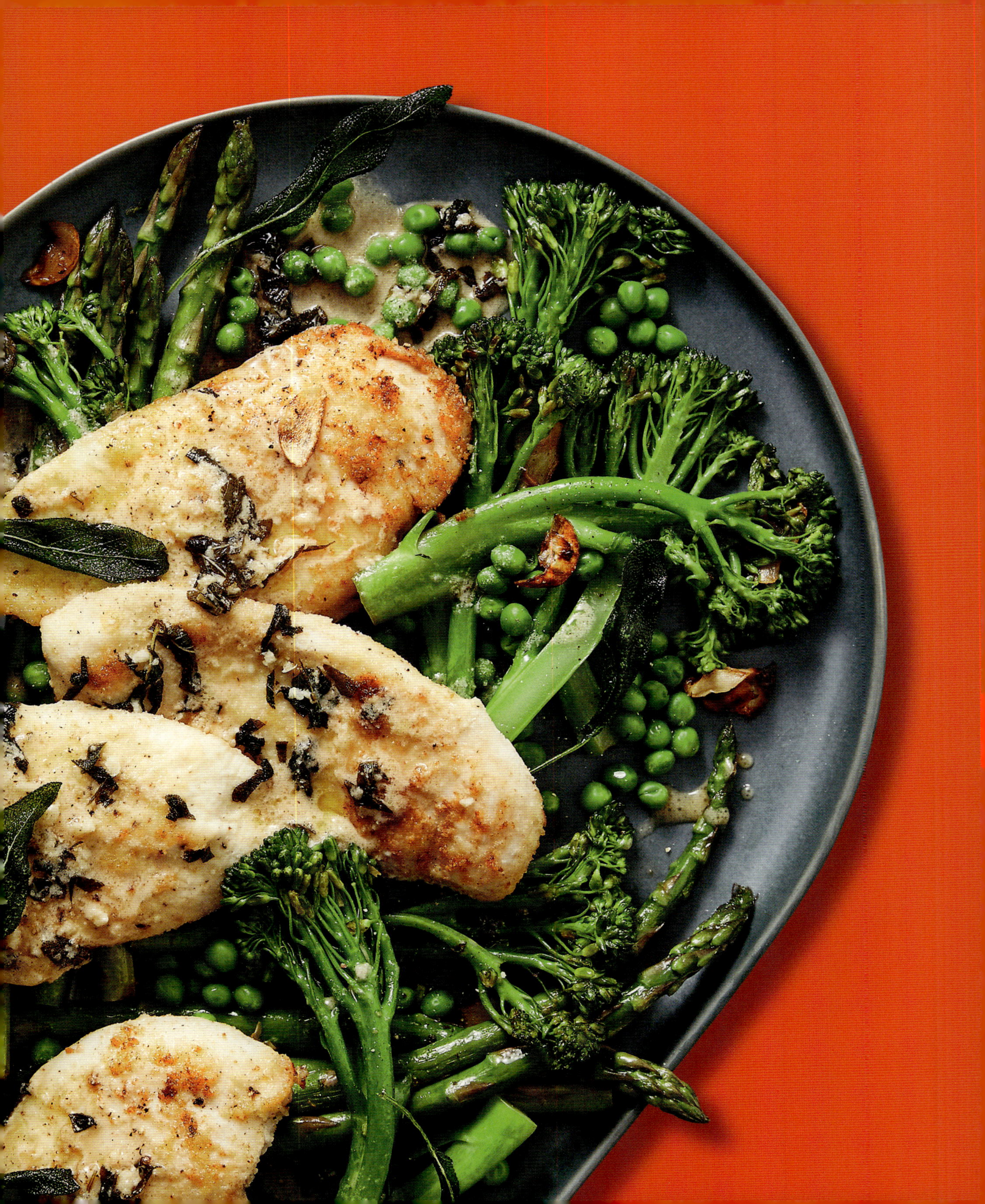

04.

Mains

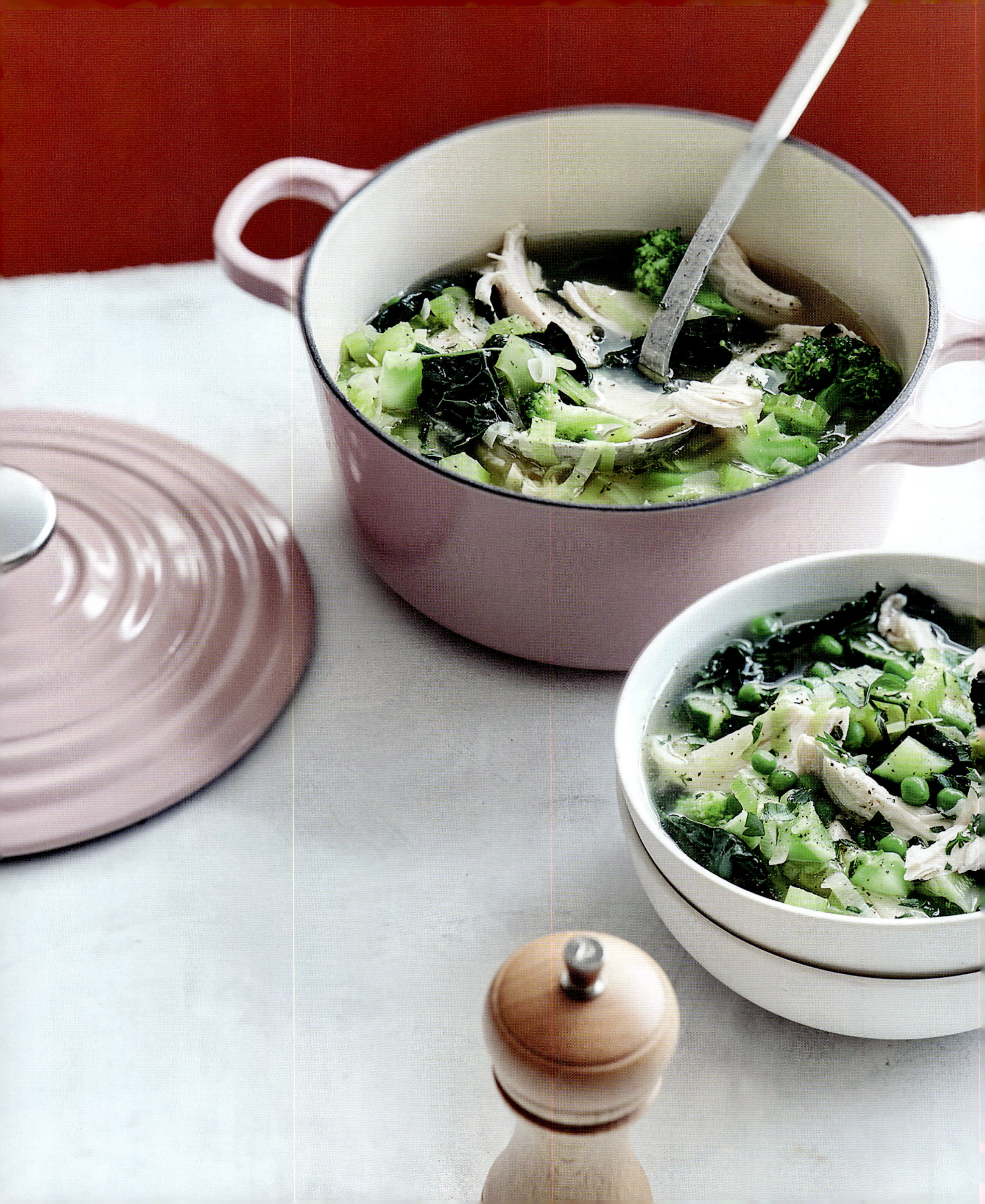

UNITS PER SERVE:	
Breads, Cereals, Legumes, Starchy Veg	0
Dairy	0
Lean Meat, Fish, Poultry, Eggs, Tofu	1.5
Low–Moderate Carbohydrate Veg	3
Healthy Fats	2

Chicken Soup with Spring Greens

CARBS 15g PER SERVE

SERVES: 4 | PREPARATION: 20 MINUTES | COOKING: 2 HOURS 20 MINS

2 tablespoons extra virgin olive oil
1 leek, thinly sliced
1 large zucchini, diced
2 sticks celery, diced
1 large head broccoli, stems diced and florets chopped into 2 cm pieces (use the florets for the stock, below)
4 cloves garlic, thinly sliced
2 cm piece of ginger, finely grated
5 sprigs thyme, leaves picked
1.5 litres (6 cups) Salt-reduced Chicken Stock (see recipe below)
3 cups shredded chicken meat (left over from chicken stock recipe below)
4 cups Tuscan kale leaves, stalks removed (see notes)
½ cup (75 g) frozen green peas
Juice of 1 lemon
½ cup chopped flat-leaf parsley

SALT-REDUCED CHICKEN STOCK

1 large (1.5 kg) whole chicken
Florets from 1 head broccoli (see above)
1 tablespoon apple cider vinegar
1 small onion, sliced into wedges
4 cloves garlic, smashed with the side of a knife
1 stick celery, diced
2 bay leaves
1 tablespoon whole black peppercorns

1. To make the chicken stock, add all the ingredients to a large stockpot and cover with water. Place over high heat and bring to the boil. Reduce the heat, cover and simmer for 1½ hours.
2. Carefully remove the whole chicken from the pot and remove the skin. Discard the chicken carcass and skin. Shred the meat using two forks. You should have roughly 600 g of meat – set this aside for the soup. Drain the stock through a sieve into a bowl. Discard the vegetables.
3. Place the same pot over medium–high heat and add the olive oil. Add the leek, zucchini, celery and the broccoli stems. Cook, stirring, for 5–6 minutes until softened. Add the garlic, ginger and thyme and cook, stirring, for another 1 minute until fragrant. Return the stock to the pan, then simmer for 10 minutes, allowing the flavours to come together.
4. Add the shredded chicken, kale and frozen peas and stir for 1–2 minutes until the kale has wilted and the chicken and peas are warmed through. Remove from the heat and stir the lemon juice and parsley into the soup.
5. Divide the soup between four bowls and serve seasoned with ¼ teaspoon freshly ground black pepper.

Notes

Tuscan kale, also known as cavolo nero, has flat dark leaves. You can use curly kale instead.

To freeze, divide the soup into individual portions in airtight containers or glass jars. Freeze for up to 3 months.

UNITS PER SERVE:	
Breads, Cereals, Legumes, Starchy Veg	0
Dairy	0.5
Lean Meat, Fish, Poultry, Eggs, Tofu	1.5
Low–Moderate Carbohydrate Veg	4
Healthy Fats	3

Cumin Chicken with Pumpkin and Garlic Yoghurt

CARBS 19g PER SERVE

SERVES: 4 | PREPARATION: 15 MINUTES | COOKING: 30 MINUTES

300 g peeled butternut pumpkin, chopped into 3 cm chunks
2 teaspoons ground cumin
1 tablespoon extra virgin olive oil
⅓ cup (40 g) walnuts
600 g chicken tenderloins
2 teaspoons ground coriander

GARLIC YOGHURT

2 cloves garlic, skins left on
¾ cup (200 g) natural yoghurt

KALE SALAD

1 tablespoon extra virgin olive oil
2 bunches broccolini, chopped into 5 cm pieces
4 cups kale leaves, stalks removed, roughly chopped
2 teaspoons Dijon mustard
Juice of ½ lemon

1. Preheat the oven to 200°C (180°C fan-forced).
2. Place the pumpkin and garlic cloves (for the garlic yoghurt) on a baking tray. Sprinkle 1 teaspoon of the cumin and 1 teaspoon of the olive oil over and toss the pumpkin and garlic in the oil. Spread the pumpkin and garlic out on the tray and bake in the oven for 25 minutes until the pumpkin is golden on the edges and tender. For the last 5 minutes of cooking, place the walnuts on the tray to lightly toast them.
3. To make the kale salad, heat ½ teaspoon of the olive oil in a large frying pan over medium–high heat. Add the broccolini and cook, tossing occasionally, for 3 minutes, until bright green and slightly tender. Add to a large bowl with the kale.
4. Place the mustard, remaining olive oil and the lemon juice in a small bowl and mix to combine. Add the mixture to the bowl with the greens and toss to coat.
5. Place the chicken in a large bowl with the remaining cumin, the coriander, ½ teaspoon freshly ground black pepper and 1 teaspoon of the olive oil. Return the frying pan to the heat and add the remaining olive oil. Add the chicken and cook for 3 minutes on each side until browned and cooked through.
6. For the garlic yoghurt, remove the skins from the garlic and place the garlic in a bowl. Mash with a fork, then add the yoghurt to the bowl and stir to combine.
7. Divide the roasted pumpkin, chicken and kale salad between four bowls. Serve with the garlic yoghurt, and the walnuts crumbled over the top.

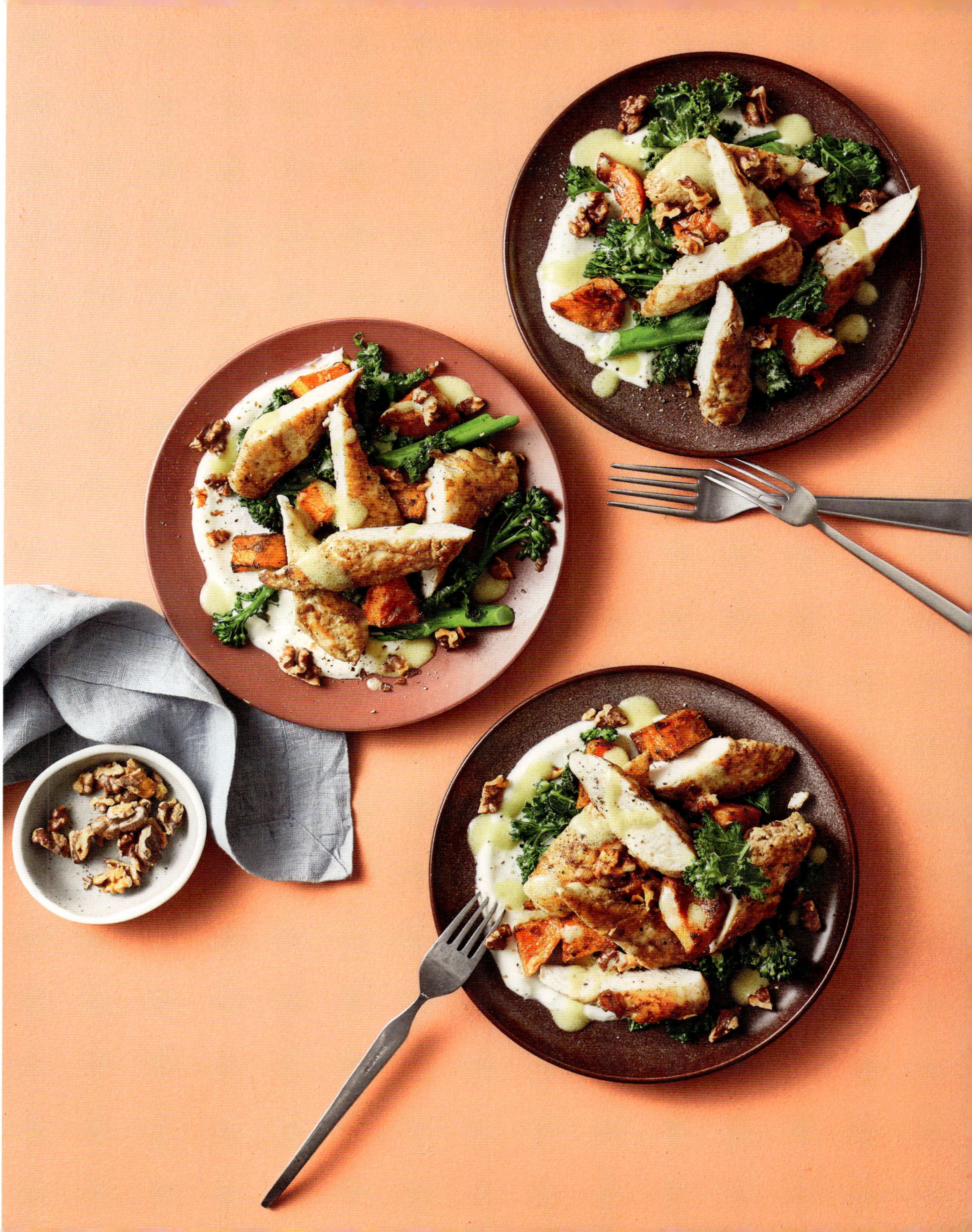

UNITS PER SERVE:	
Breads, Cereals, Legumes, Starchy Veg	0.5
Dairy	0
Lean Meat, Fish, Poultry, Eggs, Tofu	1.5
Low–Moderate Carbohydrate Veg	2
Healthy Fats	3

Satay Chicken and Asparagus Stir-fry

CARBS 8g PER SERVE

SERVES: 4 | PREPARATION: 10 MINUTES | COOKING: 12 MINUTES

600 g chicken thigh fillets, visible fat removed, chopped into 2 cm pieces
2 tablespoons cornflour
1 teaspoon ground turmeric
1 tablespoon sesame oil
3 bunches asparagus, woody ends trimmed, thinly sliced
2 teaspoons rice vinegar
4 cups baby spinach leaves
1 Lebanese cucumber, thinly sliced

SATAY SAUCE

2 tablespoons crunchy peanut butter (see notes)
1 tablespoon coconut milk
½ teaspoon curry powder
Juice of ½ lime
2 teaspoons salt-reduced tamari (see notes)

1. To make the satay sauce, place all the ingredients in a bowl and mix to combine. Add 2 tablespoons room temperature water to thin the sauce out to a drizzling consistency. Set aside.
2. Place the chicken, cornflour, turmeric and ¼ teaspoon freshly ground black pepper in a bowl and toss to coat the chicken.
3. Heat half the sesame oil in a large frying pan over medium–high heat. Add half the chicken pieces, allowing them space in the pan to sear and cook for 4 minutes, turning to brown all sides. Transfer to a bowl. Repeat with the remaining sesame oil and chicken.
4. Return all the chicken to the pan with the asparagus and cook, tossing occasionally, for 3 minutes, until the asparagus is tender and the chicken is cooked through. Add the rice vinegar and cook for 1 minute, using a spatula to scrape up any bits caught on the bottom of the pan.
5. Divide the chicken and asparagus between four bowls, add the spinach and cucumber, drizzle over the satay sauce and serve.

Notes

When purchasing nut butters, it is important to look at the food label. Ensure your nut butter has no added sugar or salt.

Tamari is a higher-salt product, so ideally use low-salt or no-added-salt alternatives. If you are following a low-sodium diet, omit this ingredient.

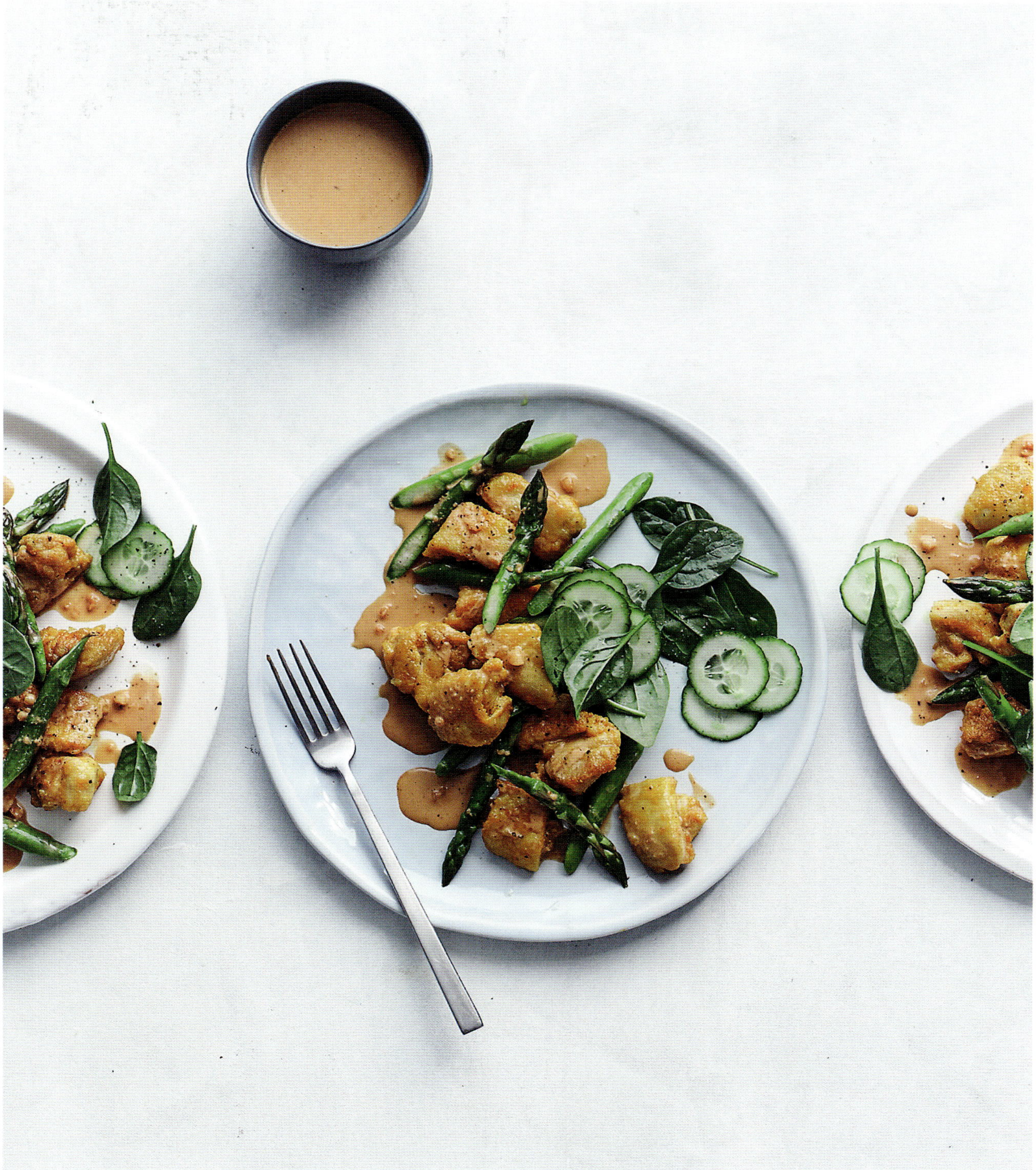

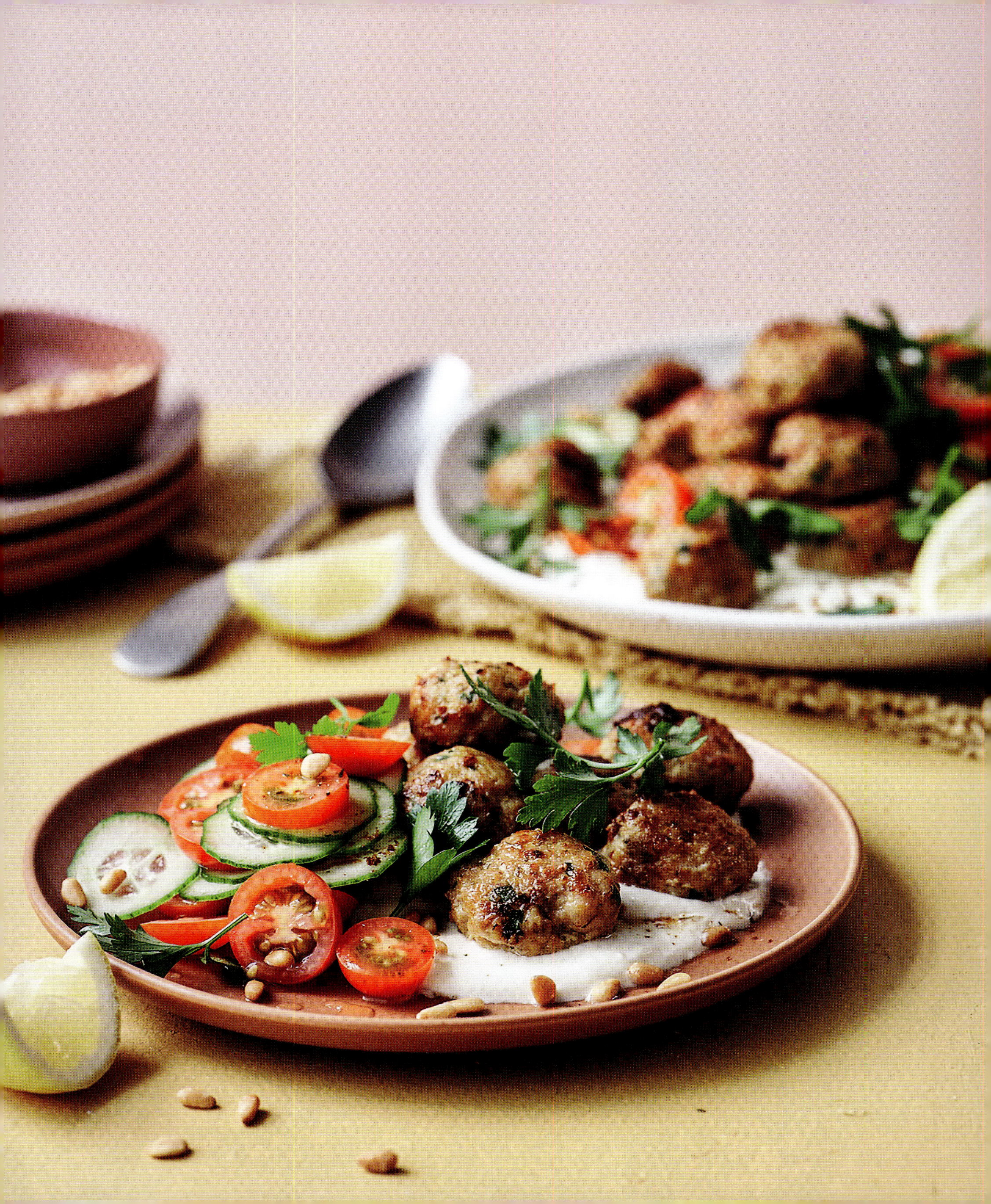

UNITS PER SERVE:	
Breads, Cereals, Legumes, Starchy Veg	0
Dairy	1
Lean Meat, Fish, Poultry, Eggs, Tofu	1.5
Low–Moderate Carbohydrate Veg	3
Healthy Fats	2

Moroccan Chicken Meatballs

CARBS 13 g PER SERVE

SERVES: 4 | PREPARATION: 10 MINUTES | COOKING: 15 MINUTES

2 tablespoons pine nuts
1 tablespoon extra virgin olive oil
40 g reduced-fat Danish feta
¾ cup (200 g) reduced-fat natural yoghurt
1 lemon, halved, one half cut into wedges
500 g cherry tomatoes, halved
2 Lebanese cucumbers, thinly sliced

MEATBALLS

550 g lean chicken mince
1 × 55 g free-range egg
2 tablespoons almond meal
3 cloves garlic, crushed
¼ cup flat-leaf parsley, finely chopped, plus extra for garnishing
1 tablespoon Moroccan spice blend (no added sugar or salt)

1. To make the meatballs, place the chicken mince, egg, almond meal, garlic, parsley and Moroccan spice blend in a bowl, then use your hands to combine the mixture really well. Scoop up 1 tablespoon amounts of the mixture and roll into balls.
2. Place a frying pan over medium–high heat and toast the pine nuts, tossing occasionally, for 1–2 minutes until lightly golden. Transfer to a plate and set aside.
3. Heat the olive oil in the same frying pan, then cook the meatballs, tossing occasionally, for 1–2 minutes, to brown the outside. Reduce the heat to medium and continue cooking and tossing regularly for 5–6 minutes, until the meatballs are cooked through. Remove from the heat.
4. Place the feta in a small bowl and mash with the back of a fork. Add the yoghurt and the juice from half the lemon and mix together until smooth.
5. Spread the yoghurt across four serving plates. Top with the meatballs, toasted pine nuts, tomatoes and cucumber. Top with more parsley leaves and serve with the lemon wedges on the side.

Note

To freeze, make the meatball mixture and roll it into balls, then place the balls in a single layer on a baking tray. Place in the freezer overnight. Once frozen, transfer to a large ziplock bag or container and freeze for up to 2 months.

UNITS PER SERVE:	
Breads, Cereals, Legumes, Starchy Veg	0
Dairy	0
Lean Meat, Fish, Poultry, Eggs, Tofu	1.5
Low–Moderate Carbohydrate Veg	3
Healthy Fats	3

Chicken with Chimichurri Sauce

CARBS 8 g PER SERVE

SERVES: 4 | PREPARATION: 30 MINUTES + 20 MINUTES–24 HOURS MARINATING | COOKING: 15 MINUTES

2 × 300 g chicken breast fillets, visible fat removed, sliced in half horizontally to make 4 thin steaks
3 zucchini, sliced lengthways

CHIMICHURRI SAUCE

½ cup finely chopped oregano
1 bunch flat-leaf parsley, roughly chopped
5 cloves garlic, crushed
1 teaspoon sweet paprika
½ teaspoon ground cumin
Pinch dried chilli flakes
¼ cup (60 ml) red wine vinegar
2 tablespoons extra virgin olive oil

TOMATO SALAD

500 g tomatoes, cut into wedges
½ small red onion, thinly sliced
1 tablespoon red wine vinegar
1 tablespoon extra virgin olive oil
¼ teaspoon freshly ground black pepper

1. To make the chimichurri sauce, add all the ingredients to a food processor and blitz for about 2 minutes until finely chopped and well combined. Allow to sit for 20 minutes, or up to overnight, in the refrigerator to allow the flavours to develop.
2. To make the tomato salad, place all the ingredients in a bowl and toss to combine. Set aside to marinate.
3. Place half the chimichurri sauce in a large bowl with the chicken steaks and toss to coat.
4. Preheat a barbecue grill plate to high or a chargrill pan on the stovetop over high heat. Cook the chicken steaks for 4 minutes on each side, or until cooked through and charred. Set aside to rest, loosely covered with foil. Add the zucchini slices to the barbecue or pan and cook for 2 minutes on each side until charred and softened.
5. Divide the chicken, zucchini and tomato salad between four plates, spoon over the remaining chimichurri sauce and serve.

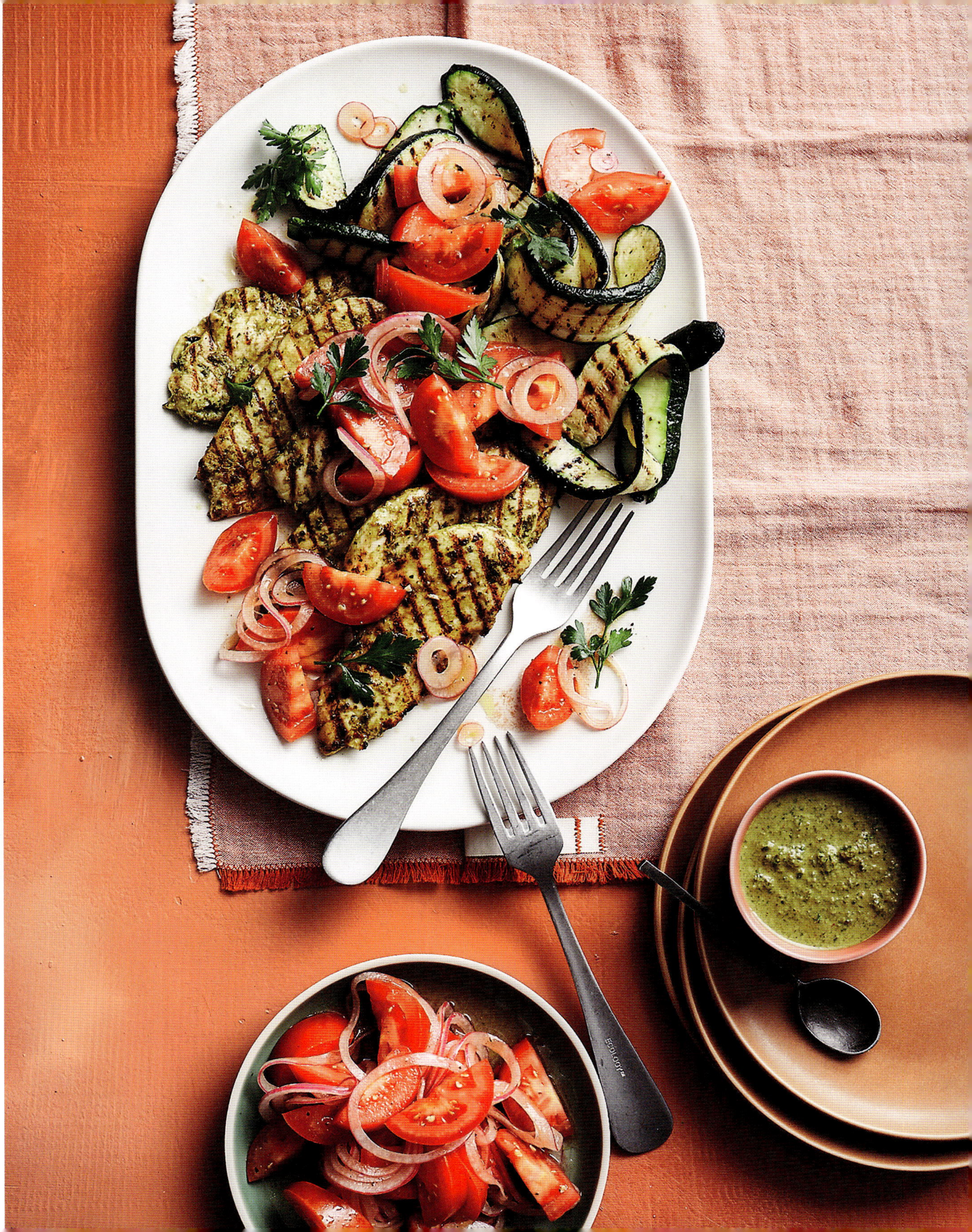

UNITS PER SERVE:	
Breads, Cereals, Legumes, Starchy Veg	0
Dairy	0
Lean Meat, Fish, Poultry, Eggs, Tofu	1.5
Low–Moderate Carbohydrate Veg	3
Healthy Fats	2.5

Chicken Puttanesca with Broccolini

CARBS 9g PER SERVE

SERVES: 4 | PREPARATION: 10 MINUTES | COOKING: 25 MINUTES

2 tablespoons extra virgin olive oil
600 g chicken thigh fillets, visible fat removed
2 zucchini, finely diced
6 cloves garlic, sliced
2 anchovy fillets, finely chopped
⅓ cup (about 8) green olives, pitted
1 tablespoon capers, drained
¼ teaspoon dried chilli flakes
2 tablespoons white wine vinegar
1 cup (250 ml) tomato passata (no added sugar or salt)
½ cup roughly chopped flat-leaf parsley
3 bunches broccolini, trimmed

1. Preheat the oven to 200°C (180°C fan-forced).
2. Heat the olive oil in a large ovenproof frying pan over medium–high heat. Add the chicken and cook for 2 minutes on each side until golden brown (the meat will still be raw inside). Transfer to a plate and set aside.
3. In the same pan, cook the zucchini for 3 minutes, until softened. Add the garlic, anchovy, olives, capers and chilli flakes and cook for another 1–2 minutes until fragrant.
4. Add the vinegar and use a spatula to scrape off any bits caught on the bottom of the pan. Add the passata and ¼ cup (60 ml) water and mix to combine, then return the chicken to the pan. Bring to the boil, then remove from the heat, cover and transfer to the oven. Bake for 15 minutes until the chicken is cooked through. Remove the pan from the oven, add the parsley and stir it through.
5. Bring a medium saucepan of water to the boil. Add the broccolini and boil for 5 minutes, until tender. Drain.
6. Divide the broccolini, chicken and puttanesca sauce between four plates and serve.

Note

To freeze, divide the chicken into individual portions in airtight containers and freeze for up to 3 months. Cook the broccolini fresh.

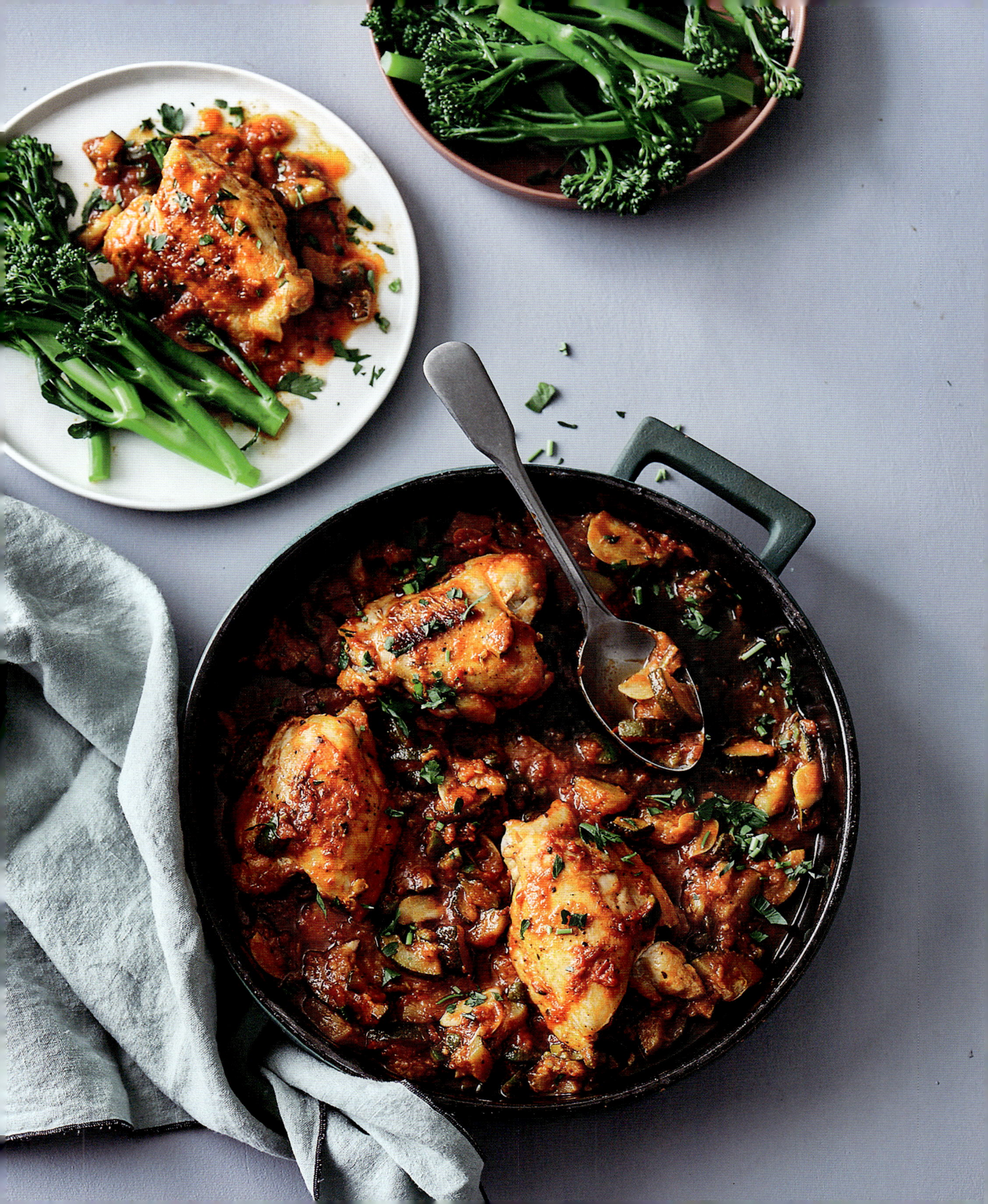

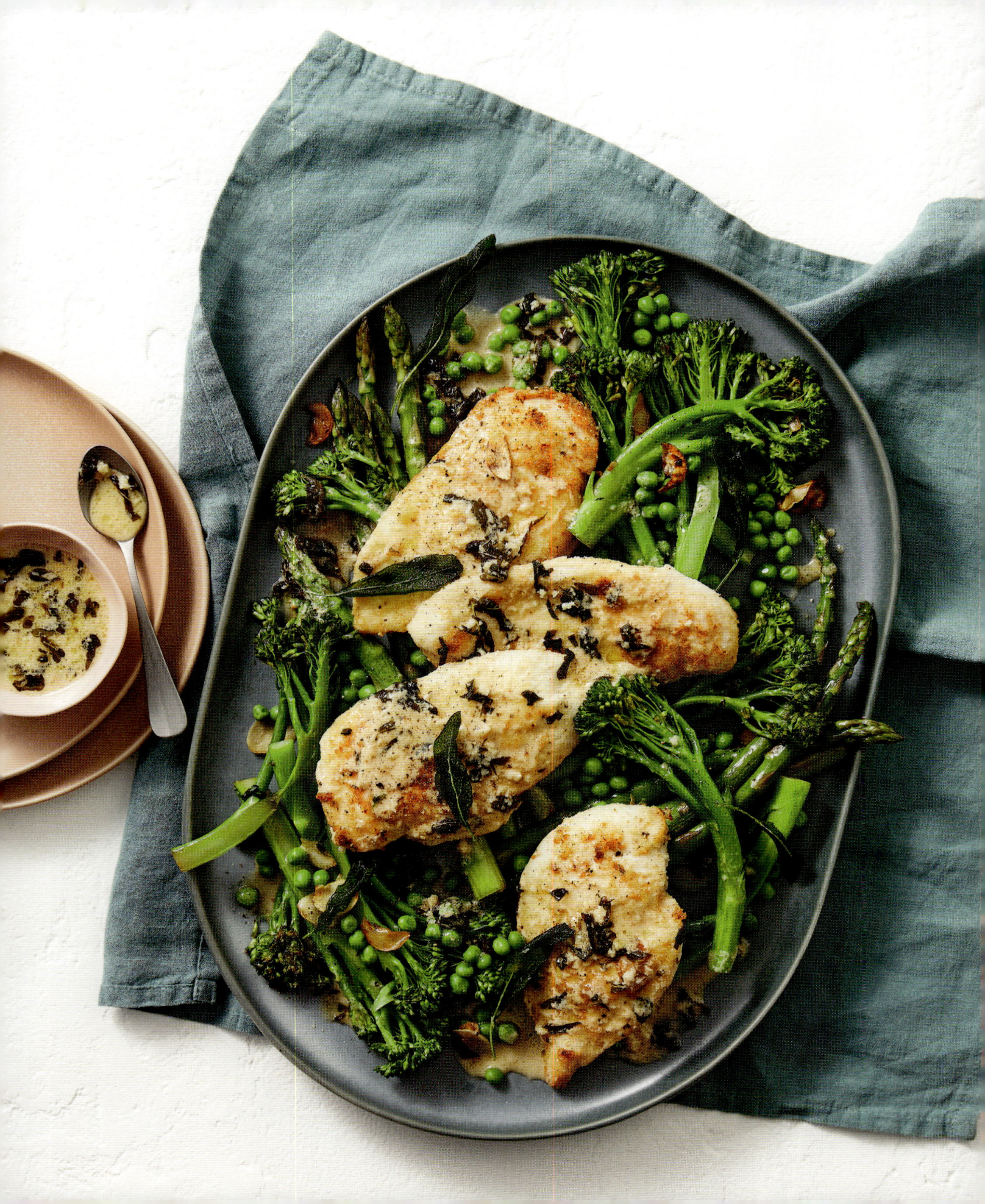

UNITS PER SERVE:	
Breads, Cereals, Legumes, Starchy Veg	0
Dairy	0
Lean Meat, Fish, Poultry, Eggs, Tofu	1.5
Low–Moderate Carbohydrate Veg	2
Healthy Fats	2.5

Garlic Sage Chicken Steaks

CARBS 15 g PER SERVE

SERVES: 4 | PREPARATION: 10 MINUTES | COOKING: 25 MINUTES

35 g fine almond flour
2 × 300 g chicken breast fillets, visible fat removed, sliced in half horizontally to make 4 thin steaks
1 tablespoon extra virgin olive oil
4 cloves garlic, crushed
1 bunch sage, leaves picked and roughly chopped
Juice of ½ lemon
1¾ cup (435 ml) salt-reduced chicken stock (see note)
½ cup (125 ml) full-fat cow's milk

GREEN VEGGIES

3 teaspoons extra virgin olive oil
2 cloves garlic, sliced
3 bunches broccolini
2 bunches asparagus, woody ends trimmed
½ cup (75 g) frozen green peas

1. Mix the almond flour and ¼ teaspoon freshly ground black pepper in a small bowl. Lay the chicken steaks flat on a plate and sprinkle the seasoned almond flour over the top, pressing it into the chicken to lightly coat. Flip and repeat on the other side.
2. Heat a drizzle of the olive oil in a large frying pan over medium–high heat. Add two chicken steaks (depending on how big your pan is) and cook for 4 minutes on each side, or until golden brown and the juices run clear. Set the chicken aside on a plate and continue with the remaining chicken steaks.
3. In the same frying pan, cook the garlic and sage, stirring, for 1 minute until fragrant. Add the lemon juice, chicken stock and milk. Reduce the heat slightly and simmer gently for 2 minutes to infuse the flavours. Return the chicken steaks and any resting juices to the pan and stir them through, then remove the pan from the heat. Set aside and cover with a lid to keep warm.
4. For the green veggies, heat the olive oil and garlic in a large frying pan with a lid over medium–high heat. In batches, add the broccolini, asparagus and peas and cook, tossing occasionally, for 2–3 minutes, then cover and steam for 1 minute. Uncover and toss again for 1–2 minutes until tender and lightly charred.
5. Divide the green veggies between four plates, top with the chicken steaks and spoon over the garlic sage sauce. Season with freshly ground black pepper and serve.

Note

Commercial chicken stock is usually very high in sodium. We recommend shopping for 'chicken broth', which is a similar product you can find in the refrigerator section of supermarkets and grocers. Broth is sold in small batches and contains less sodium. Check the label to ensure your stock contains less than 50 mg sodium per 100 g. Alternatively, if you'd like to make your own homemade stock, see the recipe on page 131.

UNITS PER SERVE:	
Breads, Cereals, Legumes, Starchy Veg	0
Dairy	1
Lean Meat, Fish, Poultry, Eggs, Tofu	1.5
Low–Moderate Carbohydrate Veg	3
Healthy Fats	2

Greek Oregano and Capsicum Chicken Skewers

CARBS 13 g PER SERVE

SERVES: 4 | PREPARATION: 15 MINUTES + 20 MINUTES–24 HOURS MARINATING | COOKING: 10 MINUTES

½ cup (130 g) natural Greek-style yoghurt
6 cloves garlic, crushed
2 tablespoons dried oregano
1 teaspoon smoked paprika
600 g chicken thigh fillets, visible fat removed, cut into 2 cm chunks
8 wooden skewers, soaked in water for 10 minutes
2 red capsicums, seeded and chopped into 3 cm chunks

CUCUMBER ASPARAGUS SALAD

2 Lebanese cucumbers
2 cups baby spinach leaves
1 bunch thin asparagus, woody ends trimmed, finely chopped
3 spring onions, finely chopped
Juice of 1 lemon
2 tablespoons extra virgin olive oil
40 g reduced-fat Greek feta, crumbled

1. Place the yoghurt, garlic, oregano, paprika and ½ teaspoon freshly ground black pepper in a large bowl and mix to combine. Add the chicken and toss to coat. Set aside to marinate for 20 minutes, covered, at room temperature, or up to 24 hours, covered, in the refrigerator.
2. For the cucumber asparagus salad, place the cucumbers on a chopping board. Use a rolling pin to bash them lightly, then roughly chop. Place in a bowl with the spinach, asparagus, spring onion, lemon juice and olive oil and toss to combine. Add the feta and toss it gently through the salad.
3. Thread the chicken and capsicum onto the skewers.
4. Heat a barbecue flat plate to high. Cook the chicken skewers for 3–4 minutes on each side until the capsicum is charred and the chicken is cooked through.
5. Divide the chicken skewers and cucumber and asparagus salad between four plates and serve.

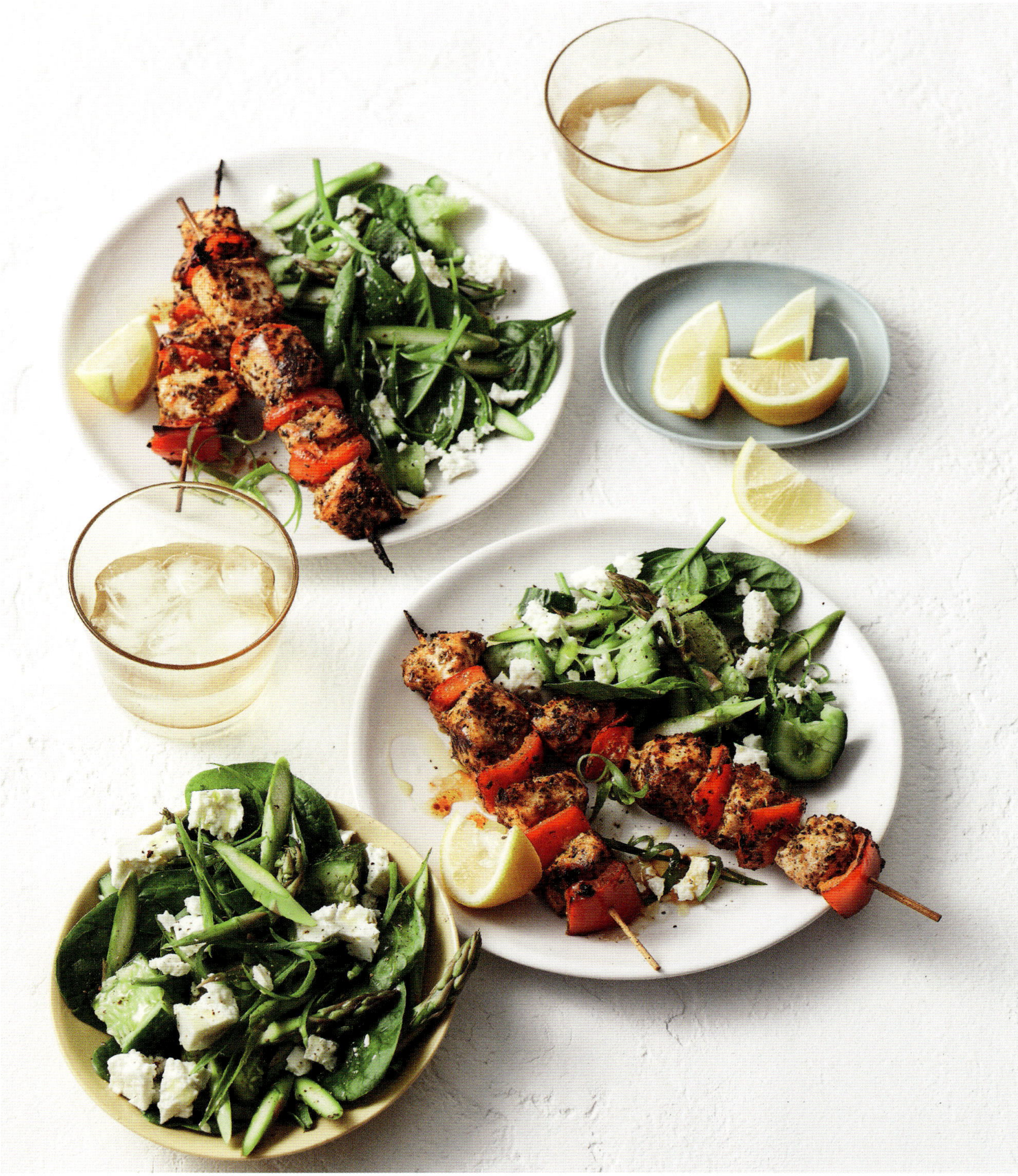

UNITS PER SERVE:	
Breads, Cereals, Legumes, Starchy Veg	0
Dairy	0
Lean Meat, Fish, Poultry, Eggs, Tofu	1.5
Low–Moderate Carbohydrate Veg	3.5
Healthy Fats	2

Chicken with Mushroom Sauce and Broccolini

CARBS 9g PER SERVE

SERVES: 4 | PREPARATION: 10 MINUTES | COOKING: 15 MINUTES

- 2 tablespoons extra virgin olive oil
- 600 g chicken thigh fillets, visible fat removed
- 1 tablespoon cornflour
- 2 golden shallots, thinly sliced
- 2 cloves garlic, thinly sliced
- 600 g sliced Swiss brown mushrooms
- 1 tablespoon white wine vinegar
- 1½ cups (375 ml) salt-reduced chicken stock (see note)
- 3 bunches broccolini
- ½ cup (75 g) frozen green peas

1. Heat half the olive oil in a large frying pan over medium–high heat. Dust the chicken in the cornflour, then add to the pan and cook for 3 minutes on each side until browned. Transfer the chicken to a plate and set aside.
2. To the same pan, add the remaining olive oil and cook the shallot and garlic for 1 minute. Add the mushrooms and cook for 4–5 minutes, until softened and most of the excess liquid from the mushrooms has evaporated. Add the vinegar and cook for 1 minute, using a spatula to scrape up any bits caught on the bottom of the pan. Add the stock and return the chicken to the pan. Simmer for 15 minutes until the chicken is cooked through.
3. Bring a large saucepan of water to the boil over high heat and cook the broccolini and peas for 5 minutes, until bright green and tender. Drain.
4. Divide the broccolini, peas, chicken and mushroom sauce between four plates and serve.

Note

Commercial chicken stock is usually very high in sodium. We recommend shopping for 'chicken broth', which is a similar product you can find in the refrigerator section of supermarkets and grocers. Broth is sold in small batches and contains less sodium. Check the label to ensure your stock contains less than 50 mg sodium per 100 g. Alternatively, if you'd like to make your own homemade stock, see the recipe on page 131.

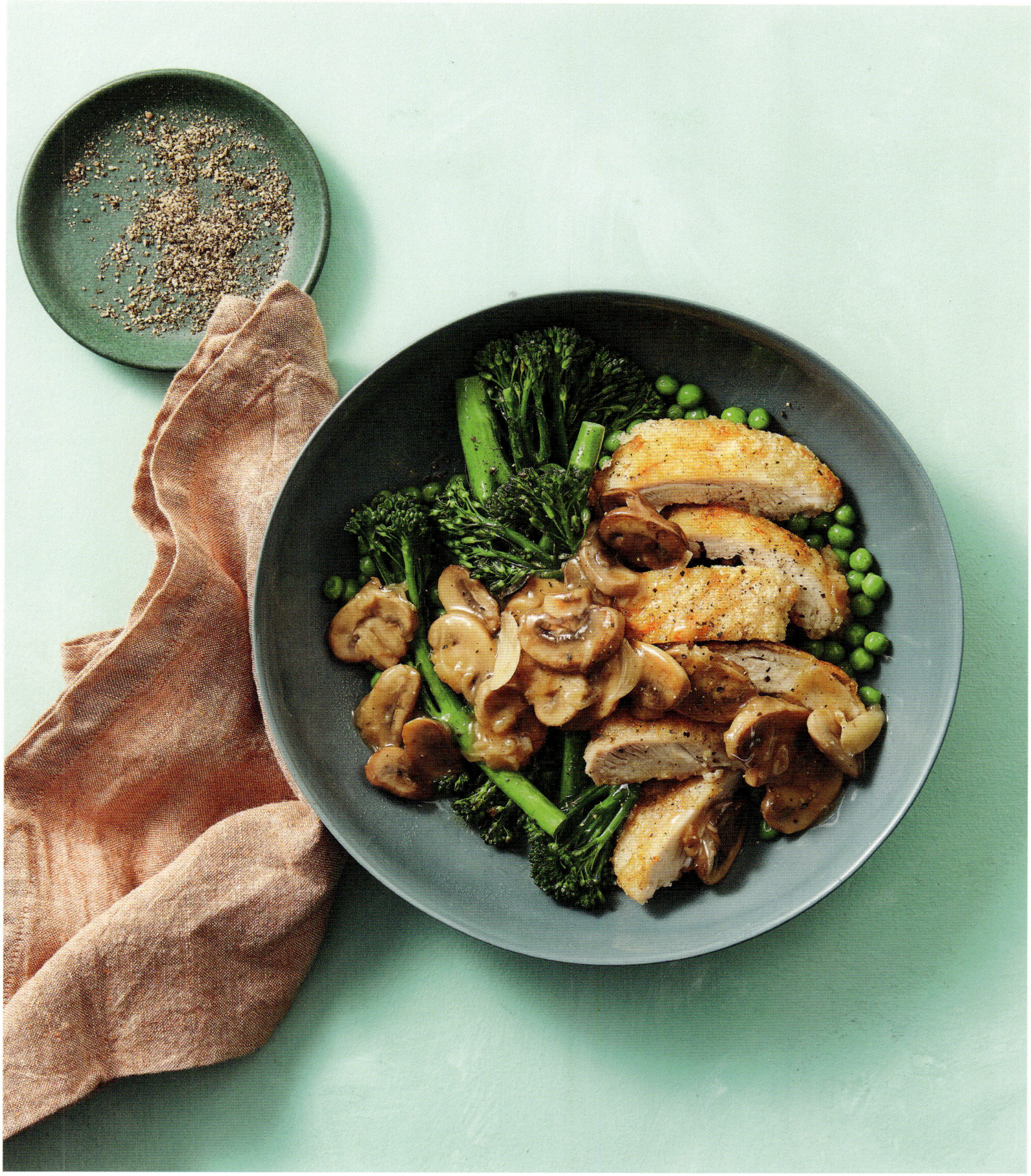

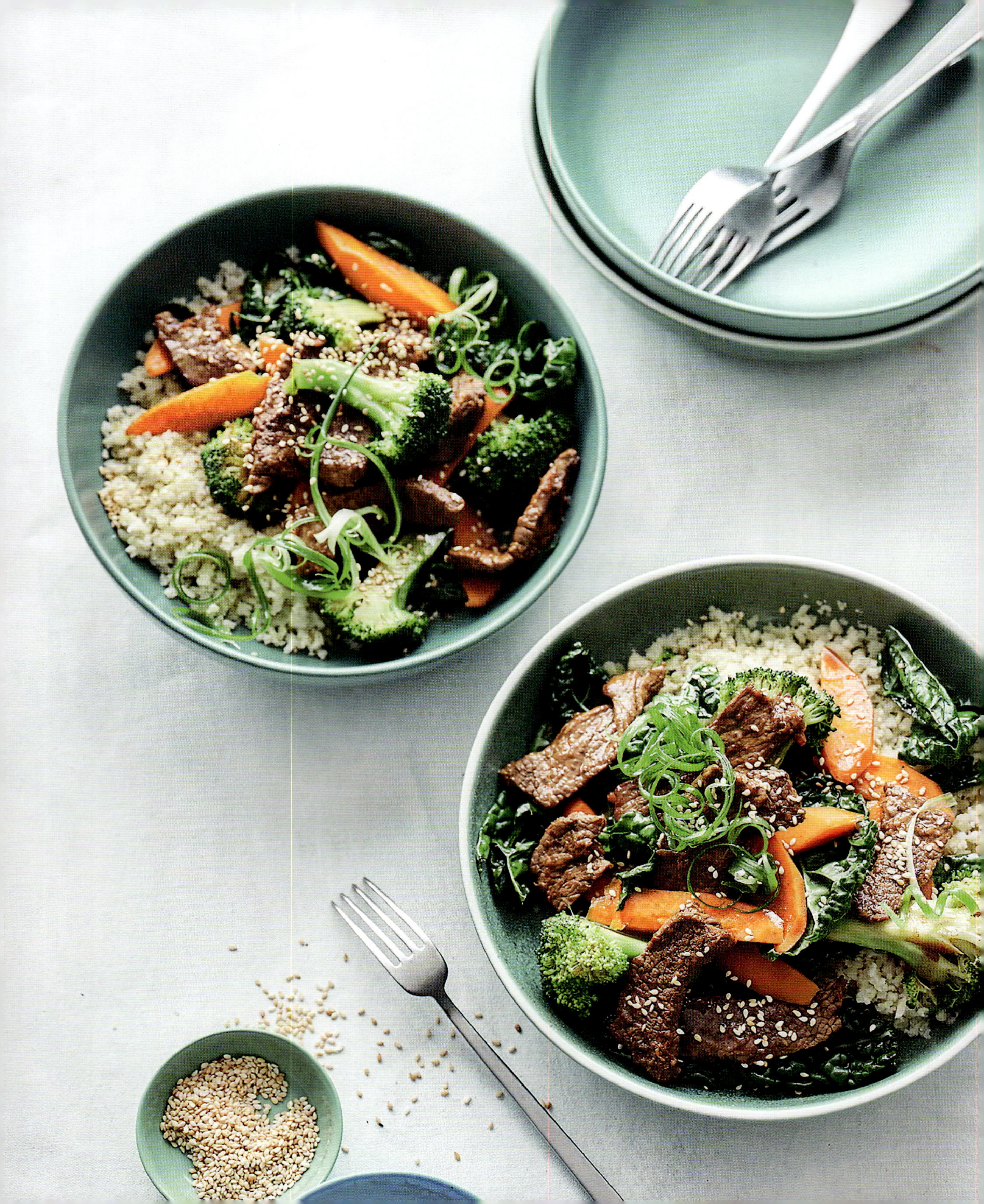

UNITS PER SERVE:	
Breads, Cereals, Legumes, Starchy Veg	0
Dairy	0
Lean Meat, Fish, Poultry, Eggs, Tofu	1.5
Low–Moderate Carbohydrate Veg	3
Healthy Fats	2.5

Korean Beef Bulgogi Bowl with Sriracha Drizzle

CARBS 17 g PER SERVE

SERVES: 4 | PREPARATION: 15 MINUTES | COOKING: 12 MINUTES

- 3 teaspoons salt-reduced tamari (see notes)
- 4 cloves garlic, crushed
- 3 cm piece of ginger, finely grated
- 1 tablespoon sesame oil
- 1 tablespoon rice wine vinegar
- 600 g lean beef stir-fry strips
- 1 large carrot, thinly sliced
- 2 heads broccoli, roughly chopped
- 1 bunch Tuscan kale, stalks removed, leaves roughly chopped (see notes)
- 450 g cauliflower rice, heated according to the packet instructions (see notes)
- 2 teaspoons sesame seeds
- 2 spring onions, finely chopped

SRIRACHA DRIZZLE

- 1 tablespoon sriracha
- 1½ tablespoons whole-egg mayonnaise
- 2 teaspoons rice wine vinegar
- 2 teaspoons water

1. For the sriracha drizzle, combine all the ingredients in a small bowl, then set aside.
2. In a small bowl, mix the tamari, garlic, ginger and half the sesame oil and the rice wine vinegar.
3. In a large frying pan over high heat, heat the remaining sesame oil and add half the beef strips, spreading them out in the pan. Cook the beef for 1 minute, undisturbed, until browned on the bottom but still slightly pink in the centre. Set aside and repeat with the remaining beef strips. Return all the beef to the pan along with the tamari and garlic sauce mixture. Cook, tossing the beef in the sauce for 2 minutes until fragrant. Transfer the beef to a bowl and cover loosely with foil.
4. In the same frying pan, place the carrot, broccoli and ¼ cup (60 ml) water. Cover the pan and cook for 5 minutes, tossing the veggies at 2 minutes, until tender. Transfer to a bowl and set aside.
5. Add the kale to the pan and cook, tossing occasionally, for 1–2 minutes until wilted.
6. Divide the heated cauliflower rice between four bowls and top with the beef, carrot, broccoli and kale. Add the sriracha drizzle, sprinkle over the sesame seeds and spring onion and serve.

Notes

Tamari is a higher-salt product, so ideally use low-salt or no-added-salt alternatives. If you are following a low-sodium diet, omit this ingredient.

Tuscan kale, also known as cavolo nero, has flat dark leaves. You can use curly kale instead.

You can find fresh cauliflower rice in the fresh produce section at your local supermarket. If unavailable, use the frozen variety instead.

UNITS PER SERVE:	
Breads, Cereals, Legumes, Starchy Veg	0
Dairy	1
Lean Meat, Fish, Poultry, Eggs, Tofu	1.5
Low–Moderate Carbohydrate Veg	3
Healthy Fats	2

Beef and Mushroom Bolognese with Broccoli

CARBS 9g PER SERVE

SERVES: 4 | PREPARATION: 10 MINUTES | COOKING: 60 MINUTES

1 tablespoon extra virgin olive oil
1 onion, finely diced
1 zucchini, finely diced
600 g lean beef mince
300 g sliced Swiss brown mushrooms
5 cloves garlic, crushed
½ bunch oregano, leaves picked (or 2 teaspoons dried oregano)
3 tablespoons tomato paste (no added sugar or salt)
2 tablespoons red wine vinegar
1 cup (250 ml) salt-reduced chicken stock (see notes)
400 g tinned diced tomatoes (no added sugar or salt)
3 heads broccoli, stems and florets chopped into 2 cm pieces separately
60 g parmesan, shaved

1. Place half the olive oil in a large, deep frying pan over medium–high heat and cook the onion and zucchini, stirring, for 5 minutes, until translucent and soft. Add the beef mince and cook, breaking it up with a wooden spoon, for 3–4 minutes until mostly browned. Add the remaining olive oil, the mushrooms, garlic and oregano and cook, stirring, for 3–5 minutes until the mushrooms are wilted and the excess liquid has evaporated.
2. Add the tomato paste to the pan and stir it through for 1 minute until it sticks to the bottom of the pan. Add the red wine vinegar and cook for 1 minute, using a spatula to scrape up any bits caught on the bottom of the pan. Add the chicken stock and diced tomatoes and bring to the boil. Reduce the heat to low–medium and cook, partially covered, for 30–40 minutes, or until thickened. Add ½ cup (125 ml) of water at a time, as needed, to keep the sauce from sticking to the bottom of the pan and thickening too much.
3. Once the bolognese has 10 minutes to go, bring a saucepan of water to the boil. Add the broccoli stems and cook for 3 minutes, then add the florets and cook for a further 2 minutes, until softened. Drain.
4. Divide the broccoli and bolognese between four bowls and serve with the parmesan and some freshly ground black pepper.

Notes

Commercial chicken stock is usually very high in sodium. We recommend shopping for 'chicken broth', which is a similar product you can find in the refrigerator section of supermarkets and grocers. Broth is sold in small batches and contains less sodium. Check the label to ensure your stock contains less than 50 mg sodium per 100 g. Alternatively, if you'd like to make your own homemade stock, see the recipe on page 131.

To freeze, divide the bolognese and broccoli into individual portions and freeze in airtight containers for up to 3 months.

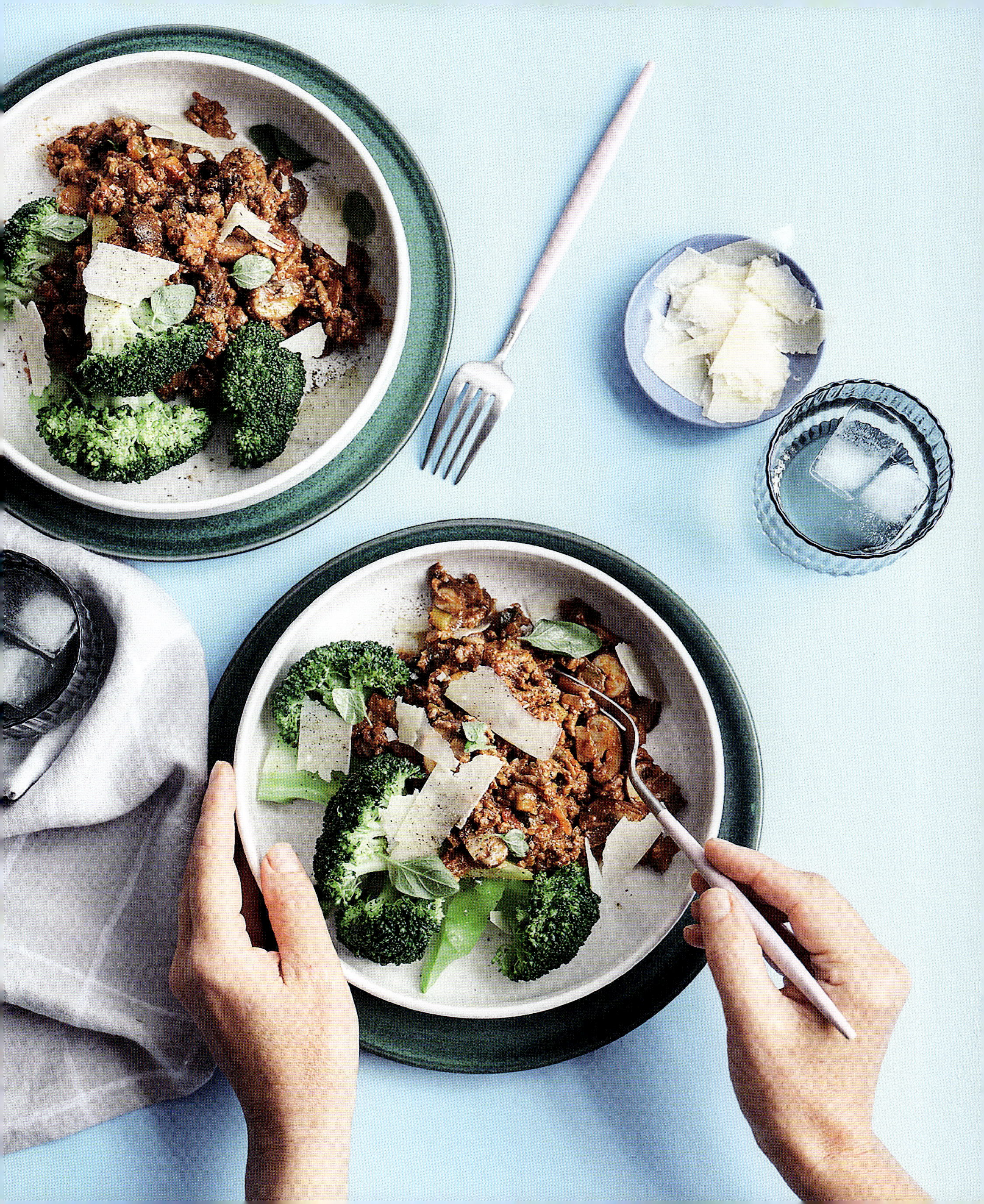

UNITS PER SERVE:	
Breads, Cereals, Legumes, Starchy Veg	0
Dairy	1
Lean Meat, Fish, Poultry, Eggs, Tofu	1.5
Low–Moderate Carbohydrate Veg	3
Healthy Fats	3

Slow-cooked Mexican Brisket

CARBS 8g PER SERVE

SERVES: 4 | PREPARATION: 20 MINUTES + 30 MINUTES–1 HOUR MARINATING | COOKING: 8 HOURS 10 MINUTES

1 teaspoon garlic powder
1 teaspoon ground cumin
2 tablespoons smoked paprika
1 tablespoon dried oregano
1 tablespoon extra virgin olive oil
1 kg beef brisket, visible fat removed (150 g meat per serve)
1 onion, sliced
2 tablespoons tomato paste (no added sugar or salt)
1 cup salt-reduced chicken stock (see note)
Juice of 1 lime
Coriander leaves, for garnishing

HERBY TOMATOES

400 g tomatoes (use a mix of varieties, such as regular, cherry, roma etc.)
2 tablespoons red wine vinegar
1 small clove garlic, crushed
½ cup chopped flat-leaf parsley
½ cup chopped coriander leaves

AVOCADO CUCUMBER SALAD

1 avocado, sliced
1 telegraph cucumber, sliced
1 baby cos lettuce, leaves roughly chopped
Juice of ½ lemon
60 g Danish feta, crumbled

1. Place the garlic powder, cumin, paprika, oregano and 2 teaspoons of the olive oil in a small bowl and mix to combine. Massage the mixture all over the brisket to coat it well.
2. Heat the remaining 2 teaspoons of olive oil in a large frying pan over medium–high heat. Add the brisket and sear on all sides.
3. Place the onion in a slow cooker and place the brisket on top.
4. Combine the tomato paste, stock and lime juice in a jug, then pour the mixture over the brisket. Put the lid on the slow cooker and cook on high for 8 hours until the meat is very tender and pulls apart easily with a fork.
5. Shred the brisket in the slow cooker using two forks. Stir the meat into the sauce to combine. Transfer to a platter and scatter with the coriander leaves.
6. Meanwhile, for the herby tomatoes, place all the ingredients in a bowl and toss to combine. Allow to marinate for 30 minutes to 1 hour before serving.
7. To make the avocado cucumber salad, place all the ingredients in a large bowl and toss to combine.
8. Place the Mexican brisket and the two salads in the centre of the table and let everyone serve themselves.

Note

Commercial chicken stock is usually very high in sodium. We recommend shopping for 'chicken broth', which is a similar product you can find in the refrigerator section of supermarkets and grocers. Broth is sold in small batches and contains less sodium. Check the label to ensure your stock contains less than 50 mg sodium per 100 g. Alternatively, if you'd like to make your own homemade stock, see the recipe on page 131.

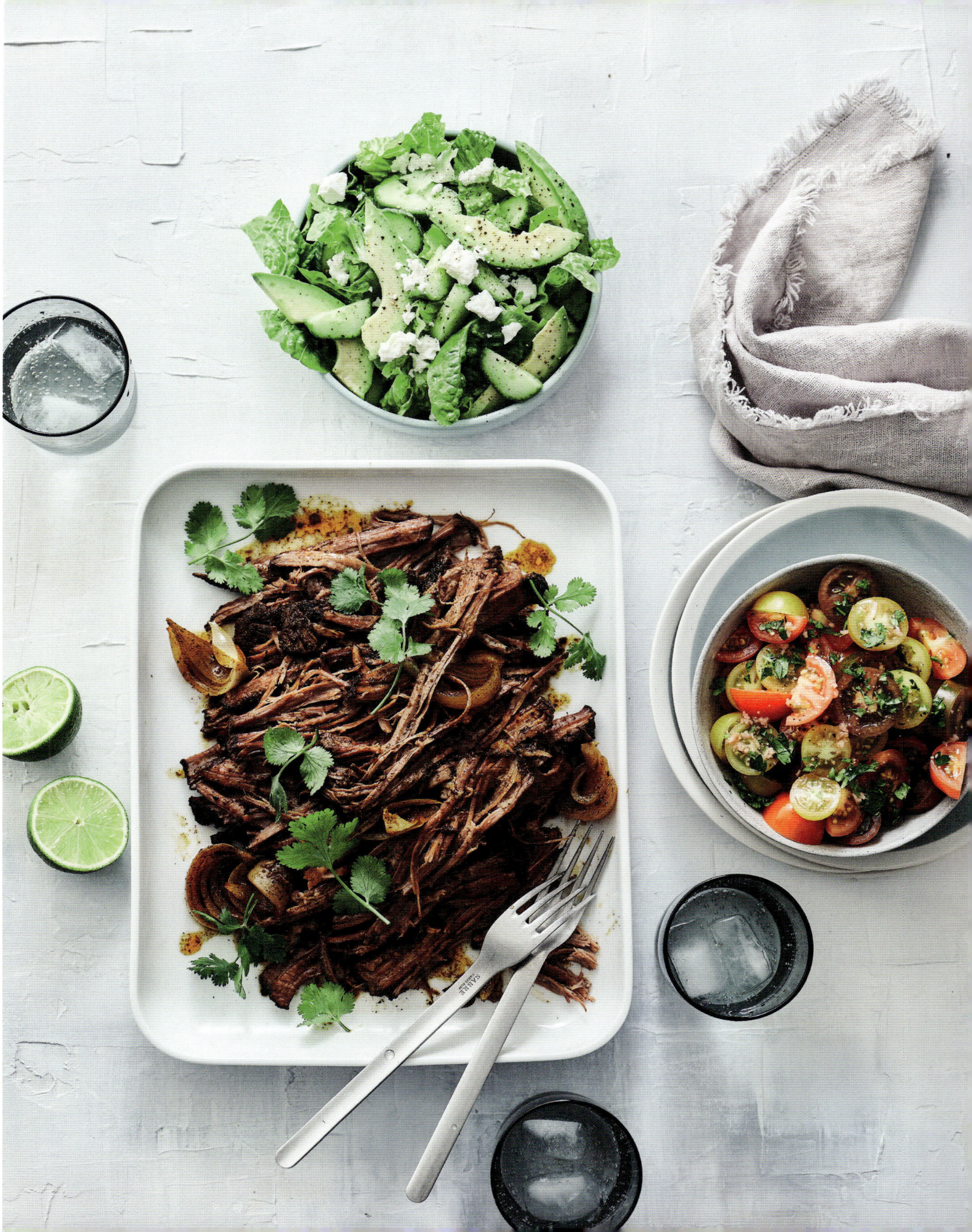

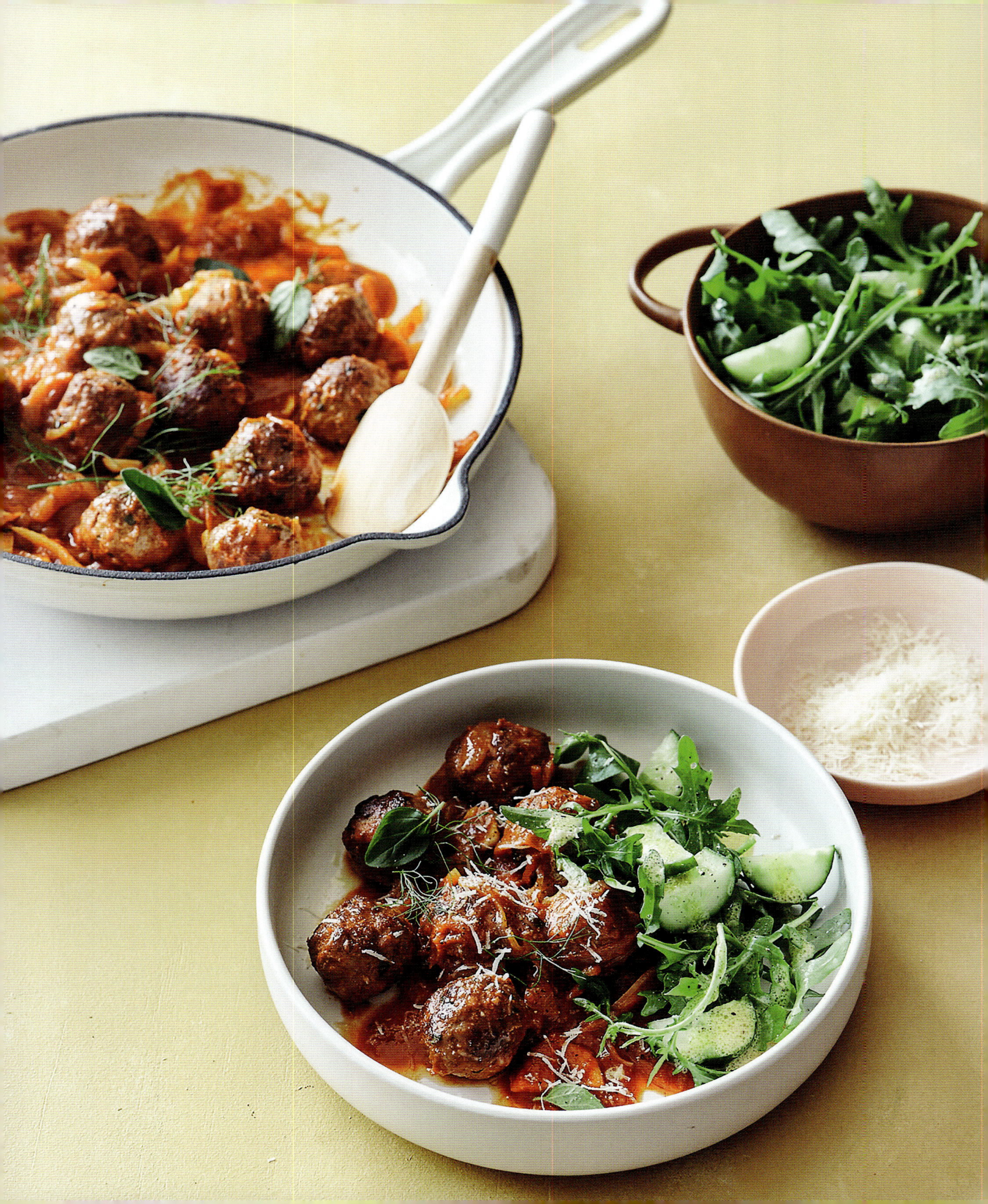

UNITS PER SERVE:	
Breads, Cereals, Legumes, Starchy Veg	0
Dairy	0.5
Lean Meat, Fish, Poultry, Eggs, Tofu	1.5
Low–Moderate Carbohydrate Veg	2.5
Healthy Fats	2

Meatballs in Fennel Tomato Sauce with Rocket Salad

CARBS 12g PER SERVE

SERVES: 4 | PREPARATION: 10 MINUTES | COOKING: 20 MINUTES

550 g extra-lean beef mince
1 × 55 g free-range egg
¼ cup (25 g) almond meal
6 sprigs oregano, leaves picked
1 tablespoon extra virgin olive oil
2 golden shallots, thinly sliced
1 small bulb fennel, trimmed and sliced
4 cloves garlic, thinly sliced
2 tablespoons white wine vinegar
1½ cups (375 ml) tomato passata (no added sugar or salt)
1 cup (250 ml) salt-reduced chicken broth
40 g parmesan, shaved

ROCKET SALAD

1 teaspoon Dijon mustard
2 teaspoons white wine vinegar
2 teaspoons extra virgin olive oil
4 cups rocket leaves
1 Lebanese cucumber, cut into half moons

1. Place the beef, egg, almond meal and half the oregano in a large bowl and use your hands to combine the mixture really well. Scoop out tablespoon amounts of the mixture and roll into balls.
2. Heat half the olive oil in a large frying pan over medium–high heat. Add the meatballs and cook, tossing occasionally, for 6 minutes until browned all over and cooked through. Transfer to a bowl and set aside.
3. Add the remaining olive oil to the same pan over medium heat. Add the shallot and fennel and cook, stirring, for 3–4 minutes until tender and golden brown. Add the garlic and remaining oregano and continue stirring for 1 minute until fragrant. Add the vinegar to the pan and cook for 1 minute, using a spatula to scrape up any bits stuck to the bottom of the pan.
4. Return the meatballs to the pan along with the passata and chicken broth. Stir for 1–2 minutes to bring everything together.
5. To make the rocket salad, place the Dijon mustard, vinegar and olive oil in a large bowl and stir to combine. Add the rocket leaves and cucumber and toss gently to incorporate.
6. Divide the meatballs and sauce between four bowls. Top with the parmesan, season with freshly ground black pepper and serve with the rocket salad.

UNITS PER SERVE:	
Breads, Cereals, Legumes, Starchy Veg	0
Dairy	0
Lean Meat, Fish, Poultry, Eggs, Tofu	1.5
Low–Moderate Carbohydrate Veg	2
Healthy Fats	2

Steak with Herby Mushroom Gravy

CARBS 5g PER SERVE

SERVES: 4 | PREPARATION: 10 MINUTES | COOKING: 20 MINUTES

4 × 150 g beef steaks (sirloin, porterhouse, rump or hanger steak), visible fat removed
2 tablespoons extra virgin olive oil
3 bunches broccolini
3 cloves garlic, thinly sliced
6 sprigs thyme, leaves picked
700 g mixed mushrooms, sliced (try a mix of enoki, shiitake, king brown and Swiss brown)
1½ cups (375 ml) salt-reduced chicken stock (see note)
1 tablespoon cornflour (or tapioca starch)

1. Season both sides of the steaks with freshly ground black pepper.
2. Heat half the olive oil in a large frying pan over medium–high heat. Add the steaks, two at a time, and cook for 3 minutes on each side. Transfer to a plate, cover loosely with foil and set aside.
3. In the same pan, cook the broccolini for 5 minutes, tossing until tender and charred in spots. Transfer to a plate and set aside.
4. Add the remaining olive oil to the frying pan, add the garlic, thyme and mushrooms and cook for 2 minutes until the mushrooms are tender.
5. In a small bowl, whisk together 2 tablespoons of the stock and the cornflour, then add the mixture to the pan with the mushrooms along with the remaining stock. Stir to combine, then reduce the heat and simmer for 2–3 minutes until the mixture thickens slightly.
6. Divide the steak and broccolini between four plates. Spoon over the mushrooms and sauce, season generously with freshly ground black pepper and serve.

Note

Commercial chicken stock is usually very high in sodium. We recommend shopping for 'chicken broth', which is a similar product you can find in the refrigerator section of supermarkets and grocers. Broth is sold in small batches and contains less sodium. Check the label to ensure your stock contains less than 50 mg sodium per 100 g. Alternatively, if you'd like to make your own homemade stock, see the recipe on page 131.

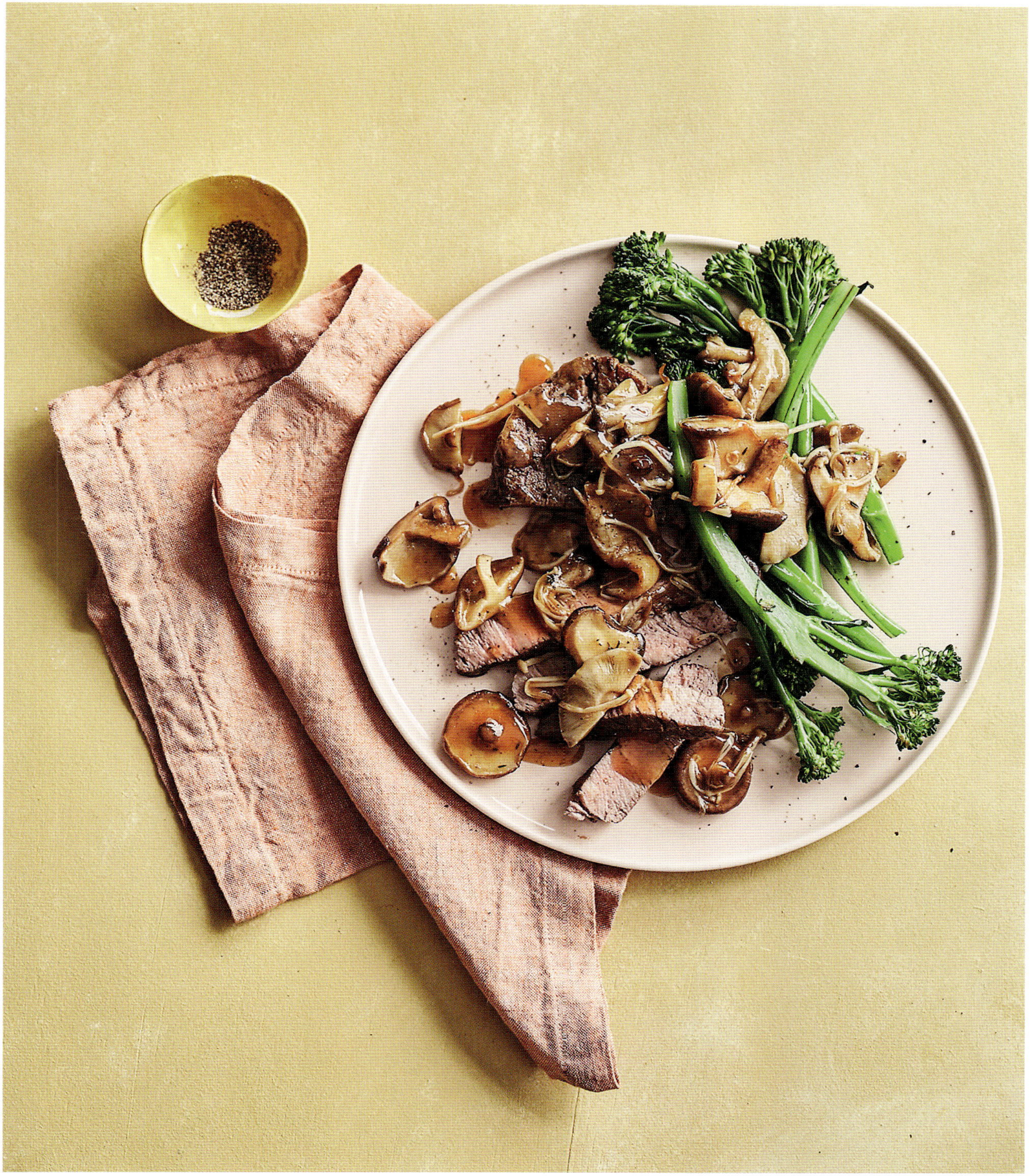

UNITS PER SERVE:	
Breads, Cereals, Legumes, Starchy Veg	0
Dairy	0
Lean Meat, Fish, Poultry, Eggs, Tofu	1.5
Low–Moderate Carbohydrate Veg	3.5
Healthy Fats	2.5

Osso Buco with Parsnip Cauli Mash

CARBS 18 g PER SERVE

SERVES: 4 | PREPARATION: 15 MINUTES | COOKING: 2 HOURS

1 tablespoon arrowroot flour
1.2 kg oxtail osso buco pieces (if you can't find it at the supermarket, ask your butcher to cut it for you)
2 tablespoons extra virgin olive oil
1 onion, diced
1 zucchini, finely diced
2 sticks celery, diced
½ cup flat-leaf parsley, leaves and stems roughly chopped separately
6 cloves garlic, crushed
4 sprigs thyme, leaves picked
¼ cup (60 ml) apple cider vinegar
2 cups (500 ml) salt-reduced beef or chicken stock (see notes)
400 g tinned diced tomatoes
½ bunch kale, stalks removed, leaves roughly torn

PARSNIP CAULI MASH

2 parsnips, peeled and chopped into 3 cm chunks
½ head cauliflower, chopped into 3 cm pieces
2 tablespoons full-fat cow's milk
2 teaspoons Nuttelex or light canola margarine

1. Preheat the oven to 180°C (160°C fan-forced).
2. Sprinkle the arrowroot and some freshly ground black pepper over the osso buco.
3. Heat half the olive oil in a large, deep cast-iron pot over high heat. Add the osso bucco pieces and sear on each side for 2 minutes, until golden brown. Remove from the pan and set aside.
4. Reduce the heat to medium and add the remaining olive oil, the onion, zucchini, celery and parsley stems. Saute for 10 minutes until softened. Add the garlic and thyme and cook for another 1 minute until fragrant. Add the apple cider vinegar and use a spatula to scrape up any bits stuck to the bottom of the pan. Cook for about 1 minute until the vinegar evaporates.
5. Add the stock and diced tomatoes, stirring to combine. Return the osso bucco to the pan and bring to the boil. Place a lid on the pan, transfer to the oven and cook for 1½ hours until the meat is falling off the bone.
6. Remove the pot from the oven, remove the lid and place the kale on top of the osso buco. Place the lid back on and allow the kale to steam and wilt in the residual heat for 5 minutes.
7. To make the mash, place the parsnip and cauliflower in a large saucepan and cover with water. Bring to the boil over high heat and cook for 15 minutes until the veggies are soft. Drain the vegetables, then return to the pan with the milk, Nuttelex and ¼ teaspoon freshly ground black pepper and mash with a fork.
8. Divide the osso buco, kale and parsnip cauli mash between four bowls and serve.

Notes

Commercial stock is usually very high in sodium. We recommend shopping for 'chicken broth', which is a similar product you can find in the refrigerator section of supermarkets and grocers. Broth is sold in small batches and contains less sodium. Check the label to ensure your stock contains less than 50 mg sodium per 100 g. Alternatively, if you'd like to make your own homemade stock, see the recipe on page 131.

To freeze, shred the meat and stir it through the sauce. Divide between four airtight containers and freeze for up to 3 months. Thaw in the refrigerator and reheat in a saucepan for 5 minutes until warmed through.

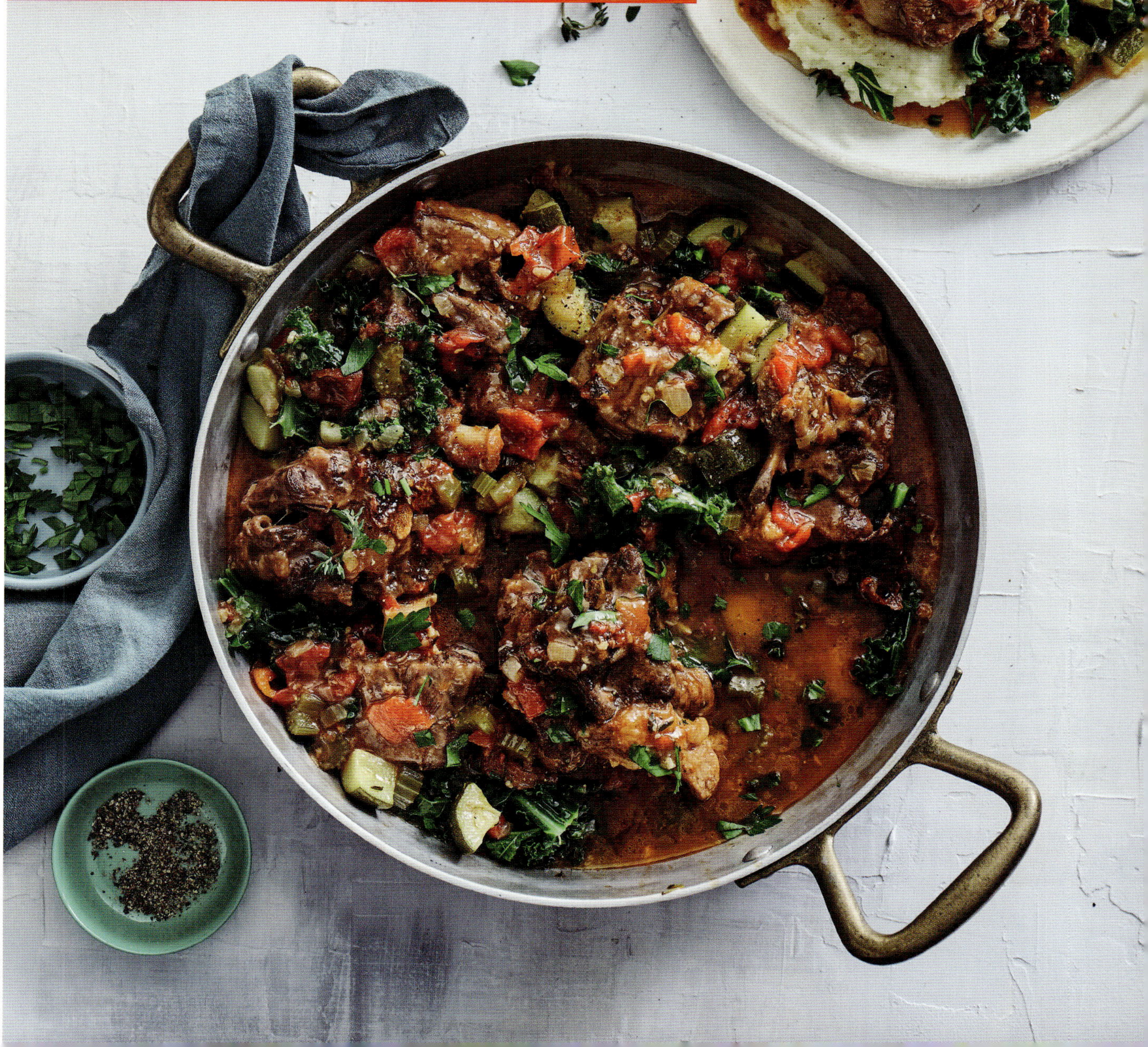

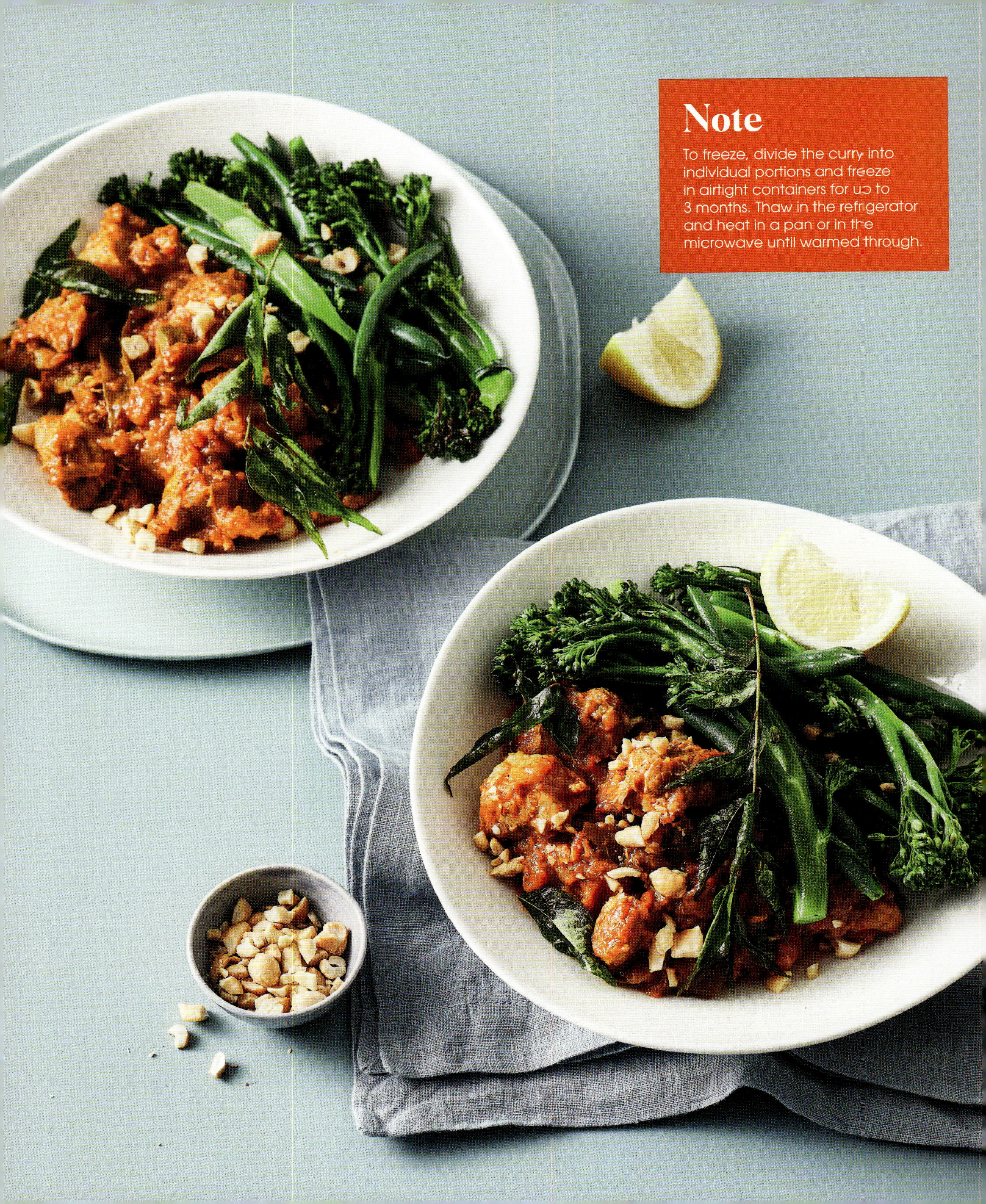

Note

To freeze, divide the curry into individual portions and freeze in airtight containers for up to 3 months. Thaw in the refrigerator and heat in a pan or in the microwave until warmed through.

UNITS PER SERVE:	
Breads, Cereals, Legumes, Starchy Veg	0
Dairy	0
Lean Meat, Fish, Poultry, Eggs, Tofu	1.5
Low–Moderate Carbohydrate Veg	3
Healthy Fats	3

Slow-cooked Pork Curry with Lemony Greens

CARBS 15g PER SERVE

SERVES: 4 | PREPARATION: 10 MINUTES | COOKING: 1 HOUR 20 MINUTES

2 tablespoons extra virgin olive oil
600 g pork shoulder, excess fat removed, cut into 3 cm pieces
2 onions, finely diced
1 zucchini, finely diced
2 cm piece of ginger, finely grated
5 cloves garlic
15 curry leaves
1 tablespoon white wine vinegar
250 g tinned finely chopped tomatoes
Lemon wedges, to serve

SPICE BLEND

1 teaspoon brown mustard seeds
1 teaspoon ground turmeric
1 teaspoon cumin seeds
2 teaspoons coriander seeds
2 whole cloves
½ cinnamon stick
1 teaspoon fennel seeds
2 teaspoons whole black peppercorns

LEMONY GREENS

2 teaspoons extra virgin olive oil
2 bunches broccolini
150 g green beans, ends trimmed
2 tablespoons roasted unsalted cashews, finely chopped
Juice of ½ lemon

1. Heat a deep cast-iron pot over medium–high heat. Add all the ingredients for the spice blend and toast for 3 minutes until the spices are aromatic and lightly browned. Transfer to a mortar and pestle and grind to a powder.
2. Heat half the olive oil in the same pot, add the pork and sear on all sides for 3 minutes, then toss and cook for another 3 minutes until browned. Transfer the pork to a bowl and set aside.
3. Add the onion and zucchini to the pan and cook, stirring, for 5 minutes until golden brown. Add the remaining olive oil, ginger, garlic, curry leaves and the spice blend and cook, stirring, for 2 minutes until fragrant. Add the vinegar and cook for about 1 minute, using a spatula to scrape up any bits caught on the bottom of the pan. Add the chopped tomatoes and cook, stirring, for 10 minutes, until the vegetables and spices form a thick paste. Return the pork to the pan and stir to coat in the spice paste.
4. Add 2 cups (500 ml) water to the pan and stir to combine. Bring to the boil, then reduce the heat to low, cover and simmer for 45–60 minutes, stirring every now and then and adding another ¼ cup (60 ml) water when needed to keep the sauce from burning on the bottom of the pan. (This curry is meant to be quite thick.)
5. For the lemony greens, heat the olive oil in a large frying pan over medium heat. Add the broccolini and green beans and cook, tossing occasionally, for 1 minute to coat the veggies in the oil. Cover the pan with a lid and steam for 5–6 minutes, shaking the pan every few minutes to move the greens around until they're charred and tender. Remove the lid, add the cashews and toss for another 1 minute until golden brown. Remove the pan from the heat and squeeze over the lemon juice.
6. Divide the pork curry and lemony greens between four bowls and serve with the lemon wedges on the side.

UNITS PER SERVE:	
Breads, Cereals, Legumes, Starchy Veg	0
Dairy	0
Lean Meat, Fish, Poultry, Eggs, Tofu	1.5
Low–Moderate Carbohydrate Veg	3
Healthy Fats	3

Smoked Pulled Pork Shoulder with Asparagus Slaw

CARBS 10 g PER SERVE

SERVES: 4 | PREPARATION: 10 MINUTES | COOKING: 4 HOURS 30 MINUTES

2 teaspoons fennel seeds
1 teaspoon ground cumin
1 tablespoon smoked paprika
1 teaspoon ground cinnamon
1 teaspoon chilli powder
5 cloves garlic, crushed
1 tablespoon extra virgin olive oil
1.5 kg lean boneless pork shoulder, fat on top trimmed (150 g meat per serve)
½ cup (125 ml) tomato passata (no added sugar or salt)
½ cup (125 ml) salt-reduced chicken stock (see notes)
2 tablespoons apple cider vinegar
2 bay leaves

ASPARAGUS SLAW

2 bunches thin asparagus, woody ends trimmed, cut into 1 cm pieces
1 small bulb fennel, trimmed and thinly sliced, fronds reserved for serving
1 small avocado, thinly sliced lengthways
2 tablespoons chopped roasted unsalted almonds
1 cup chopped coriander leaves
Juice of ½ lemon
2 teaspoons extra virgin olive oil

CHARRED BROCCOLINI

2 teaspoons extra virgin olive oil
2 bunches broccolini

1. Preheat the oven to 180°C (160°C fan-forced).
2. Place the fennel seeds, cumin, paprika, cinnamon, chilli powder and 1 teaspoon freshly ground black pepper in a bowl and mix to combine. Add the garlic and olive oil and mix into a paste. Stir in 1–2 teaspoons water to thin the paste out a little.
3. Place the pork shoulder in a roasting dish and cover with the spice paste, massaging it into the meat well.
4. In a small bowl, mix together the passata, stock and vinegar, then pour the mixture into the base of the roasting dish. Add the bay leaves, cover the dish with foil (or a lid) and roast the pork in the oven for 3½–4 hours until the meat is very tender and pulls apart easily with a fork. Remove the foil and roughly tear up the pork in the dish using two forks. Return the pork to the oven and cook, uncovered, for 30 minutes, until slightly browned on top.
5. For the asparagus slaw, place all the ingredients in a bowl and toss together to combine. Top with the reserved fennel fronds.
6. For the charred broccolini, heat half the olive oil in a large frying pan over medium–high heat. Add half the broccolini and cook for 5 minutes, tossing occasionally, until the broccolini is tender and charred in spots. Set aside and repeat with the remaining olive oil and broccolini.
7. Place the pulled pork in the centre of the table with the asparagus slaw and charred broccolini on the side.

Notes

Commercial chicken stock is usually very high in sodium. We recommend shopping for 'chicken broth', which is a similar product you can find in the refrigerator section of supermarkets and grocers. Broth is sold in small batches and contains less sodium. Check the label to ensure your stock contains less than 50 mg sodium per 100 g. Alternatively, if you'd like to make your own homemade stock, see the recipe on page 131.

To freeze, cool the pulled pork to room temperature and shred the meat. Divide between four ziplock bags or airtight containers and freeze for up to 3 months.

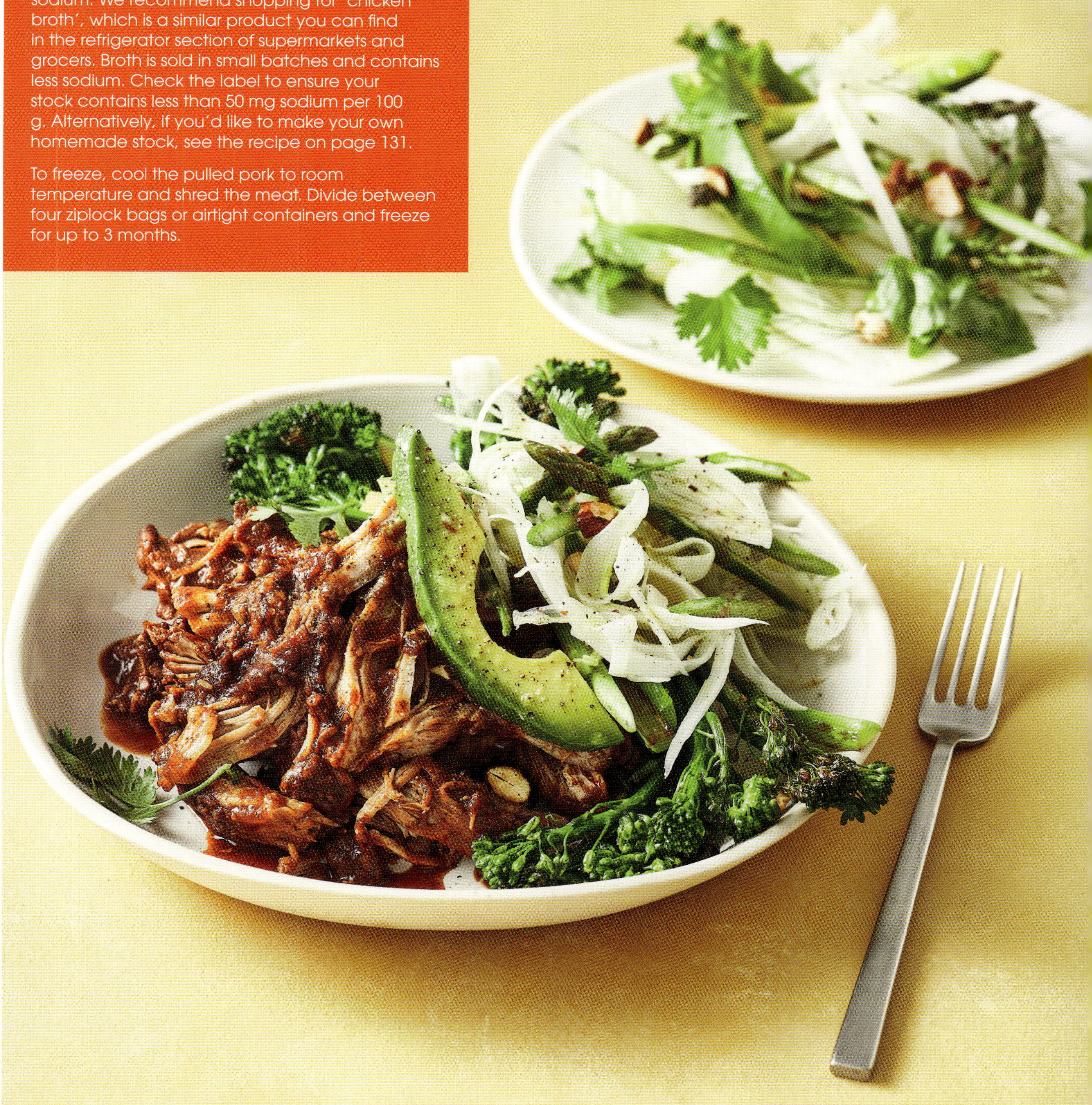

UNITS PER SERVE:	
Breads, Cereals, Legumes, Starchy Veg	0
Dairy	0
Lean Meat, Fish, Poultry, Eggs, Tofu	1.5
Low–Moderate Carbohydrate Veg	3
Healthy Fats	2.5

Spiced Pork and Mushroom Stir-fry

CARBS 14 g PER SERVE

SERVES: 4 | PREPARATION: 10 MINUTES | COOKING: 20 MINUTES

- 1 tablespoon sesame oil
- 8 spring onions, thinly sliced, white and green parts separate
- 450 g Swiss brown mushrooms, sliced
- 600 g lean pork mince
- 3 teaspoons Chinese five-spice powder
- 3 cm piece of ginger, finely grated
- 3 cloves garlic, crushed
- Pinch dried chilli flakes
- ½ cup (60 g) roasted unsalted cashews, roughly chopped
- 2 tablespoons rice wine vinegar
- 4 bunches broccolini, chopped into 2 cm pieces
- 1 tablespoon salt-reduced tamari (see notes)
- 1 cup (250 ml) salt-reduced chicken stock (see notes)
- 4 cups (400 g) cauliflower rice, heated according to the packet instructions (see notes)

1. Heat the sesame oil in a large, deep frying pan over medium–high heat. Add the white part of the spring onion and the mushrooms and cook, stirring, for 2 minutes until golden. Push the mushroom and spring onion to the side of the pan and add the pork mince. Cook for 4–5 minutes, breaking it up with a wooden spoon and tossing occasionally, until brown and cooked through. Mix the pork, mushrooms and spring onion together, then cover the pan with a lid. Steam for 2 minutes – this will help reduce the veggies without using a lot of oil. Remove the lid and continue cooking for 5 minutes until the excess liquid has evaporated.
2. Add the Chinese five-spice powder, ginger, garlic, chilli flakes and half the cashews and cook for 2–3 minutes, until fragrant. Add the vinegar and cook for 1 minute, using a spatula to scrape up any pieces stuck to the bottom of the pan. Add the broccolini, tamari and chicken stock. Simmer for 2–3 minutes until the liquid has reduced by half and the broccolini has softened.
3. Divide the heated cauliflower rice and the pork and mushroom stir-fry between four bowls, top with the spring onion greens and the remaining cashews and serve.

Notes

Tamari is a higher-salt product, so ideally use low-salt or no-added-salt alternatives. If you are following a low-sodium diet, omit this ingredient.

Commercial chicken stock is usually very high in sodium. We recommend shopping for 'chicken broth', which is a similar product you can find in the refrigerator section of supermarkets and grocers. Broth is sold in small batches and contains less sodium. Check the label to ensure your stock contains less than 50 mg sodium per 100 g. Alternatively, if you'd like to make your own homemade stock, see the recipe on page 131.

You can find fresh cauliflower rice in the fresh produce section at your local supermarket. If unavailable, use the frozen variety instead.

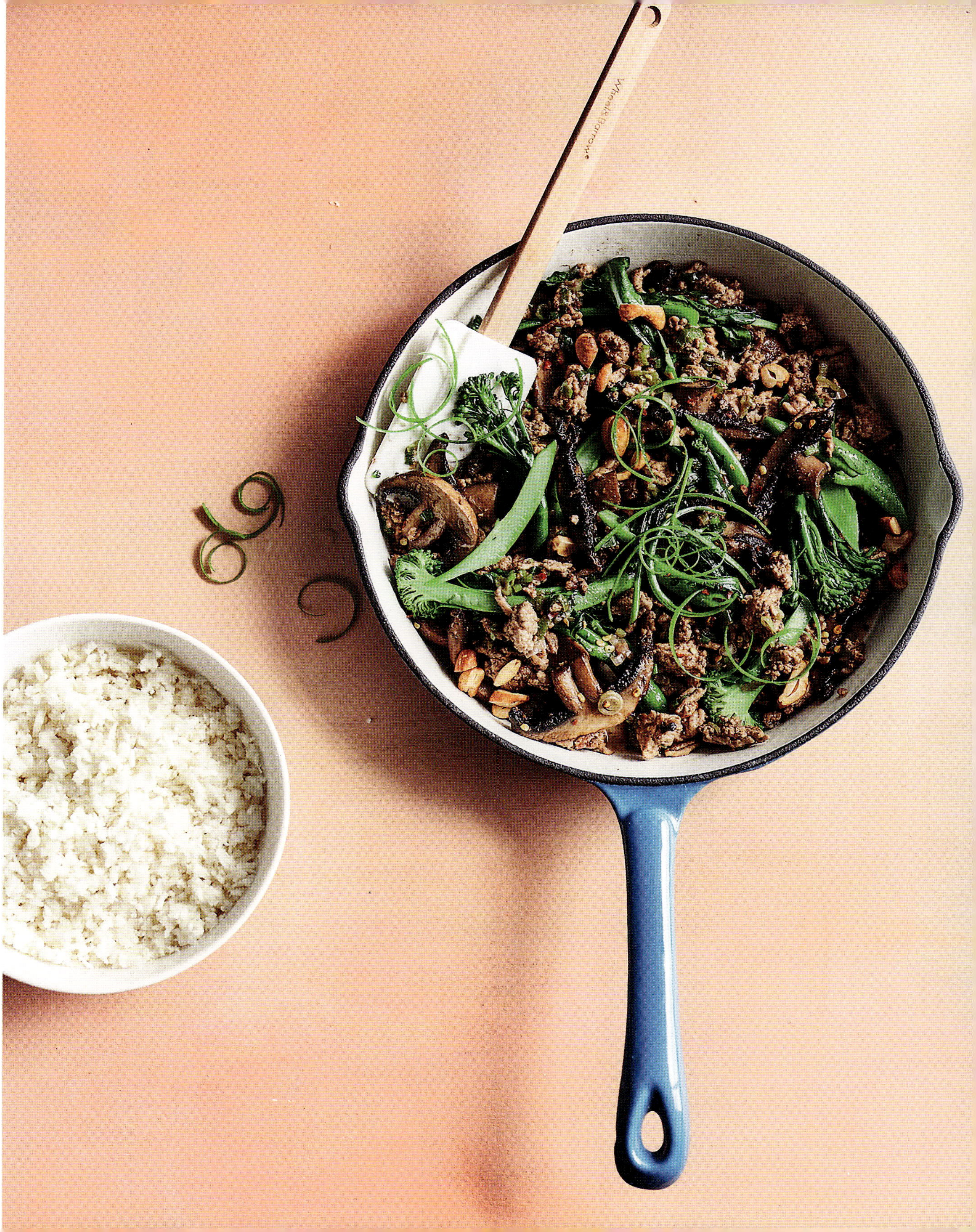

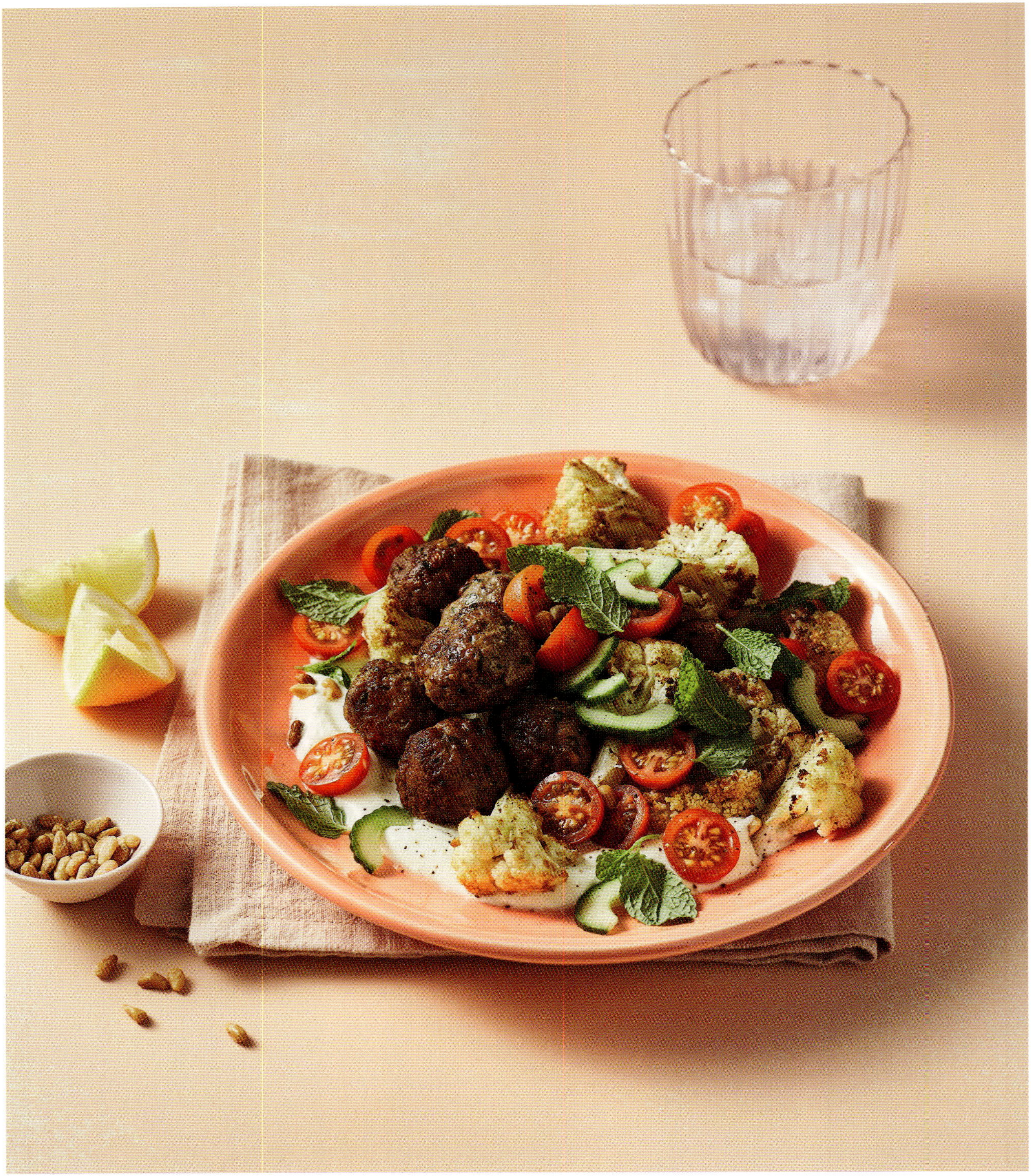

UNITS PER SERVE:	
Breads, Cereals, Legumes, Starchy Veg	0
Dairy	1
Lean Meat, Fish, Poultry, Eggs, Tofu	1.5
Low–Moderate Carbohydrate Veg	3
Healthy Fats	3

Pistachio Lamb Meatballs with Feta Sauce

CARBS 12g PER SERVE

SERVES: 4 | PREPARATION: 15 MINUTES | COOKING: 25 MINUTES

550 g extra-lean lamb mince
1 × 55 g free-range egg
¼ cup (25 g) almond meal
2 tablespoons raw unsalted pistachios, finely chopped
½ cup flat-leaf parsley, finely chopped
1 teaspoon extra virgin olive oil

ROASTED CAULIFLOWER

1 small head cauliflower, chopped into 2–3 cm chunks
1 teaspoon ground coriander
1 teaspoon ground cumin
2 teaspoons extra virgin olive oil

FETA SAUCE

¾ cup (200 g) natural yoghurt
40 g reduced-fat Danish goat's feta

SALAD

1½ tablespoons pine nuts
½ cup mint leaves
400 g cherry tomatoes, halved
1 telegraph cucumber, cut into half moons
Juice of ½ lemon
3 teaspoons extra virgin olive oil

1. Preheat the oven to 200°C (180°C fan-forced).
2. For the roasted cauliflower, place the cauliflower on a baking tray and sprinkle with the coriander and cumin. Drizzle the olive oil over and toss to coat the cauliflower in the oil. Bake in the oven for 25 minutes until tender and browned on the edges.
3. Meanwhile, place the lamb mince, egg, almond meal, pistachios and parsley in a large bowl and use your hands to combine the mixture really well. Scoop out tablespoon-sized amounts of the mixture and roll into balls.
4. Heat the olive oil in a large frying pan over medium–high heat. Add the meatballs and cook, tossing regularly, for 7–8 minutes until they're brown all over and cooked through. Set aside.
5. To make the feta sauce, place the yoghurt and feta in a bowl and mash together with a fork until smooth.
6. For the salad, place a non-stick frying pan over medium heat. Add the pine nuts and toast for 2–3 minutes, tossing, until golden brown. Transfer to a bowl with the remaining salad ingredients and toss to combine.
7. Divide the feta sauce between four shallow bowls. Top with the roasted cauliflower, the meatballs and serve with the salad.

UNITS PER SERVE:	
Breads, Cereals, Legumes, Starchy Veg	0
Dairy	0.5
Lean Meat, Fish, Poultry, Eggs, Tofu	1.5
Low–Moderate Carbohydrate Veg	2.5
Healthy Fats	2.5

Spiced Lamb Chops with Green Beans and Herby Salad

CARBS 7g PER SERVE

SERVES: 4 | PREPARATION: 10 MINUTES | COOKING: 17 MINUTES

4 x 150 g lamb loin chops, visible fat removed
2 teaspoons ground cumin
4 cloves garlic, crushed
1 tablespoon extra virgin olive oil
100 g green beans, ends trimmed, halved
2 zucchini, cut into 1 cm thick slices
10 green olives, pitted

HERBY SALAD

2 Lebanese cucumbers, thinly sliced
2 tablespoons roasted unsalted almonds, roughly chopped
1 cup torn flat-leaf parsley
¼ cup torn dill
½ cup torn mint
Juice of ½ lemon
2 teaspoons extra virgin olive oil
40 g reduced-fat Greek feta

1. Place the lamb chops, cumin, half the garlic and 2 teaspoons of the olive oil in a bowl and toss to combine and coat the lamb.
2. For the herby salad, place all the ingredients in a bowl and toss to combine. Set aside.
3. Heat the remaining olive oil in a large frying pan over medium–high heat. Add the lamb chops, two at a time, cooking for 3 minutes on each side or until cooked to your liking. Transfer to a plate and set aside.
4. In the residual oil in the same pan, cook the green beans and zucchini, tossing occasionally, for 3 minutes until almost tender. Add the olives and the remaining garlic and continue cooking and tossing for 2 minutes until fragrant.
5. Divide the lamb chops, green beans, zucchini and herby salad between four plates and serve.

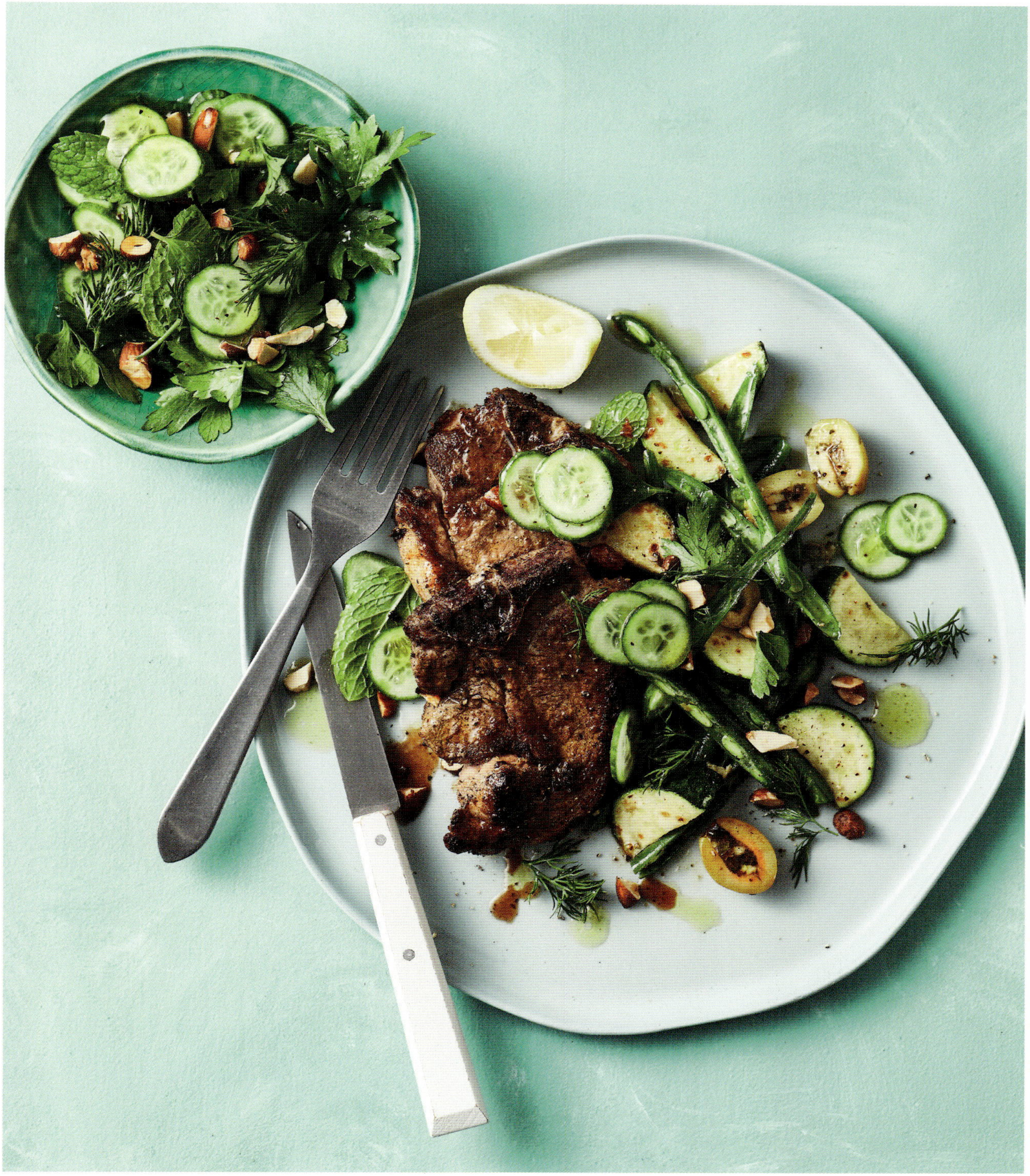

UNITS PER SERVE:	
Breads, Cereals, Legumes, Starchy Veg	0
Dairy	1
Lean Meat, Fish, Poultry, Eggs, Tofu	1.5
Low–Moderate Carbohydrate Veg	3
Healthy Fats	3

Butterflied Rosemary and Garlic Lamb

CARBS 8g PER SERVE

SERVES: 4 | PREPARATION: 20 MINUTES + 2–24 HOURS MARINATING | COOKING: 25 MINUTES

3 sprigs rosemary, leaves picked and finely chopped
5 cloves garlic, crushed
1 tablespoon lemon zest
1 tablespoon extra virgin olive oil
1 kg boneless, butterflied leg of lamb (BBQ cut) (150 g meat per serve)
4 cups rocket leaves
1 lemon, sliced into wedges

VEGGIES

1 small eggplant, cut into 1 cm thick slices
2 zucchini, thinly sliced
1 red capsicum, seeded and cut into thick strips
1 bunch asparagus, woody ends trimmed
250 g Swiss brown mushrooms
2 cloves garlic, crushed
2 tablespoons extra virgin olive oil
¼ cup flat-leaf parsley, finely chopped
60 g reduced-fat feta, crumbled

1. In a small bowl, combine the rosemary, garlic, lemon zest, olive oil and 1 teaspoon freshly ground black pepper.
2. Place the lamb in a roasting dish and smear the rosemary and garlic mixture over the lamb, massaging it into the flesh well. Cover and set aside to marinate for up to 24 hours, or a minimum of 2 hours.
3. Preheat a barbecue flat plate to high. Cook the lamb for 10 minutes on each side, then transfer to a plate, cover loosely with foil and rest for 10 minutes.
4. For the veggies, place the eggplant, zucchini, capsicum, asparagus, mushrooms, garlic and olive oil in a large mixing bowl and toss to coat. Place the veggies across the barbecue plate and cook for 1–2 minutes on each side, turning until tender and charred. Return to the large mixing bowl, along with the parsley and feta and toss to combine.
5. Slice the lamb into thin slices and serve on a large platter or divide between four plates with the grilled veggies. Serve with a handful of rocket leaves and the lemon wedges to squeeze over the whole meal.

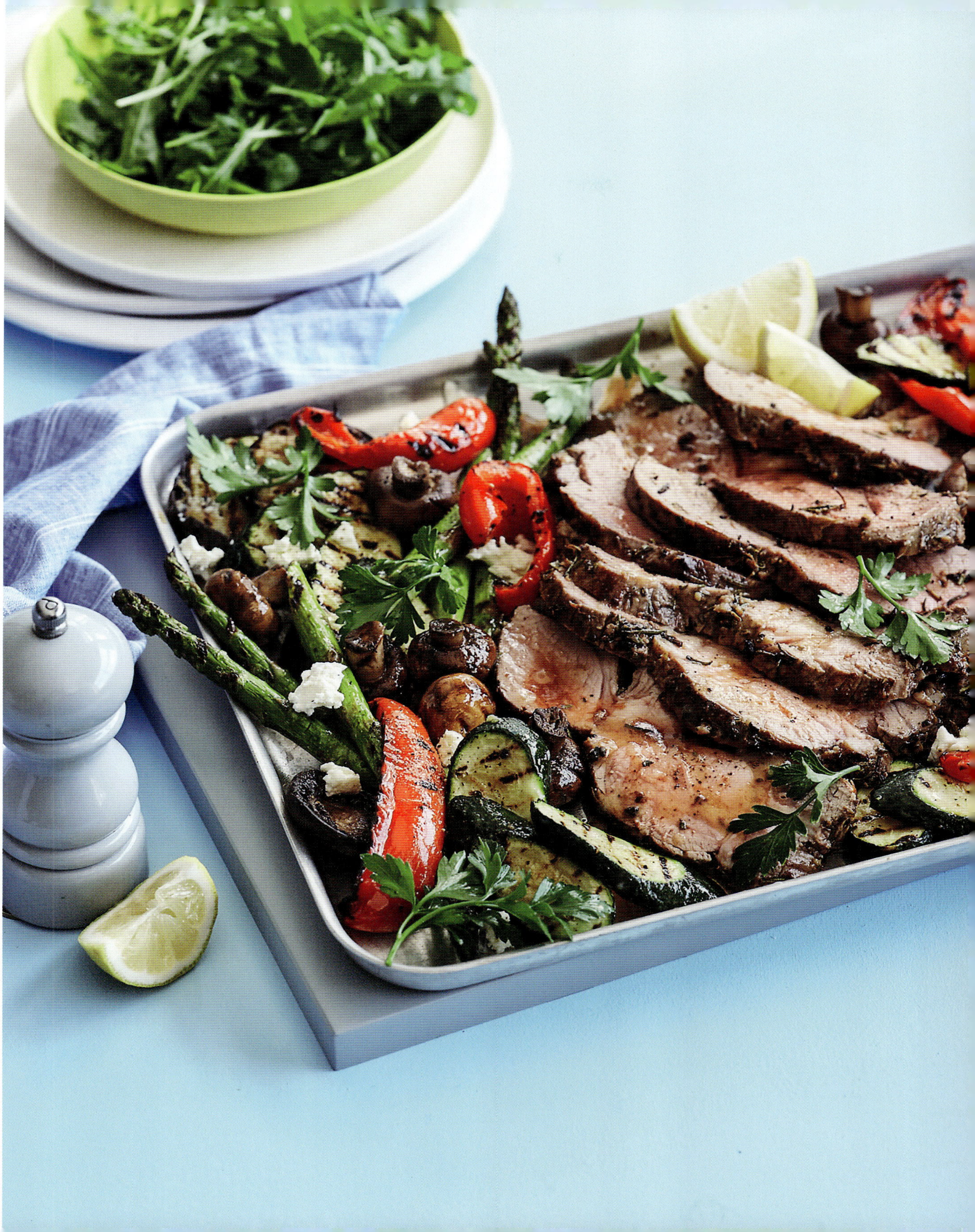

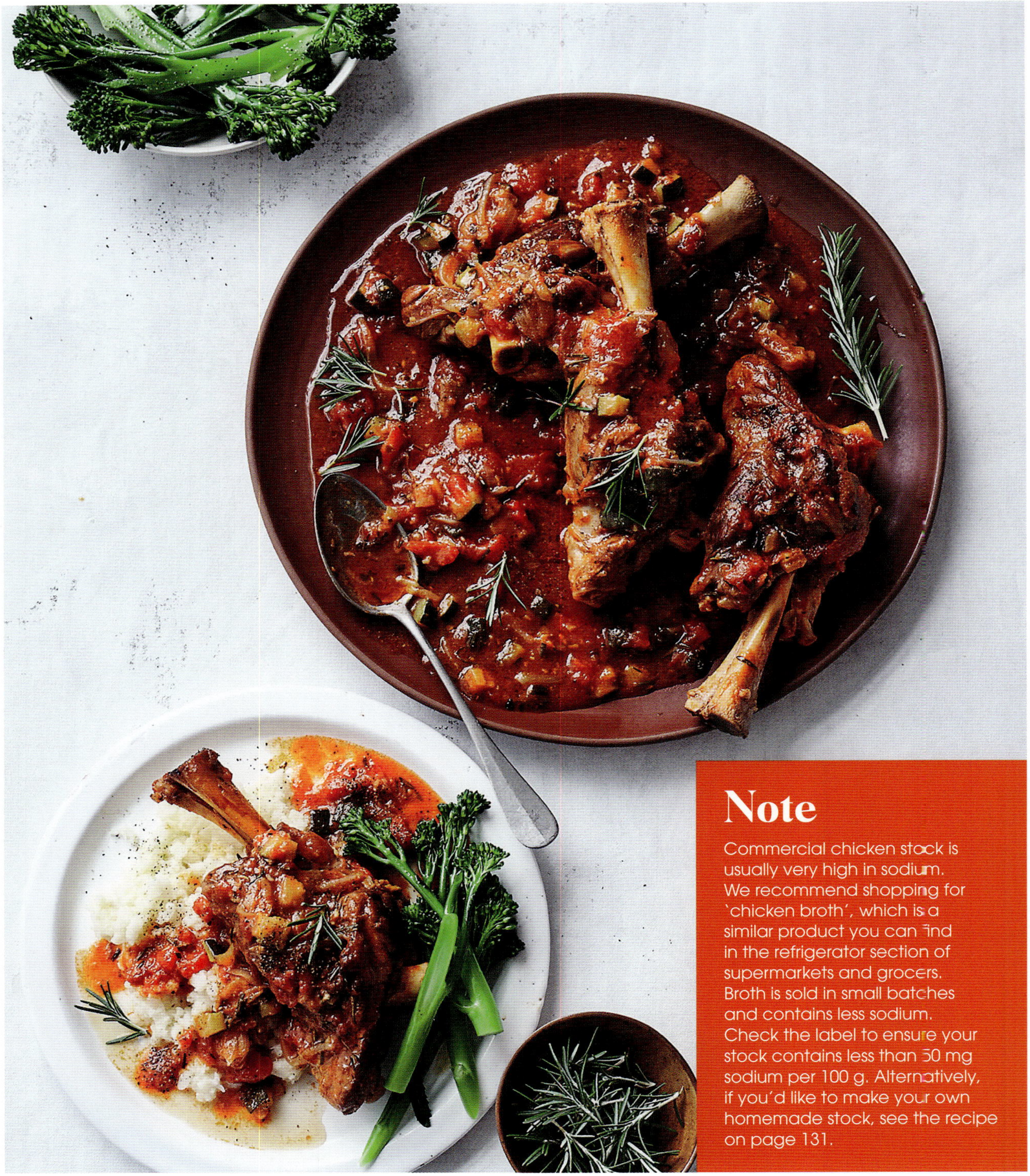

Note

Commercial chicken stock is usually very high in sodium. We recommend shopping for 'chicken broth', which is a similar product you can find in the refrigerator section of supermarkets and grocers. Broth is sold in small batches and contains less sodium. Check the label to ensure your stock contains less than 50 mg sodium per 100 g. Alternatively, if you'd like to make your own homemade stock, see the recipe on page 131.

UNITS PER SERVE:	
Breads, Cereals, Legumes, Starchy Veg	0
Dairy	0.5
Lean Meat, Fish, Poultry, Eggs, Tofu	1.5
Low–Moderate Carbohydrate Veg	3
Healthy Fats	2

Tomato-braised Lamb Shanks with Crushed Cauliflower

CARBS 14g PER SERVE

SERVES: 4 | PREPARATION: 15 MINUTES | COOKING: 2.5–3.5 HOURS

1½ tablespoons extra virgin olive oil
4 large fully trimmed lamb shanks (1.8 kg) (150 g meat per serve)
1 onion, thinly sliced
1 zucchini, finely diced
4 cloves garlic, crushed
4 sprigs thyme, leaves picked
2 sprigs rosemary, leaves picked and chopped
2 tablespoons tomato paste (no added sugar or salt)
2 tablespoons red wine vinegar
400 g tinned whole peeled tomatoes (no added sugar or salt)
2 cups (500 ml) salt-reduced chicken stock (see note)
2 bunches broccolini, trimmed

CRUSHED CAULIFLOWER

½ head cauliflower, chopped into 3 cm chunks
30 g parmesan, finely grated
2 teaspoons extra virgin olive oil

1. Preheat the oven to 200°C (180°C fan-forced).
2. Heat the olive oil in a large heavy-based casserole dish over medium–high heat. Add the lamb shanks in batches, and cook, turning, for 4–5 minutes until browned. Transfer to a plate and set aside.
3. To the same casserole dish, add the onion, zucchini, garlic, thyme and rosemary and cook for 3–4 minutes until softened. Add the tomato paste and stir it through until the vegetables are well coated. Add the vinegar and use a spatula to scrape up any bits from the bottom of the pan. Cook for 1 minute until the vinegar evaporates.
4. Break up the whole peeled tomatoes using your hands (or a knife) and add them to the casserole dish, along with the stock and 1 cup (250 ml) water. Return the lamb shanks to the dish, bring to the boil, then turn off the heat and place the lid on. Bake in the oven for 2–3 hours, or until the lamb is very tender.
5. When the lamb has 20 minutes cooking time left, make the crushed cauliflower. Place the cauliflower in a large saucepan over high heat and cover with water. Bring to the boil and cook for 10 minutes until the cauliflower is mostly tender. Add the broccolini and continue boiling for another 3 minutes, until the cauliflower is tender and the broccolini is bright green.
6. Pick out the broccolini with tongs and set aside, then drain the cauliflower and return it to the saucepan with the parmesan, olive oil and ¼ teaspoon freshly ground black pepper. Use a fork or potato masher to lightly crush the cauliflower.
7. Divide the lamb shanks, broccolini and crushed cauliflower between four bowls and spoon over the tomato sauce to serve.

UNITS PER SERVE:	
Breads, Cereals, Legumes, Starchy Veg	0
Dairy	0
Lean Meat, Fish, Poultry, Eggs, Tofu	1.5
Low–Moderate Carbohydrate Veg	2
Healthy Fats	2

Fish in Shiitake Mushroom Broth with Chinese Greens

CARBS 10g PER SERVE

SERVES: 4 | PREPARATION: 15 MINUTES | COOKING: 15 MINUTES

4 dried shiitake mushrooms
1 cup (250 ml) boiling water
2 tablespoons extra virgin olive oil
2 cm piece of ginger, julienned
2 spring onions, thinly sliced, white and green parts separated
750 g mixed mushrooms (shiitake, enoki, Swiss brown, oyster, king brown)
2 cups (500 ml) salt-reduced chicken stock (see notes)
1 tablespoon salt-reduced soy sauce
1 bunch Chinese broccoli or choy sum, trimmed
600 g boneless firm white fish fillets, such as barramundi, snapper or flathead (skin on) (see notes)

1. Place the dried shiitake mushrooms in a small bowl and cover with the boiling water. Allow to sit for 10 minutes, then drain, reserving the liquid. Slice the mushrooms into quarters.
2. Heat the olive oil in a large, deep frying pan over medium heat. Add the ginger, white part of the spring onion and all the mushrooms and cook for 2 minutes, tossing in the oil until fragrant. Add the chicken stock, reserved mushroom soaking water and the soy sauce. Stir to combine, then add the Chinese broccoli or choy sum. Place the fish on top, cover and simmer for 10 minutes, until the fish is cooked through and the Chinese greens are tender.
3. Divide the fish and vegetables between four shallow bowls. Spoon the remaining stock over the top, garnish with the green part of the spring onion and serve.

Notes

Commercial chicken stock is usually very high in sodium. We recommend shopping for 'chicken broth', which is a similar product you can find in the refrigerator section of supermarkets and grocers. Broth is sold in small batches and contains less sodium. Check the label to ensure your stock contains less than 50 mg sodium per 100 g. Alternatively, if you'd like to make your own homemade stock, see the recipe on page 131.

Seafood is an ingredient high in naturally occurring sodium. Note that this recipe contains 695 mg of sodium per serve, which is above the recommended 500 mg per meal. Please be mindful if you are following a heart-healthy diet to make sure you consider your total day's intake of sodium and that you aim to keep your sodium under 2000 mg daily.

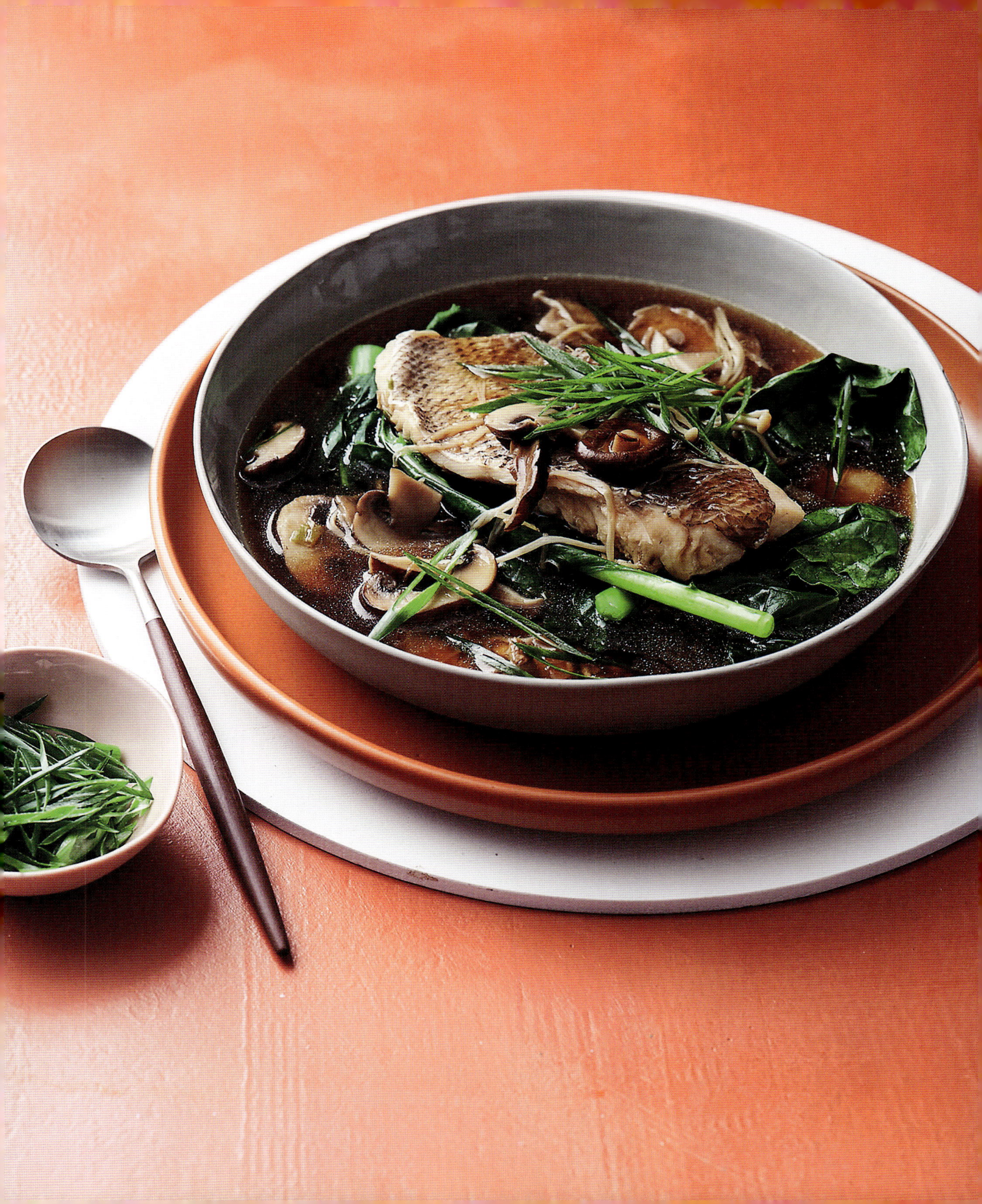

UNITS PER SERVE:	
Breads, Cereals, Legumes, Starchy Veg	0
Dairy	0
Lean Meat, Fish, Poultry, Eggs, Tofu	1.5
Low–Moderate Carbohydrate Veg	3
Healthy Fats	3

Fish with Artichoke, Cherry Tomatoes and Thyme

CARBS 16 g PER SERVE

SERVES: 4 | PREPARATION: 10 MINUTES | COOKING: 30 MINUTES

3 tablespoons extra virgin olive oil
Pinch dried chilli flakes (optional)
5 cloves garlic, thinly sliced
1 small red onion, thinly sliced
5 sprigs thyme, leaves picked, plus extra thyme leaves to serve
450 g drained artichoke hearts
750 g cherry tomatoes
2 zucchini, thinly sliced
600 g skinless, boneless firm white fish, such as snapper, barramundi or flathead (see note on page 174 regarding sodium)
2 tablespoons white wine vinegar

1. Preheat the oven to 200°C (180°C fan-forced).
2. Divide the olive oil between two medium-sized baking dishes (or one very large dish) and place in the oven for 10 minutes to heat the oil.
3. Carefully remove the baking dishes from the oven and divide the chilli flakes, garlic, onion and thyme leaves between the two dishes, tossing the ingredients together, allowing them to sizzle in the hot oil. Divide the artichoke, cherry tomatoes and zucchini between the two dishes, tossing to coat them in the oil.
4. Return the dishes to the oven and roast for 20 minutes. Carefully remove the dishes from the oven again, place the fish fillets on top and drizzle with the vinegar. Roast for a final 10 minutes until the fish is cooked through and the vegetables are very softened.
5. Divide the roasted vegetables and fish between four plates. Spoon over any sauce pooled at the bottom of the casserole dishes, sprinkle with freshly ground black pepper and the extra thyme leaves and serve.

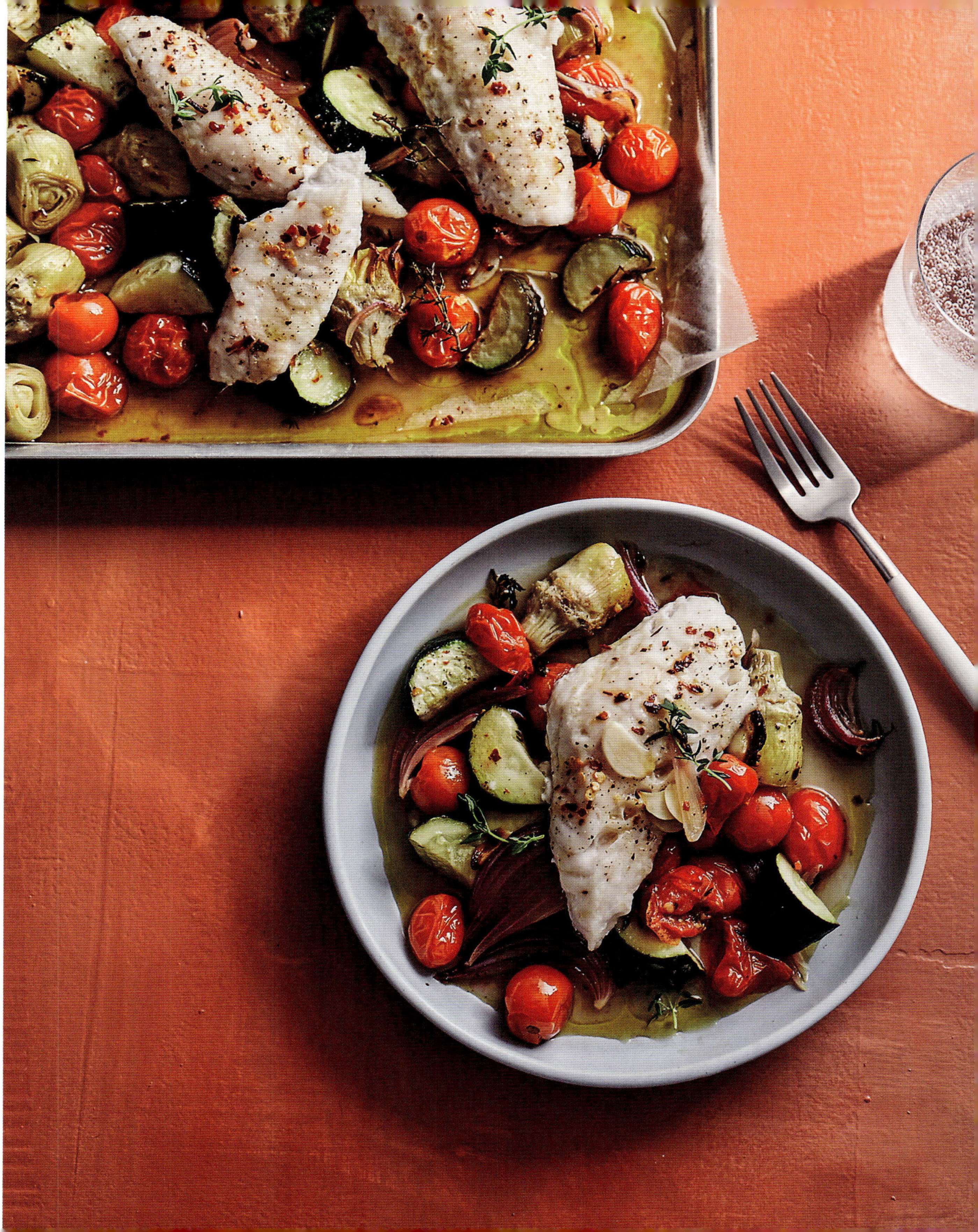

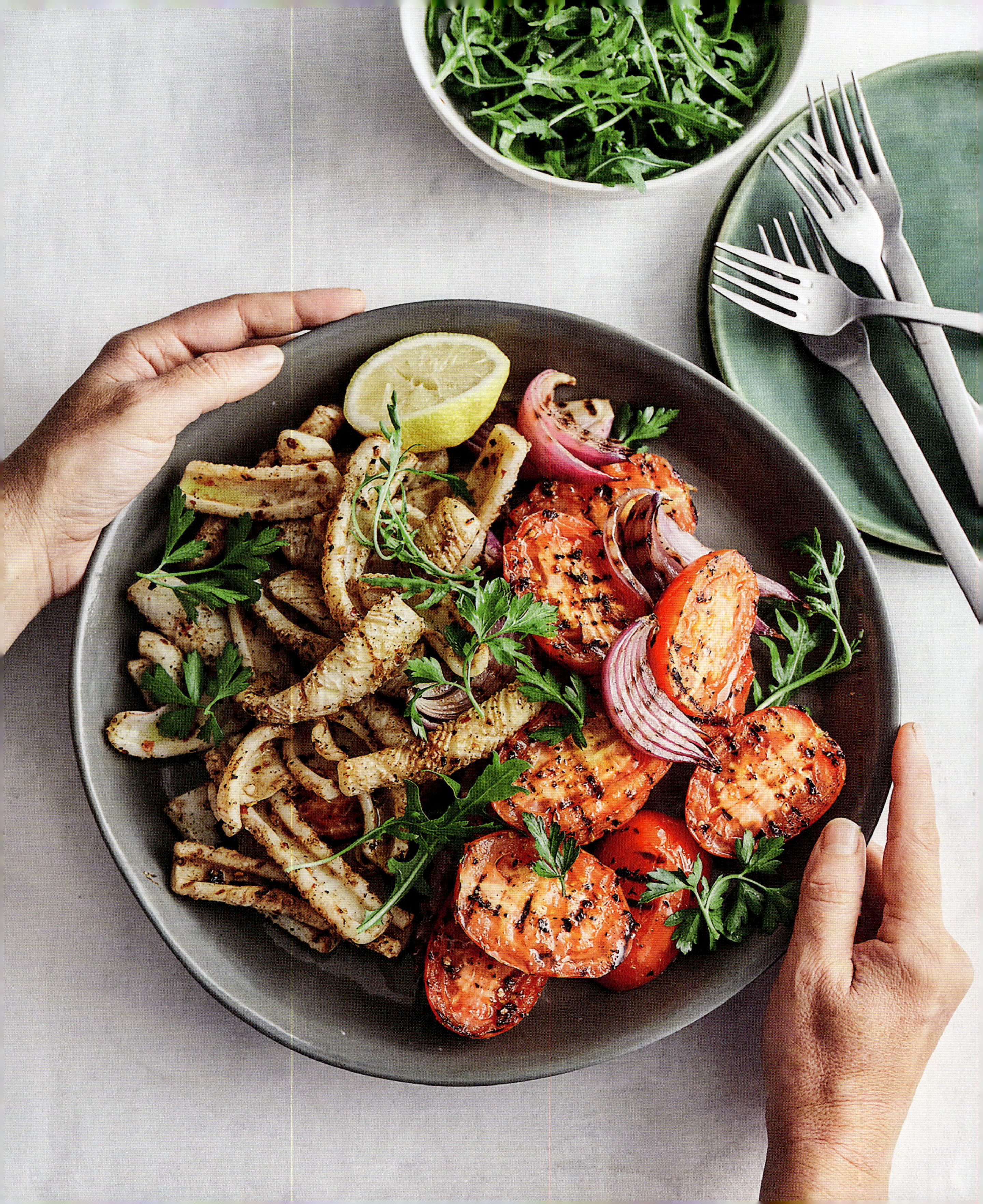

UNITS PER SERVE:	
Breads, Cereals, Legumes, Starchy Veg	0
Dairy	0
Lean Meat, Fish, Poultry, Eggs, Tofu	1.5
Low–Moderate Carbohydrate Veg	2
Healthy Fats	3

Chargrilled Chilli Squid with Rocket Salad

CARBS 7g PER SERVE

SERVES: 4 | PREPARATION: 15 MINUTES | COOKING: 15 MINUTES

600 g cleaned squid hoods (see note, and also note on page 174 regarding sodium)
1 tablespoon extra virgin olive oil
Juice of 1 lemon
2 cloves garlic, crushed
1 teaspoon dried chilli flakes
6 roma tomatoes, halved
1 small red onion, cut into 8 wedges
½ cup flat-leaf parsley leaves
1 tablespoon red wine vinegar
1½ tablespoons oil-based basil pesto

ROCKET SALAD

4 cups rocket leaves
2 teaspoons extra virgin olive oil
1 teaspoon white wine vinegar

1. Preheat a barbecue flat plate to high or heat a chargrill pan on the stovetop over high heat.
2. Slice the squid hoods open, then lightly score the front and back with small knife strokes – this makes the squid cook more evenly. Chop the squid into 3 cm lengths and place it in a bowl.
3. Add half the olive oil, half the lemon juice, the garlic, ¼ teaspoon freshly ground black pepper and the chilli flakes to the bowl and toss until the squid is well coated.
4. When the barbecue or chargrill pan is hot, place the tomato and onion in a bowl with the remaining olive oil, toss to coat, then place the tomato and onion directly on the grill (or in the pan), cut side down. Cook for 5 minutes, turning as they char, until softened. Add to a large bowl with the remaining lemon juice, the parsley, red wine vinegar and pesto, toss to combine and allow to marinate.
5. Place the squid on the barbecue plate or chargrill pan and cook for 1–2 minutes on each side until curled up and no longer translucent.
6. To make the rocket salad, place all the ingredients in a large bowl and toss to combine.
7. Divide the squid between four bowls, along with the tomato, onion and rocket salad and serve.

Note

Buy white, cleaned squid hoods, or ask your fishmonger to gut and clean them for you.

UNITS PER SERVE:	
Breads, Cereals, Legumes, Starchy Veg	0
Dairy	1
Lean Meat, Fish, Poultry, Eggs, Tofu	1.5
Low–Moderate Carbohydrate Veg	3.5
Healthy Fats	2

Prawn Curry with Cauliflower Rice

CARBS 18 g PER SERVE

SERVES: 4 | PREPARATION: 10 MINUTES | COOKING: 25 MINUTES

2 heads broccoli, stems and florets chopped
1 tablespoon extra virgin olive oil
1 onion, finely diced
1 zucchini, thinly sliced
1 long red chilli, thinly sliced
3 cloves garlic, sliced
2 cm piece of ginger, finely grated
2 teaspoons curry powder
3 teaspoons brown mustard seeds
1 teaspoon ground turmeric
400 g tinned diced tomatoes
600 g cooked prawns, peeled and deveined, tails intact (see notes, and also note on page 174 regarding sodium)
1 cup (260 g) natural yoghurt
Juice of 1 lemon

TO SERVE

450 g cauliflower rice, heated according to the packet instructions (see notes)
2 tablespoons chopped roasted unsalted cashews
½ cup coriander leaves

1. Bring a large saucepan of water to the boil and cook the broccoli for 5 minutes until tender. Drain and set aside.
2. Heat the olive oil in a large, deep frying pan over medium heat. Add the onion and zucchini and cook, stirring occasionally, for 6–7 minutes until very softened. Add the chilli, garlic, ginger, curry powder, mustard seeds, turmeric and ¼ teaspoon freshly ground black pepper and cook, stirring, for a further 1–2 minutes until fragrant.
3. Add the diced tomatoes, 2 tablespoons water and the prawns, tossing everything together. (There won't be a lot of sauce here, so place a lid on the frying pan to help the prawns steam to cook through.) Cook, covered, for 2–3 minutes until the prawns are cooked through, then stir the yoghurt and lemon juice through.
4. Divide the cauliflower rice four between bowls, spoon the prawn curry over and add the cooked broccoli. Garnish with the cashews and coriander leaves and serve.

Notes

You can use frozen raw prawns if you prefer. But don't add the water to the frying pan as the frozen prawns will release quite a bit of moisture. You may need to simmer the sauce for an extra 2 minutes to reduce any excess liquid in your curry before serving.

You can find cauliflower rice in the fresh produce section at your local supermarket. If unavailable, use the frozen variety instead.

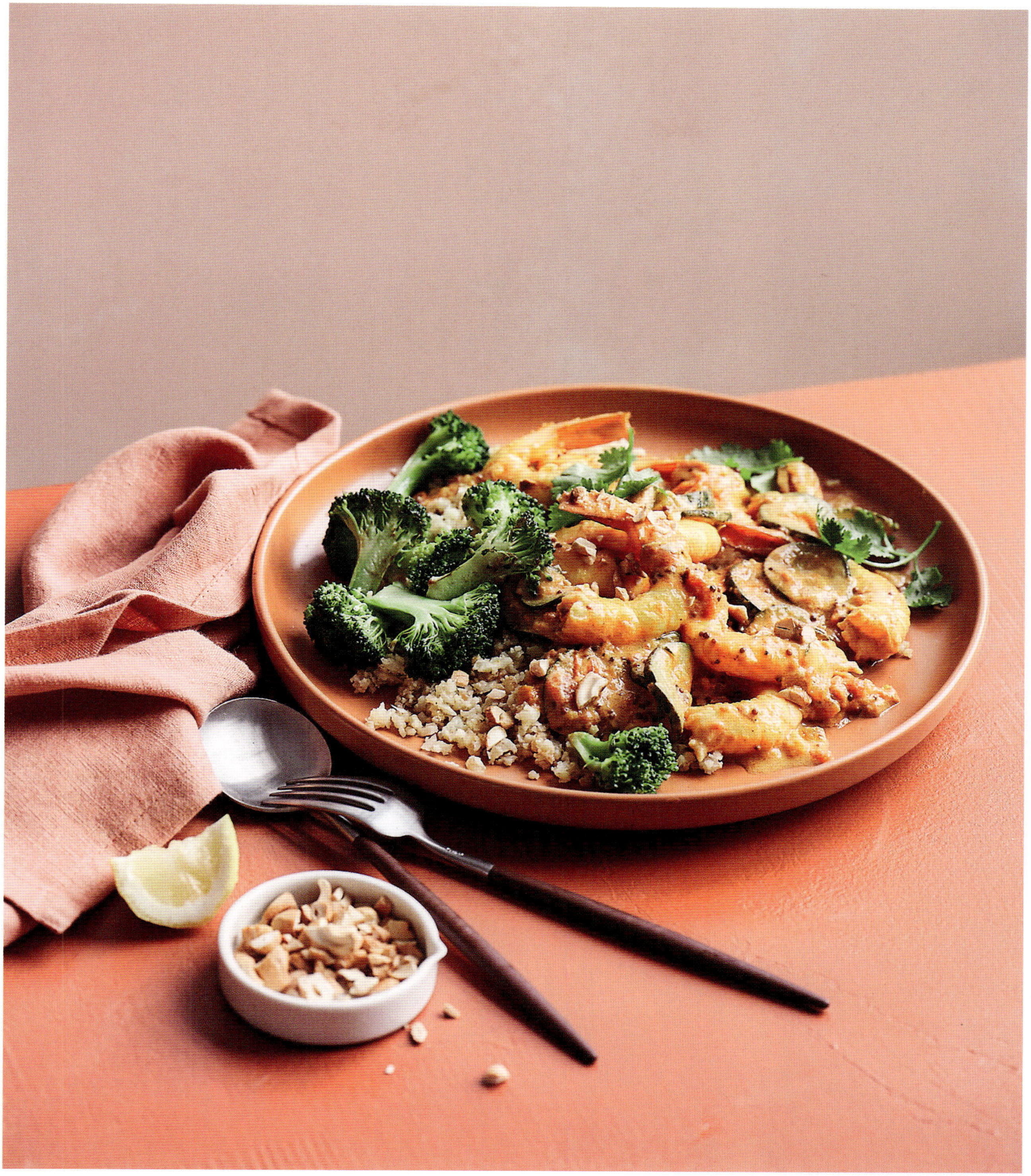

UNITS PER SERVE:	
Breads, Cereals, Legumes, Starchy Veg	0
Dairy	1
Lean Meat, Fish, Poultry, Eggs, Tofu	1.5
Low–Moderate Carbohydrate Veg	2
Healthy Fats	3

Chilli Prawn 'Linguine' with Broccoli Pesto

CARBS 5g PER SERVE

SERVES: 4 | PREPARATION: 15 MINUTES | COOKING: 25 MINUTES

2 tablespoons slivered almonds
2 teaspoons extra virgin olive oil
2 cloves garlic, crushed
Pinch dried chilli flakes
600 g raw prawns, peeled and deveined (see note on page 174 regarding sodium)
600 g zucchini noodles (see note)
40 g parmesan, grated

BROCCOLI PESTO

2 heads broccoli, florets and stems chopped into 2 cm pieces
3 cloves garlic, in their skins
2 tablespoons extra virgin olive oil
1 bunch basil, leaves picked
40 g parmesan, grated
Juice of 1 lemon

1. Preheat the oven to 200°C (180°C fan-forced).
2. To make the broccoli pesto, place the broccoli and garlic cloves on a baking tray, drizzle over 1 teaspoon of the olive oil and toss to coat. Spread the florets out on the tray, then bake for 20 minutes until charred on the edges and tender.
3. Transfer the broccoli to a food processor with the remaining pesto ingredients and blitz until a coarse paste forms.
4. Heat a large frying pan over medium heat. Add the slivered almonds and toast for 3 minutes, tossing occasionally, until golden brown. Transfer to a chopping board and chop finely.
5. Return the frying pan to the heat and add the olive oil. Add the garlic and chilli and cook for 1 minute until fragrant. Add the prawns and cook for 2 minutes until pink. Add the broccoli pesto and toss to coat all the ingredients – add a few tablespoons of water to thin out the sauce slightly.
6. Divide the zucchini noodles between four bowls and top with the prawns and broccoli pesto. Sprinkle with the parmesan and some freshly ground black pepper and serve.

Note

You'll find fresh zucchini noodles in the fresh produce section at the supermarket. If unavailable, you can simply cut 4 zucchini into thin matchsticks and use as directed in the recipe.

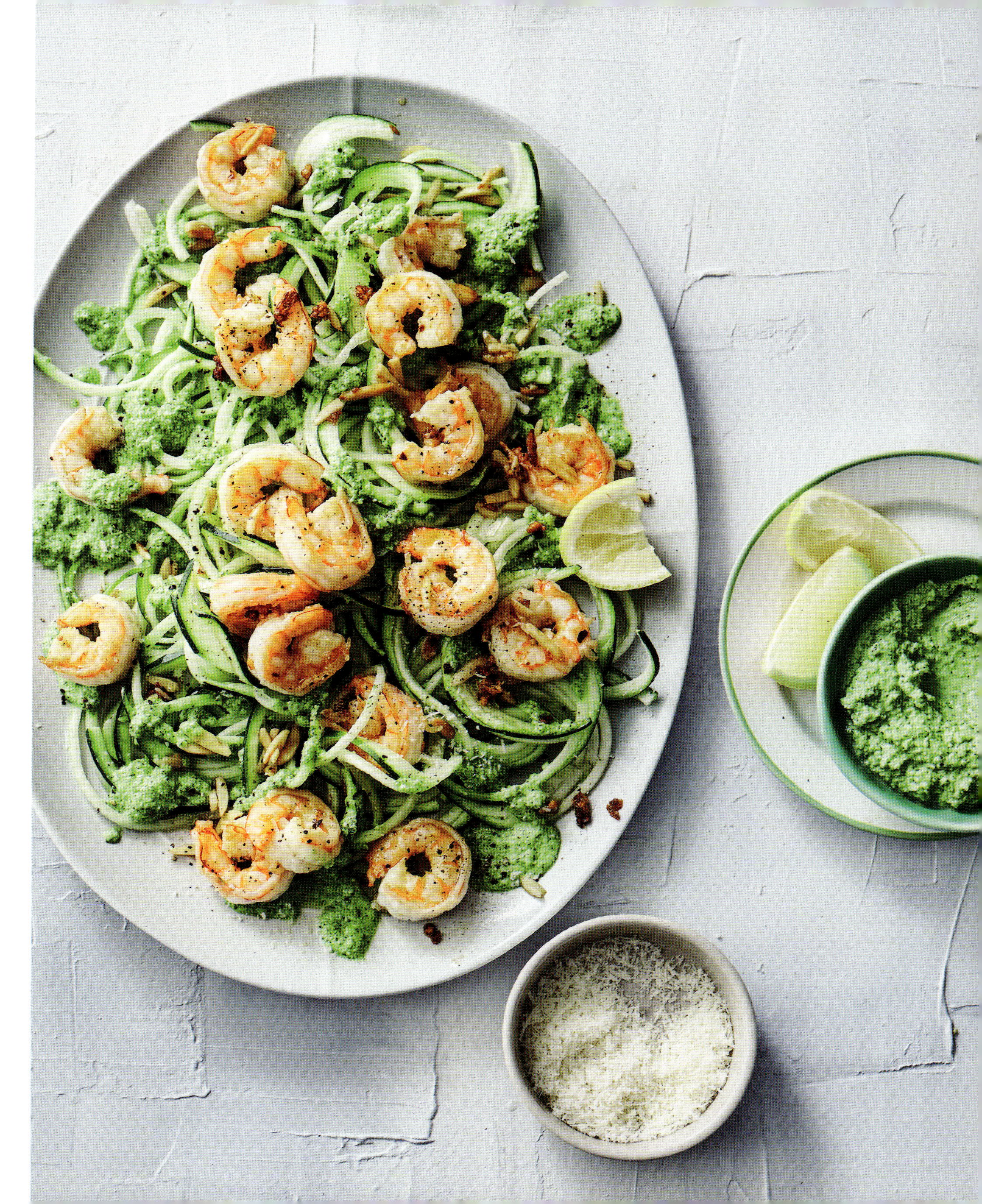

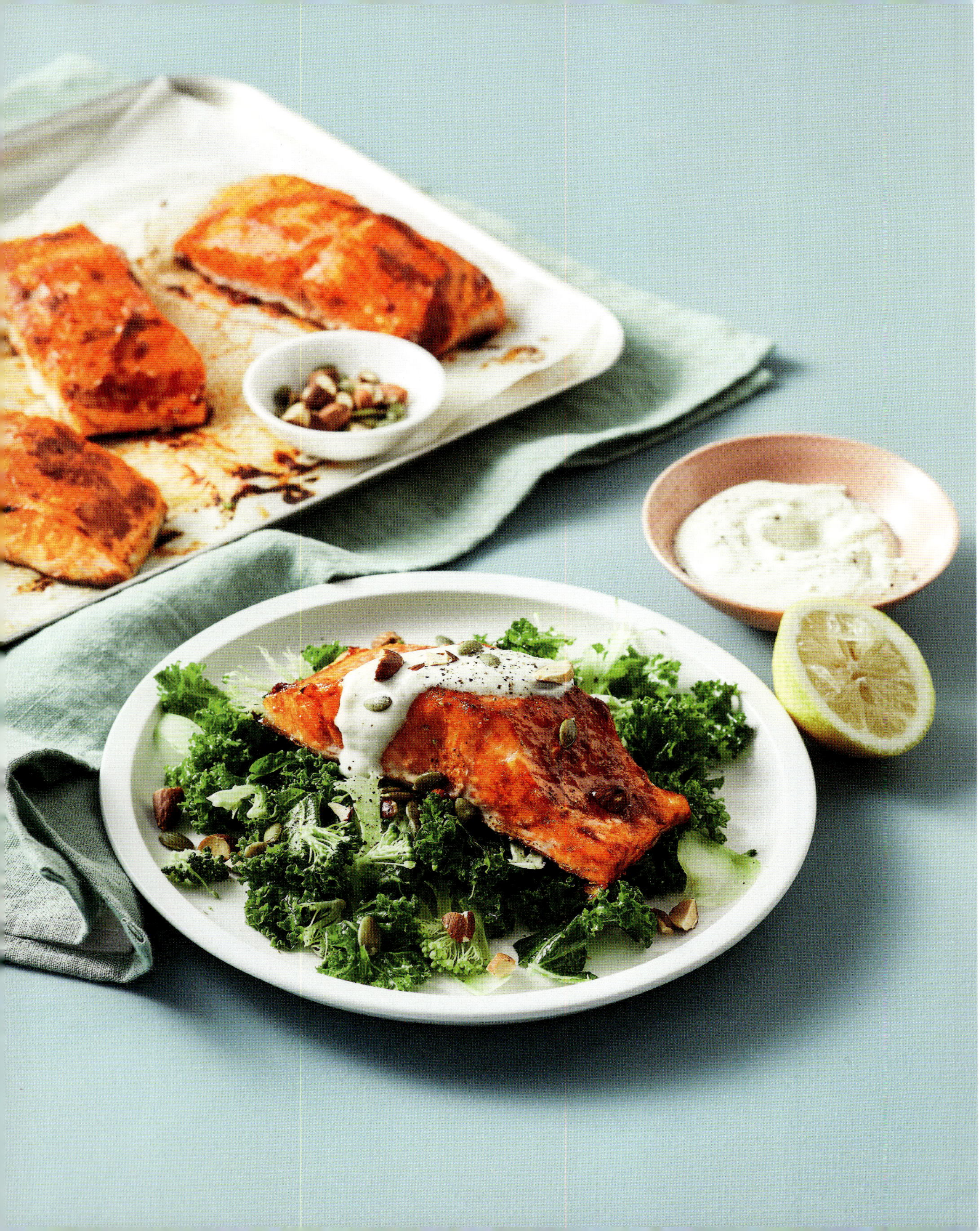

UNITS PER SERVE:	
Breads, Cereals, Legumes, Starchy Veg	0
Dairy	1
Lean Meat, Fish, Poultry, Eggs, Tofu	1.5
Low–Moderate Carbohydrate Veg	3
Healthy Fats	2.5

Harissa Roasted Salmon with Kale Broccoli Salad

CARBS 11g PER SERVE

SERVES: 4 | PREPARATION: 8 MINUTES | COOKING: 12 MINUTES

4 × 150 g boneless salmon fillets (skin on optional) (see note on page 174 regarding sodium)
2 tablespoons harissa paste
⅓ cup (40 g) roasted unsalted almonds, roughly chopped
2 tablespoons pumpkin seeds (pepitas)

KALE BROCCOLI SALAD

1 bunch kale, stalks removed, leaves roughly torn
1 small head broccoli, finely shaved (use a mandoline if you have one)
2 teaspoons extra virgin olive oil
Juice of 1 lemon

DRESSING

40 g reduced-fat Danish feta
½ cup (130 g) natural yoghurt

1. Preheat the oven to 200°C (180°C fan-forced).
2. Place the salmon on a baking tray and rub the harissa paste all over the fish. Roast in the oven for 10–12 minutes until just cooked through.
3. Meanwhile, make the salad by placing the kale and broccoli in a bowl. Drizzle in the olive oil and lemon juice, toss and massage the oil and lemon juice into the kale for about 30 seconds, so the kale wilts slightly.
4. For the dressing, mash the feta in a small bowl, then stir in the yoghurt.
5. Divide the kale broccoli salad and harissa roasted salmon between four plates. Sprinkle the almonds and pumpkin seeds over the top, drizzle with the dressing and serve.

UNITS PER SERVE:	
Breads, Cereals, Legumes, Starchy Veg	0
Dairy	0
Lean Meat, Fish, Poultry, Eggs, Tofu	1.5
Low–Moderate Carbohydrate Veg	2
Healthy Fats	2

Salmon Frittata with Dill and Chives

CARBS 4g PER SERVE

SERVES: 4 | PREPARATION: 10 MINUTES | COOKING: 1 HOUR

1 tablespoon extra virgin olive oil
3 golden shallots, thinly sliced
3 cloves garlic, thinly sliced
8 × 55 g free-range eggs
⅓ cup (80 ml) full-fat milk
1 bunch chives, finely chopped, plus extra to serve
½ cup dill leaves, finely chopped, plus extra to serve
200 g hot smoked salmon or smoked ocean trout (see note on page 174 regarding sodium)
1 bunch thin asparagus, woody ends trimmed (if you can only find thick spears, slice the spears in half lengthways)
Lemon wedges, to serve

SALAD

1 tablespoon extra virgin olive oil
Juice of 1 lemon
2 teaspoons Dijon mustard
1 butter lettuce, leaves roughly chopped
1 Lebanese cucumber, thinly sliced

1. Preheat the oven to 200°C (180°C fan-forced) and grease and line a 20 cm round cake tin.
2. Heat the olive oil in a large frying pan over medium heat. Add the shallots and garlic and cook for 4–5 minutes until golden. Set aside to cool.
3. In a large bowl, place the eggs, milk, chives, dill and ¼ teaspoon freshly ground black pepper and whisk to combine. Add half the cooked shallots and half the garlic, along with the smoked salmon and mix to combine. Pour the mixture into the prepared tin, add the asparagus spears and scatter over the remaining cooked shallots and garlic. Bake for 35–40 minutes until the egg has cooked through and the frittata is set.
4. For the salad, place the olive oil, lemon juice and mustard in a large bowl and mix to combine. Add the lettuce and cucumber and toss to coat.
5. Slice the frittata into quarters and divide between four plates. Serve with the salad, topped with the extra chives and dill and the lemon wedges on the side.

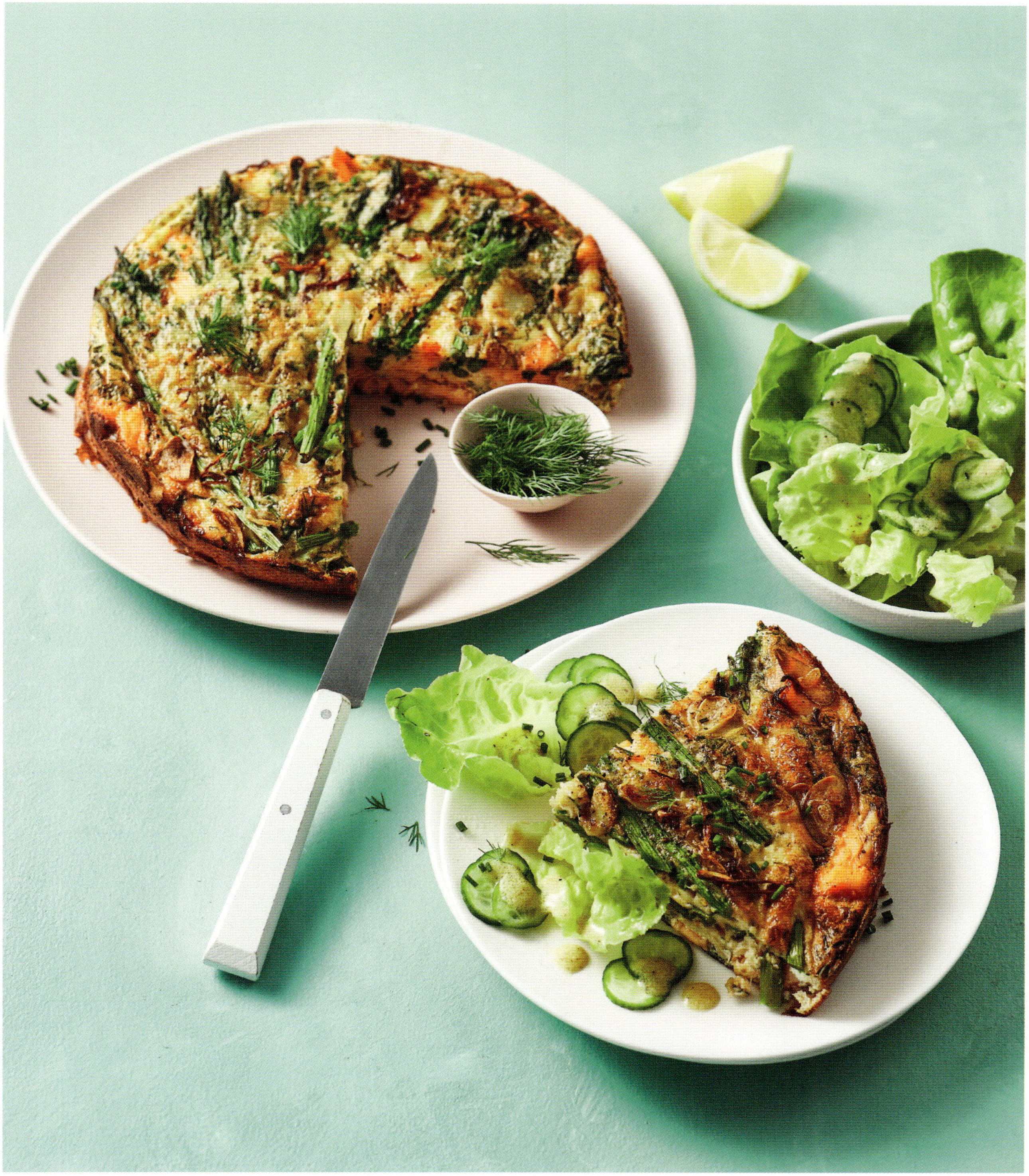

UNITS PER SERVE:	
Breads, Cereals, Legumes, Starchy Veg	0
Dairy	1
Lean Meat, Fish, Poultry, Eggs, Tofu	1.5
Low–Moderate Carbohydrate Veg	3
Healthy Fats	2.5

Tandoori Tofu Skewers with Herby Yoghurt

CARBS 18 g PER SERVE

SERVES: 4 | PREPARATION: 20 MINUTES + UP TO 24 HOURS MARINATING | COOKING: 15 MINUTES

2 tablespoons tandoori curry paste in oil
1 tablespoon tomato paste (no added sugar or salt)
⅓ cup (80 g) natural yoghurt
600 g firm tofu, cut into 3 cm dice
½ head cauliflower, florets chopped into 4 cm chunks
1 bunch broccolini, trimmed
8 stainless steel skewers, or wooden skewers soaked in water for 10 minutes

PICKLED ONION

1 small red onion, very thinly sliced
⅓ cup (80 ml) white vinegar

HERBY YOGHURT

1 cup (260 g) natural yoghurt
1 bunch coriander, washed well, roots sliced off
1 cup baby spinach leaves
Juice of ½ lemon
1 small clove garlic, crushed
½ teaspoon ground cumin

CHILLI PEANUT CUCUMBERS

1 large telegraph cucumber, sliced in half lengthways, seeded and cut into 5 mm half moons
Juice of 2 limes
¼ teaspoon dried chilli flakes
2 tablespoons roasted unsalted peanuts, finely chopped

1. Place the tandoori curry paste, tomato paste and yoghurt in a large bowl and mix to combine. Add the tofu, cauliflower and broccolini and toss gently to coat, being careful not to crumble the tofu. If you have time, set aside to marinate for up to 24 hours in the refrigerator.
2. Thread the tofu onto the skewers, leaving the veggies in the bowl.
3. To make the pickled onion, place the onion in a bowl and cover with the vinegar. Allow to sit for 10 minutes, tossing occasionally, until bright pink and softened. Drain the onion and place in a small serving bowl.
4. For the herby yoghurt, place all the ingredients in an upright blender or food processor and blitz until smooth and well combined. Pour into a small serving bowl and set aside.
5. For the chilli peanut cucumbers, place the cucumber, lime juice and chilli flakes in a serving bowl and toss to combine well, then scatter on the crushed peanuts.
6. Preheat a barbecue chargrill plate to high. Add the tofu skewers, cauliflower florets and broccolini and cook for about 10 minutes, turning every few minutes, until the tofu is charred and the cauliflower and broccolini are tender and cooked through. (Alternatively, cook in a 200°C/180°C fan-forced oven for 10–15 minutes.)
7. Serve the tandoori tofu skewers, cauliflower and broccolini in the middle of the table with the pickled onions, chilli peanut cucumbers and the herby yoghurt.

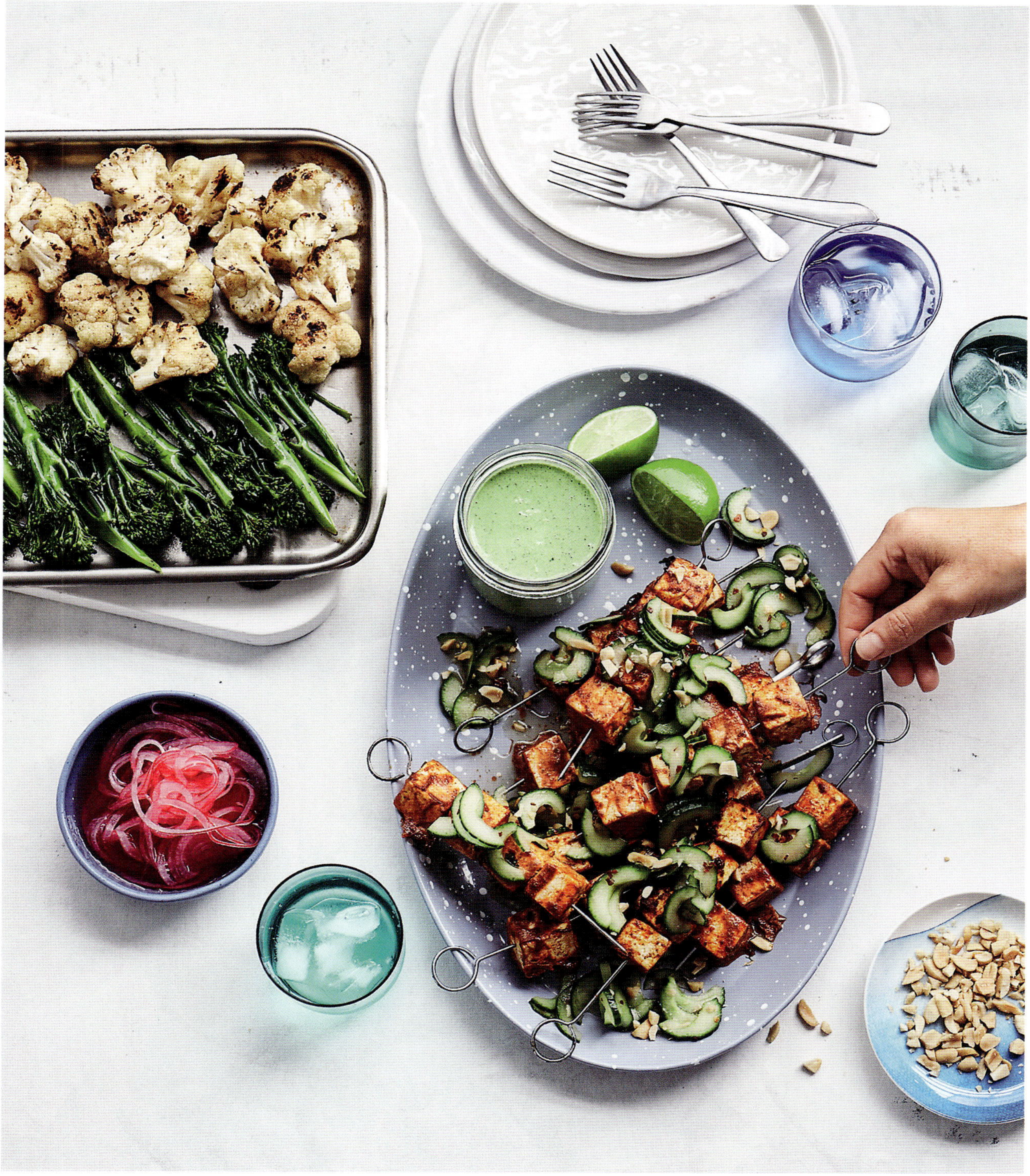

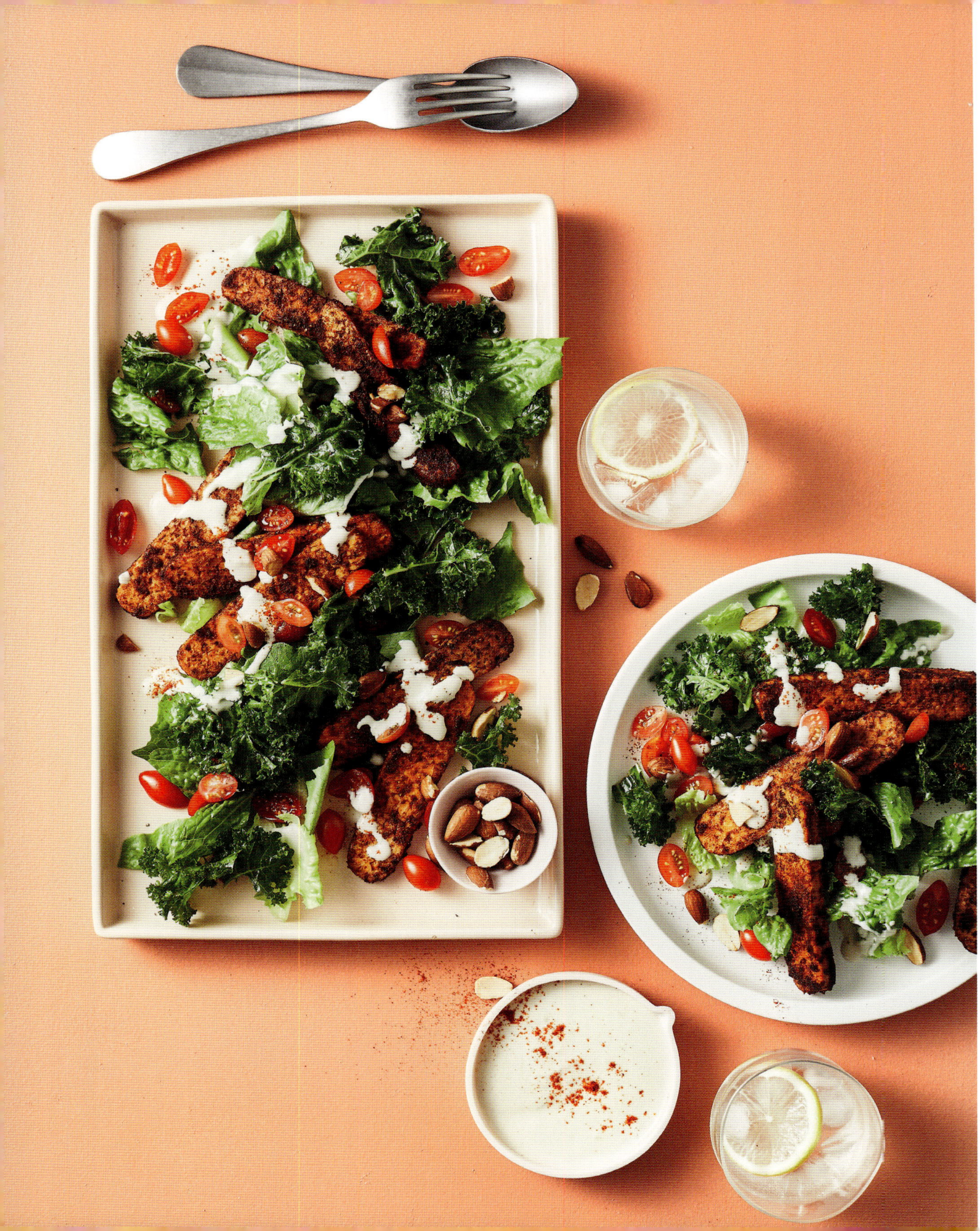

UNITS PER SERVE:	
Breads, Cereals, Legumes, Starchy Veg	0
Dairy	0
Lean Meat, Fish, Poultry, Eggs, Tofu	1.5
Low–Moderate Carbohydrate Veg	2.5
Healthy Fats	3

Tempeh 'Bacon', Lettuce and Tomato

CARBS 11g PER SERVE

SERVES: 4 | PREPARATION: 10 MINUTES | COOKING: 25 MINUTES

3 cups kale, stalks removed, leaves roughly chopped
Juice of ½ lemon
1 cos lettuce, leaves roughly chopped
250 g cherry tomatoes, halved
2 tablespoons roasted unsalted almonds, roughly chopped

TAHINI DRESSING

1½ tablespoons tahini
Juice of ½ lemon
1 small clove garlic, crushed
2 tablespoons room temperature water

TEMPEH 'BACON'

600 g unflavoured tempeh, sliced into long strips 5 mm thick
1 tablespoon smoked paprika
¼ teaspoon cayenne pepper
1 tablespoon salt-reduced tamari (see note)
1 tablespoon extra virgin olive oil

1. To make the tahini dressing, place all the ingredients in a bowl and mix to combine.
2. For the tempeh 'bacon', place the tempeh, paprika, cayenne pepper and tamari in a bowl and toss to combine. Heat 1 teaspoon of the olive oil in a large frying pan over medium–high heat. Add one-quarter of the tempeh and cook for 2–3 minutes on each side until browned. Set aside and repeat with the remaining olive oil and tempeh.
3. Place the kale in a large bowl and drizzle over the lemon juice. Massage the lemon juice into the kale for 30 seconds until the leaves are tender. Add the lettuce, tomatoes and tahini dressing and toss gently to coat the salad in the dressing.
4. Divide the salad between four bowls, top with the tempeh 'bacon', sprinkle the almonds over and serve.

Note

Tamari is a higher-salt product, so ideally use low-salt or no-added-salt alternatives. If you are following a low-sodium diet, omit this ingredient.

UNITS PER SERVE:	
Breads, Cereals, Legumes, Starchy Veg	0
Dairy	0
Lean Meat, Fish, Poultry, Eggs, Tofu	1.5
Low–Moderate Carbohydrate Veg	2.5
Healthy Fats	3

Tofu Steaks with Spring Onion Pistou

CARBS 8 g PER SERVE

SERVES: 4 | PREPARATION: 15 MINUTES | COOKING: 20 MINUTES

600 g block of firm tofu, sliced in half lengthways and widthways
2 large zucchini, thinly sliced lengthways
1 teaspoon extra virgin olive oil
400 g cherry tomatoes, halved

PISTOU

½ cup (70 g) walnuts
1 tablespoon extra virgin olive oil
2 cloves garlic, thinly sliced
Pinch dried chilli flakes
1 bunch spring onions, finely chopped
Juice of 1 lemon

1. Heat a barbecue chargrill plate to high or place a chargrill pan over high heat on the stovetop.
2. To make the pistou, heat a saucepan over medium heat. Add the walnuts and toss for 3 minutes until golden. Transfer to a board and chop roughly. Return the pan to the heat and add the olive oil, garlic and chilli flakes and cook, stirring, for 1 minute until the garlic is golden. Add the spring onion and continue to cook for 1 minute until wilted. Remove the pan from the heat and add the lemon juice and ¼ teaspoon freshly ground black pepper. Stir to combine and set aside.
3. Once the barbecue or chargrill pan is hot, brush the tofu and the zucchini lightly with the olive oil, then place them directly on the barbecue or in the chargrill pan. Cook the tofu for 3 minutes on each side until charred. Cook the zucchini for 4–5 minutes on each side until charred and tender.
4. Place the tofu, charred zucchini and cherry tomatoes on a platter. Spoon over the pistou and serve.

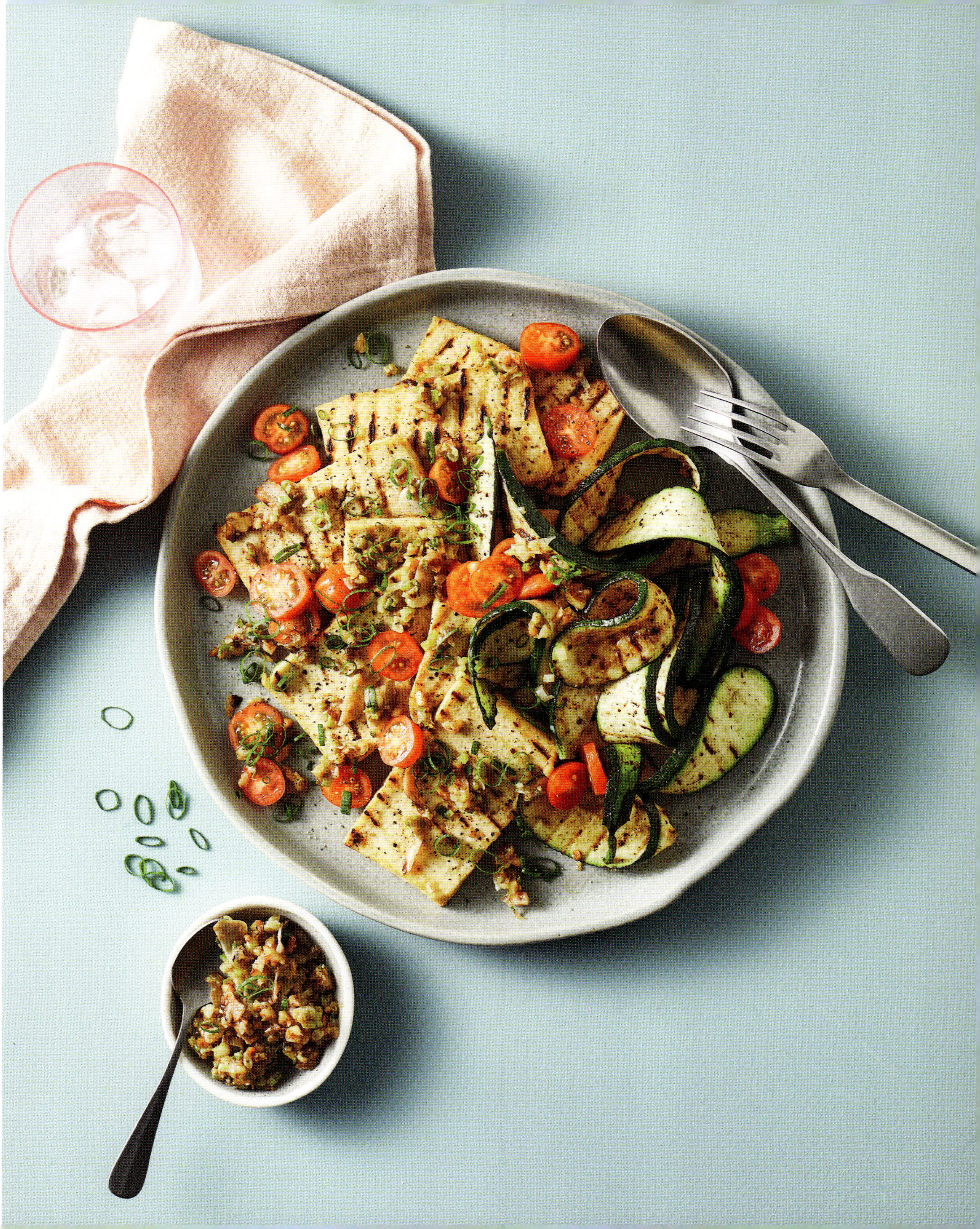

UNITS PER SERVE:	
Breads, Cereals, Legumes, Starchy Veg	0
Dairy	0
Lean Meat, Fish, Poultry, Eggs, Tofu	1.5
Low–Moderate Carbohydrate Veg	2
Healthy Fats	4

Satay Tempeh Lettuce Wraps

CARBS 10 g PER SERVE

SERVES: 4 | PREPARATION: 10 MINUTES | COOKING: 10 MINUTES

1 tablespoon extra virgin olive oil
600 g unflavoured tempeh, crumbled
300 g sliced Swiss brown mushrooms
½ bunch spring onions, finely chopped
1 teaspoon ground coriander
1 teaspoon ground cumin
Pinch dried chilli flakes
2 teaspoons salt-reduced tamari (see notes)
12 cos lettuce or butter lettuce leaf 'cups'
1 telegraph cucumber, sliced in half lengthways, seeded and cut into thin half moons
1 cup coriander, roughly chopped

SATAY SAUCE

2½ tablespoons crunchy peanut butter (see notes)
Juice of 1 lime
2 teaspoons sesame oil
1 small clove garlic, crushed
¼ cup (60 ml) warm water

1. Place all the ingredients for the satay sauce in a bowl and mix to combine.
2. Heat half the olive oil in a large frying pan over medium–high heat. Add the tempeh and cook for 4–5 minutes, tossing occasionally, until browned. Add the mushrooms and spring onion and cook, tossing occasionally, for 5 minutes until the mushrooms are browned and tender. Add the coriander, cumin and chilli flakes and toss for 1 minute until fragrant. Stir in the tamari.
3. Divide the lettuce leaves and filling between four plates. To eat, fill each lettuce leaf cup with the cucumber, the tempeh mixture and some chopped coriander and finish with a drizzle of satay sauce.

Notes

Tamari is a higher-salt product, so ideally use low-salt or no-added-salt alternatives. If you are following a low-sodium diet, omit this ingredient.

When purchasing nut butters, it is important to look at the food label. Ensure your nut butter has no added sugar or salt.

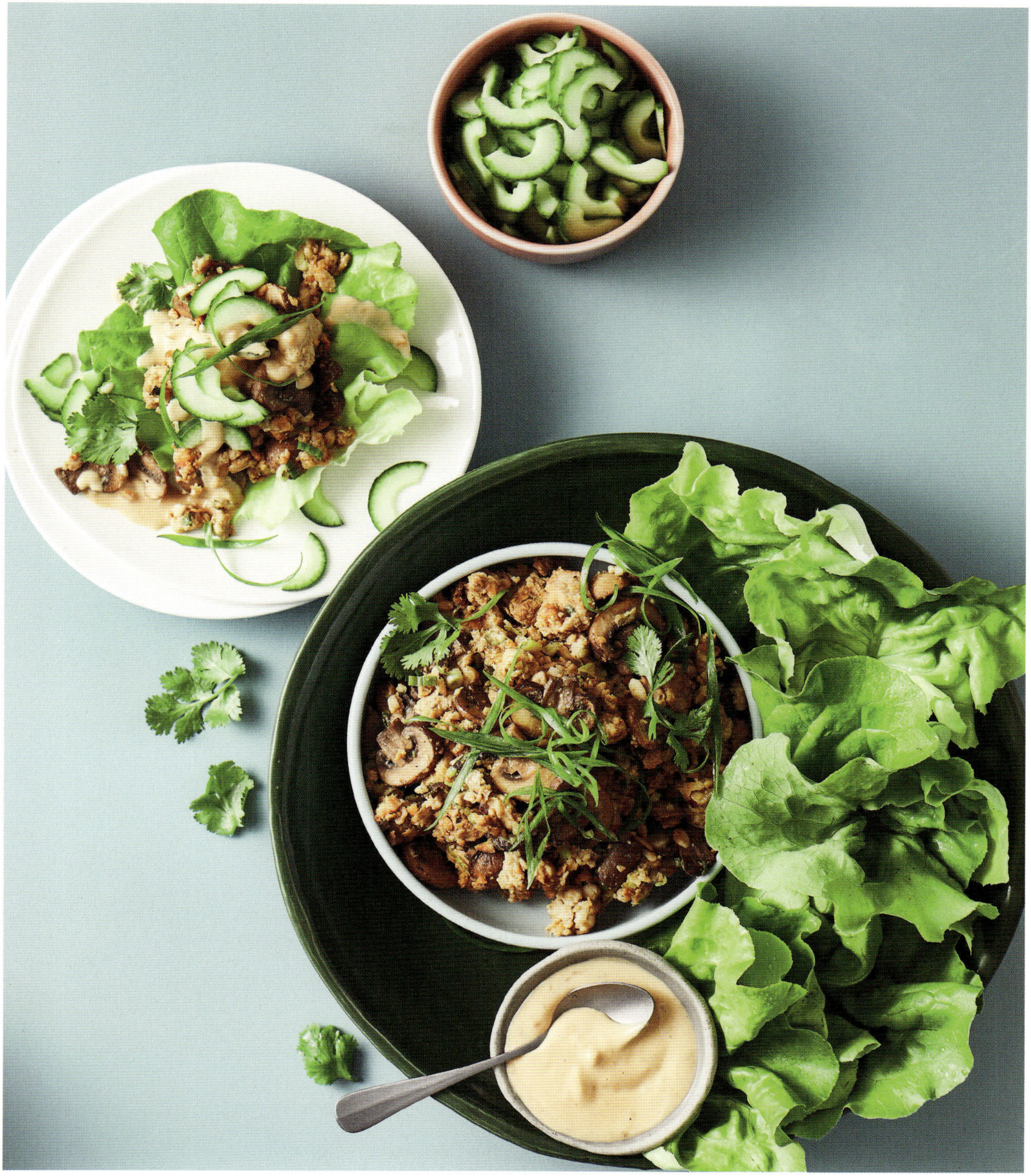

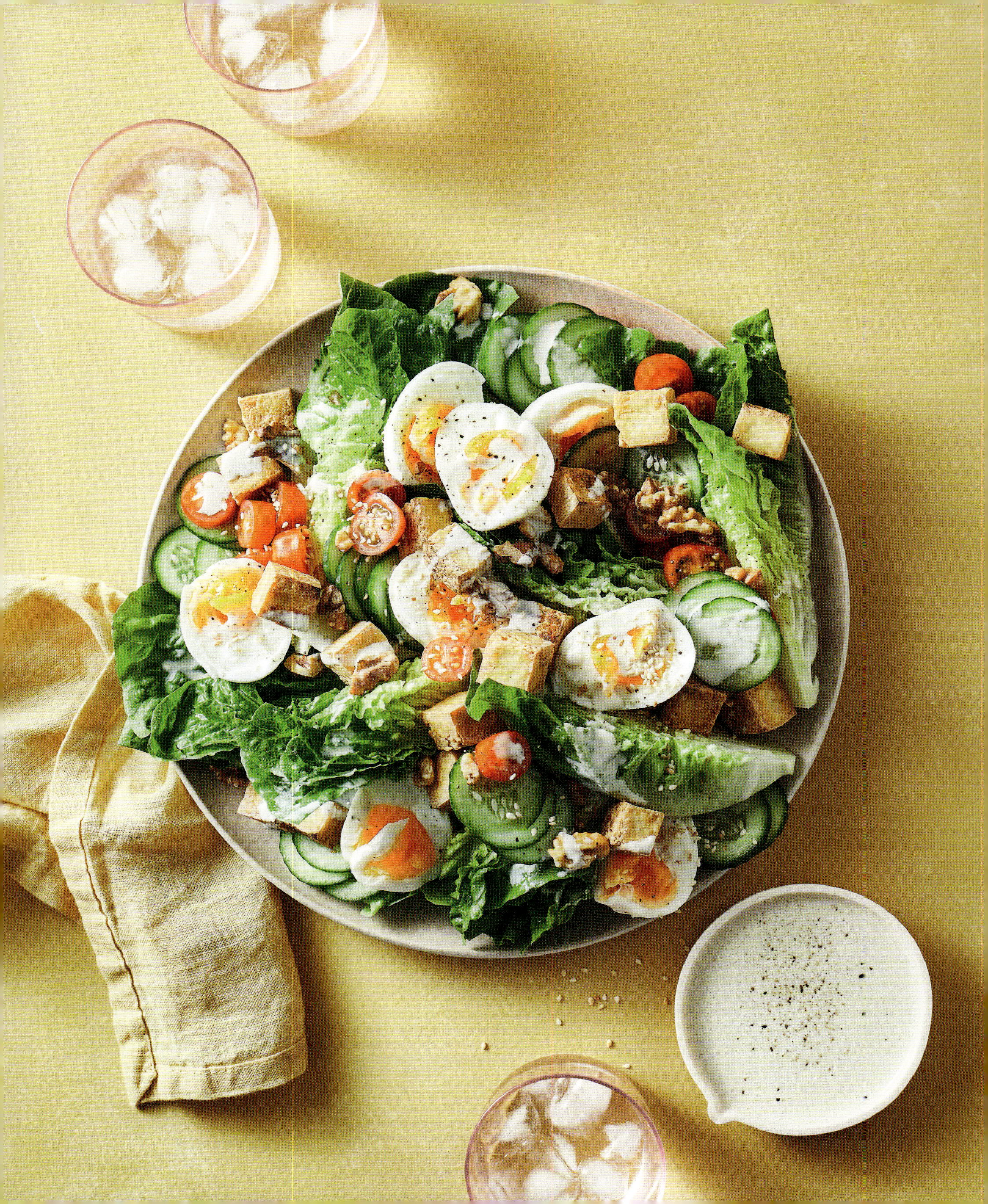

UNITS PER SERVE:	
Breads, Cereals, Legumes, Starchy Veg	0
Dairy	1
Lean Meat, Fish, Poultry, Eggs, Tofu	1.5
Low–Moderate Carbohydrate Veg	2
Healthy Fats	3

Tofu Caesar Salad

CARBS 8g PER SERVE

SERVES: 4 | PREPARATION: 10 MINUTES | COOKING: 20 MINUTES

4 x 55 g free-range eggs
½ cup (70 g) unsalted walnuts
1 tablespoon white sesame seeds
1 tablespoon extra virgin olive oil
400 g firm tofu, sliced into 2 cm cubes
2 baby cos lettuces, quartered
1 telegraph cucumber, thinly sliced
250 g cherry tomatoes, halved

CAESAR DRESSING

¾ cup (200 g) natural yoghurt
40 g parmesan, grated
1 small clove garlic, crushed
2 teaspoons Dijon mustard
2 anchovy fillets, finely chopped (optional)
¼ teaspoon freshly ground black pepper
Juice of 1 lemon

1. Bring a medium saucepan of water to the boil over high heat. Add the eggs and cook, undisturbed, for 8 minutes. Remove the eggs with a slotted spoon and run under water until cool to the touch. Peel and slice in half.
2. For the dressing, place all the ingredients in a bowl and mix to combine (or blitz in a food processor if you prefer a smoother dressing).
3. Heat a large frying pan over medium–high heat. Crumble in the walnuts and toast for 1 minute, tossing occasionally. Add the sesame seeds and continue tossing for 1 minute until the nuts and seeds are lightly toasted. Transfer to a bowl.
4. Return the frying pan to the heat with the olive oil. Add the tofu and cook for 5 minutes, tossing occasionally, until browned on all sides.
5. Place the lettuce, cucumber, tomatoes and tofu in a large bowl. Add the caesar dressing and toss gently to combine.
6. Divide the salad between four bowls. Top each bowl with two egg halves and a sprinkling of the toasted walnuts and sesame seeds and serve.

UNITS PER SERVE:	
Breads, Cereals, Legumes, Starchy Veg	0
Dairy	1
Lean Meat, Fish, Poultry, Eggs, Tofu	1.5
Low–Moderate Carbohydrate Veg	4
Healthy Fats	3

Vegetable and Walnut Bolognese with Zucchini Noodles

CARBS 14g PER SERVE

SERVES: 4 | PREPARATION: 15 MINUTES | COOKING: 1 HOUR

1 red onion, cut into 2 cm wedges
500 g roma tomatoes, quartered
1 red capsicum, sliced into 2 cm chunks
2 zucchini, cut into 1 cm thick slices
6 cloves garlic, in their skins
10 pitted green olives
1 bunch oregano, trimmed
1 bunch sage, trimmed
2 tablespoons extra virgin olive oil
¼ cup (35 g) walnuts
600 g textured vegetable protein, rehydrated according to the packet instructions (see notes)
600 g zucchini noodles (see notes)
60 g parmesan, shredded

1. Preheat the oven to 220°C (200°C fan-forced).
2. Place the onion, tomato, capsicum, zucchini, garlic and olives on two baking trays. Toss the herbs over the veggies with half the olive oil and ½ teaspoon freshly ground black pepper. Toss with your hands to coat well. Bake in the oven for 40 minutes until everything is well cooked and a little charred on the edges. In the last 5 minutes, toss the walnuts on top of the veggies and allow to toast until golden brown.
3. Transfer everything to an upright blender with ¼ cup (60 ml) water and blitz to form a chunky paste.
4. Heat the remaining olive oil in a large frying pan or wok over medium–high heat. Add the textured vegetable protein and cook for 5–6 minutes, tossing occasionally, until browned in spots.
5. Tip the vegetable puree into the pan with the textured vegetable protein and stir until well combined. Add ½ cup (125 ml) water and stir it through to thin the sauce.
6. Divide the zucchini noodles between four bowls. Top with the bolognese and sprinkle with the parmesan to serve.

Notes

We've used dehydrated Macro Textured Vegetable Protein in this recipe, found in the health food aisle of the supermarket.

You'll find zucchini noodles in the fresh produce section at the supermarket. If unavailable, you can simply cut 4 zucchini into thin matchsticks and use as directed in the recipe.

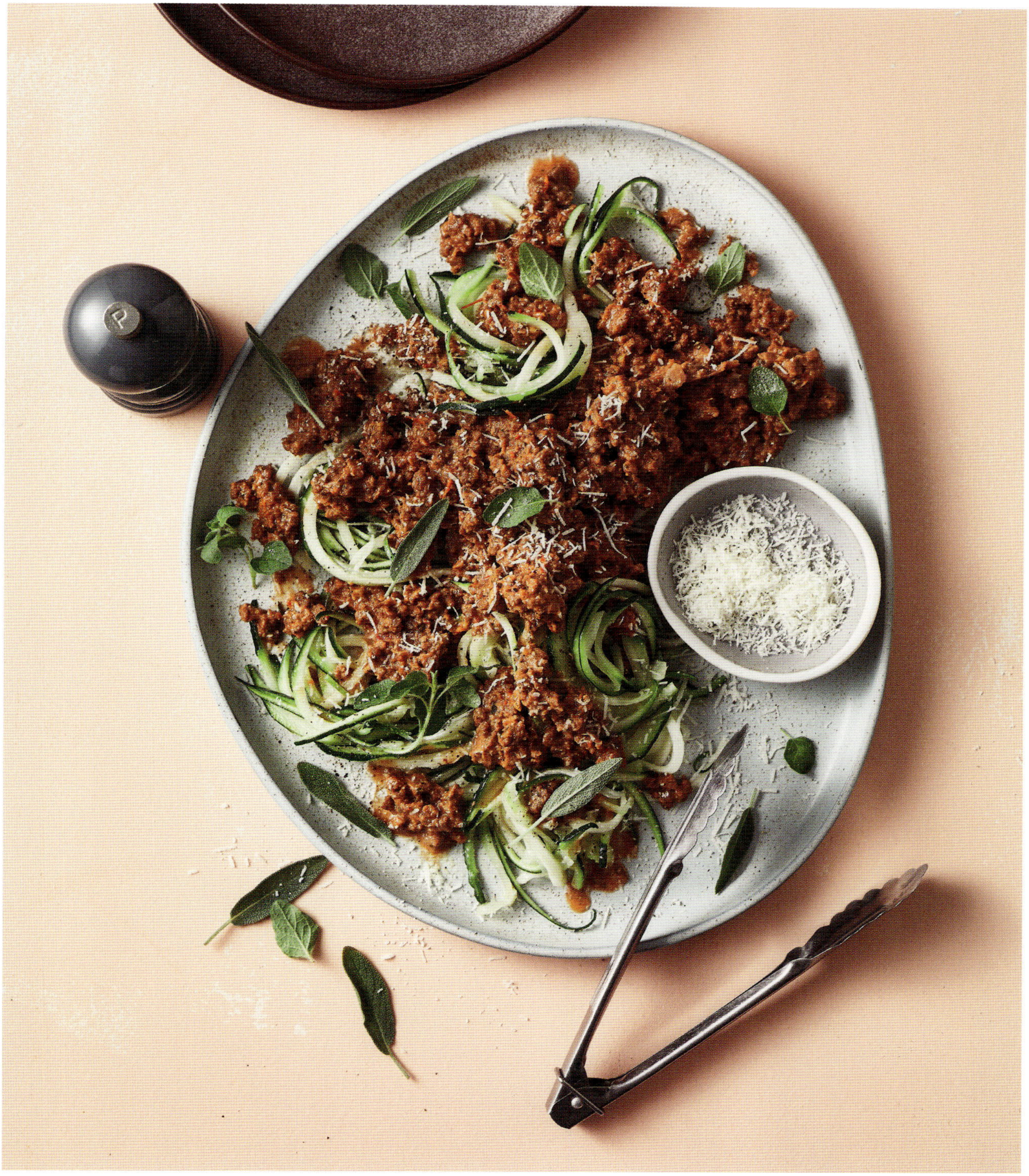

UNITS PER SERVE:	
Breads, Cereals, Legumes, Starchy Veg	0
Dairy	0.5
Lean Meat, Fish, Poultry, Eggs, Tofu	1.5
Low–Moderate Carbohydrate Veg	3
Healthy Fats	2

Tofu Saag

SERVES: 4 | PREPARATION: 15 MINUTES | COOKING: 15 MINUTES

CARBS 10 g PER SERVE

2 tablespoons extra virgin olive oil
600 g firm tofu, cut into 2 cm dice
1 onion, finely diced
1 large zucchini, finely diced
4 cloves garlic, crushed
1 teaspoon ground turmeric
1 teaspoon ground cumin
1 teaspoon garam masala
1 kg English spinach, thick stems removed (2–3 bunches)
Juice of 1 lemon
½ cup (130 g) low-fat natural yoghurt
450 g cauliflower rice, heated according to the packet instructions (see notes)

1. Heat half the olive oil in a large, deep frying pan over medium heat. Add the tofu and cook, tossing occasionally, for 5 minutes until the tofu is golden brown on most sides. Transfer to a bowl and set aside.
2. Return the frying pan to the heat with the remaining olive oil. Add the onion and zucchini and cook, stirring occasionally, for 4–5 minutes until the vegetables are golden. Add the garlic, turmeric, cumin and garam masala and stir for 1 minute until fragrant. Add the spinach leaves, a large handful at a time, and stir until wilted.
3. Transfer the mixture to an upright blender, along with the lemon juice, and process until smooth.
4. Return the pureed spinach to the frying pan, along with the tofu and the yoghurt. Stir everything together, then reduce the heat to low and cook for 1–2 minutes to warm through gently.
5. Divide the warmed cauliflower rice and tofu saag between four bowls and serve.

Notes

You can find cauliflower rice in the fresh produce section at the supermarket. If unavailable, use the frozen variety instead.

To freeze, divide individual portions of the tofu saag into containers, allow to cool, then freeze for up to 2 months. Freeze the cauliflower rice separately and heat it separately from the tofu saag.

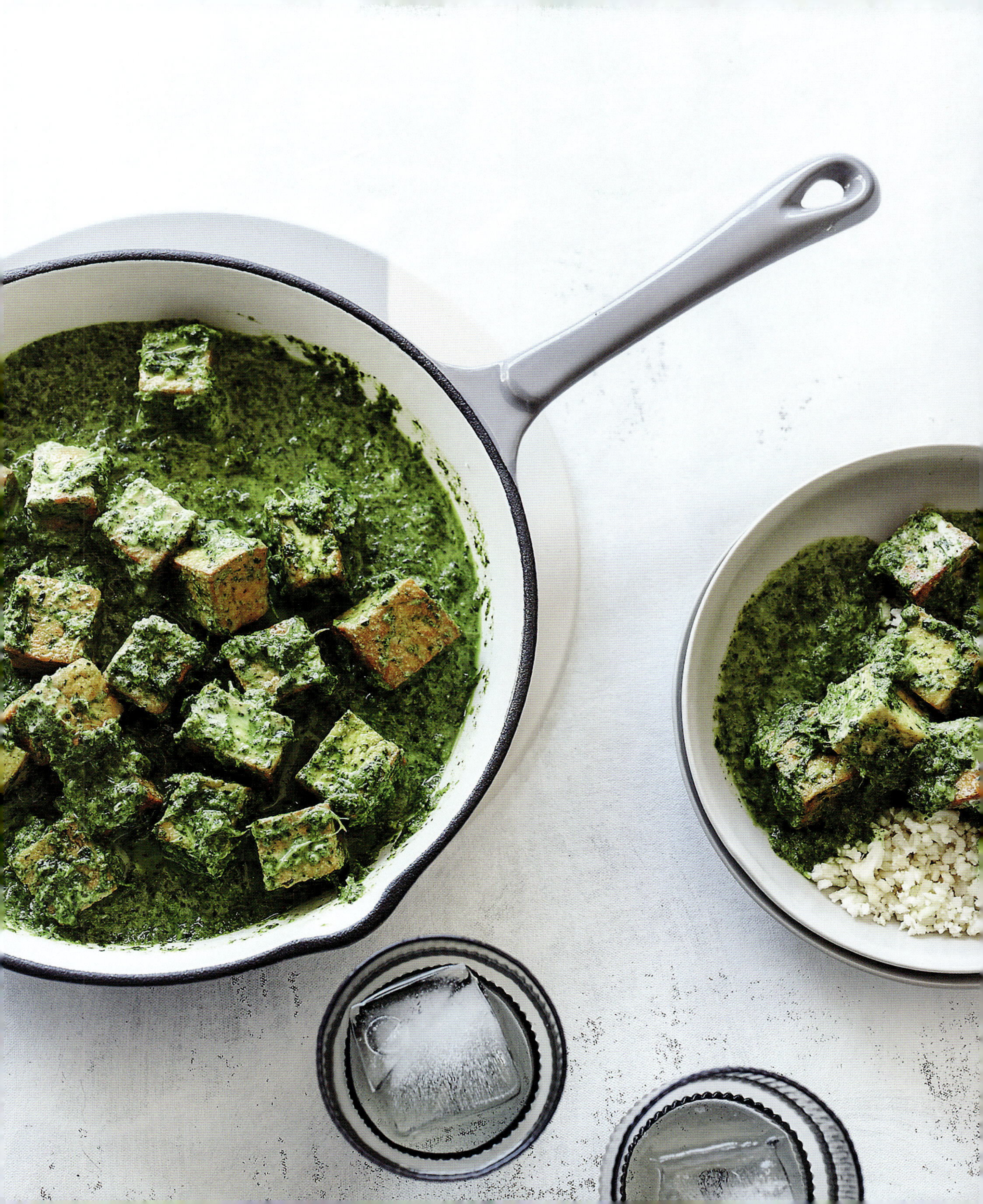

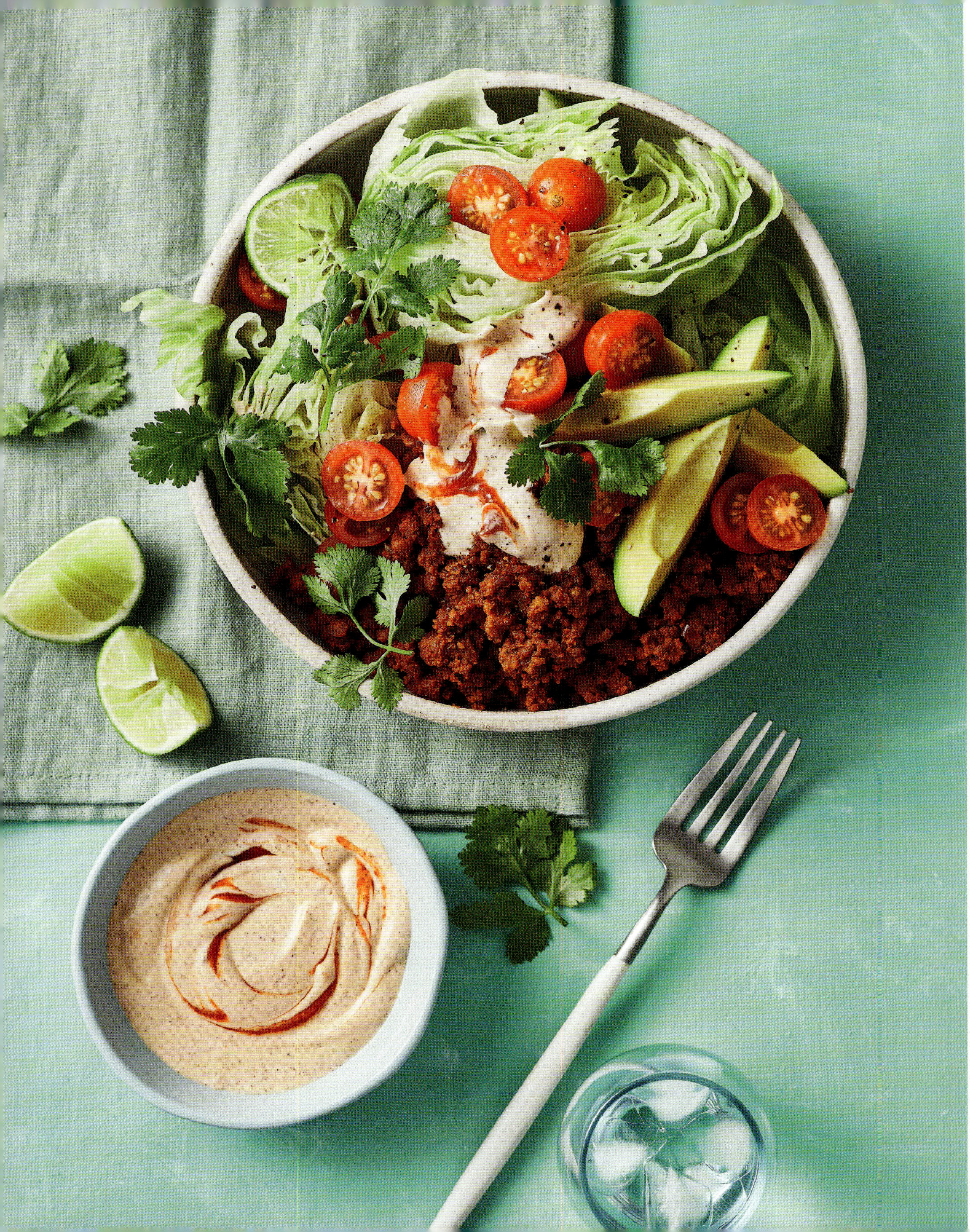

UNITS PER SERVE:	
Breads, Cereals, Legumes, Starchy Veg	0
Dairy	0
Lean Meat, Fish, Poultry, Eggs, Tofu	1.5
Low–Moderate Carbohydrate Veg	2.5
Healthy Fats	3

Vegetarian Taco Bowl with Spicy Mayonnaise

CARBS 8g PER SERVE

SERVES: 4 | PREPARATION: 20 MINUTES | COOKING: 10 MINUTES

VEGETARIAN TACO 'MEAT'

2 teaspoons extra virgin olive oil
600 g unflavoured textured vegetable protein, rehydrated according to the packet instructions (see note)
1 tablespoon smoked paprika
1 teaspoon dried oregano
1 teaspoon ground coriander
½ teaspoon ground cumin
Pinch dried chilli flakes
½ cup (125 ml) tomato passata (no added sugar or salt)

SPICY MAYONNAISE

2 teaspoons hot sauce
1 tablespoon whole-egg mayonnaise
2 tablespoons natural yoghurt
¼ teaspoon freshly ground black pepper

TO SERVE

1 iceberg lettuce, cut into wedges
250 g cherry tomatoes, halved
1 cup coriander leaves, roughly chopped
1 small avocado, sliced into wedges
1 lime, sliced into wedges

1. Place all the ingredients for the spicy mayonnaise in a small bowl and mix well to combine.
2. For the vegetarian taco 'meat', heat the olive oil in a large frying pan over medium–high heat. Add the rehydrated textured vegetable protein and cook, tossing occasionally, for 5 minutes until golden. Add the spices and cook for 1 minute until fragrant. Add the passata and stir it through for 30 seconds until everything is well coated.
3. Divide the vegetarian taco 'meat' between four bowls, then add the lettuce, tomatoes, coriander and avocado. Drizzle over the spicy mayonnaise and serve with a lime wedge to squeeze over.

Note

We've used dehydrated Macro Textured Vegetable Protein in this recipe, found in the health food aisle of the supermarket.

UNITS PER SERVE:	
Breads, Cereals, Legumes, Starchy Veg	0
Dairy	0.5
Lean Meat, Fish, Poultry, Eggs, Tofu	1.5
Low–Moderate Carbohydrate Veg	3
Healthy Fats	3

Kale and Creamy Cucumber Salad with Tempeh

CARBS 12g PER SERVE

SERVES: 4 | PREPARATION: 10 MINUTES | COOKING: 8 MINUTES

⅓ cup (80 g) natural yoghurt
¼ cup roughly chopped dill
¼ cup roughly chopped mint
2 Lebanese cucumbers, thinly sliced
2 tightly packed cups shredded green cabbage
1 bunch curly kale, stalks removed and leaves roughly chopped
1½ tablespoons extra virgin olive oil
Juice of ½ lemon
600 g unflavoured tempeh, cut into 1 cm slices lengthways
2 teaspoons smoked paprika
1 small avocado, sliced into wedges

1. Place the yoghurt, half the dill, the mint, cucumber and cabbage in a large bowl and toss to combine.
2. In another large bowl, place the kale, 2 teaspoons of the olive oil and the lemon juice. Toss the kale and massage the oil and juice into the leaves for about 30 seconds until tender.
3. Place the tempeh and paprika in a bowl and toss to combine.
4. Heat the remaining tablespoon of olive oil in a large frying pan over medium–high heat. Add the paprika-coated tempeh, in batches, and cook for 1–2 minutes on each side until golden brown.
5. Divide the kale, creamy cucumbers and tempeh between four bowls. Add a wedge of avocado, sprinkle with freshly ground black pepper and remaining dill, and serve.

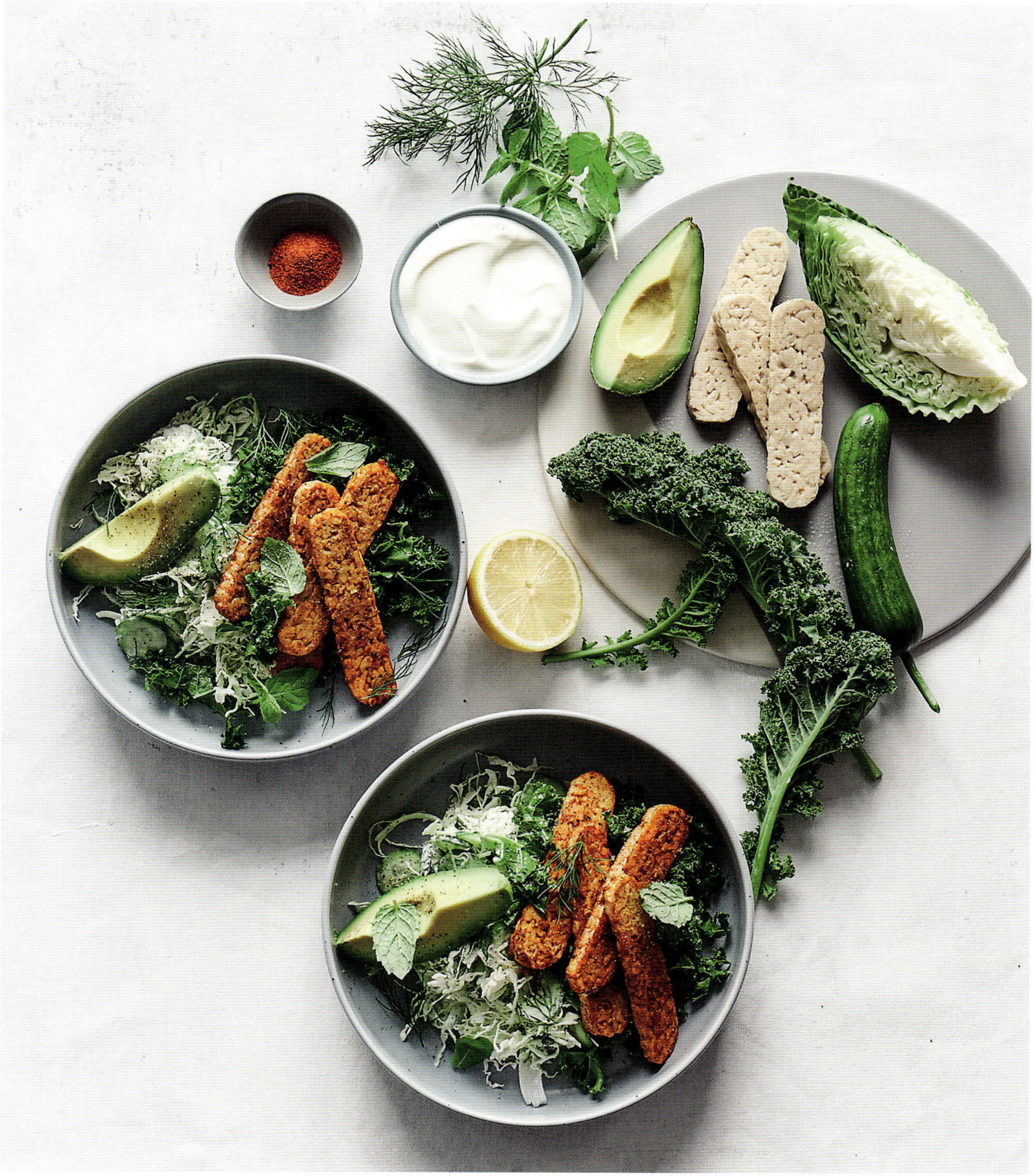

UNITS PER SERVE:	
Breads, Cereals, Legumes, Starchy Veg	0
Dairy	0.5
Lean Meat, Fish, Poultry, Eggs, Tofu	1.5
Low–Moderate Carbohydrate Veg	2.5
Healthy Fats	3

Peri Peri Tofu with Avocado Cucumber Salsa

CARBS 7g PER SERVE

SERVES: 4 | PREPARATION: 10 MINUTES | COOKING: 10 MINUTES

500 g cherry tomatoes, halved
⅓ cup (95 g) natural yoghurt

PERI PERI TOFU

600 g firm tofu
2 tablespoons smoked paprika
1 teaspoon garlic powder
¼ teaspoon freshly ground black pepper
4 sprigs thyme, leaves picked
1½ tablespoons extra virgin olive oil

AVOCADO CUCUMBER SALSA

1 small avocado, quartered lengthways
1 Lebanese cucumber, diced
1 cup coriander leaves, roughly chopped
Juice of 1 lime
40 g Danish feta, crumbled
¼ teaspoon freshly ground black pepper

1. Place all the ingredients for the peri peri tofu, except the olive oil, in a large bowl and toss to combine.
2. Heat the olive oil in a large frying pan over medium–high heat. Add the tofu mixture and cook, tossing occasionally, for 8–9 minutes until the tofu is browned on all sides.
3. For the avocado cucumber salsa, place all the ingredients in a large bowl and toss to combine.
4. Divide the peri peri tofu, cherry tomatoes and avocado cucumber salsa between four bowls and serve each with a dollop of yoghurt.

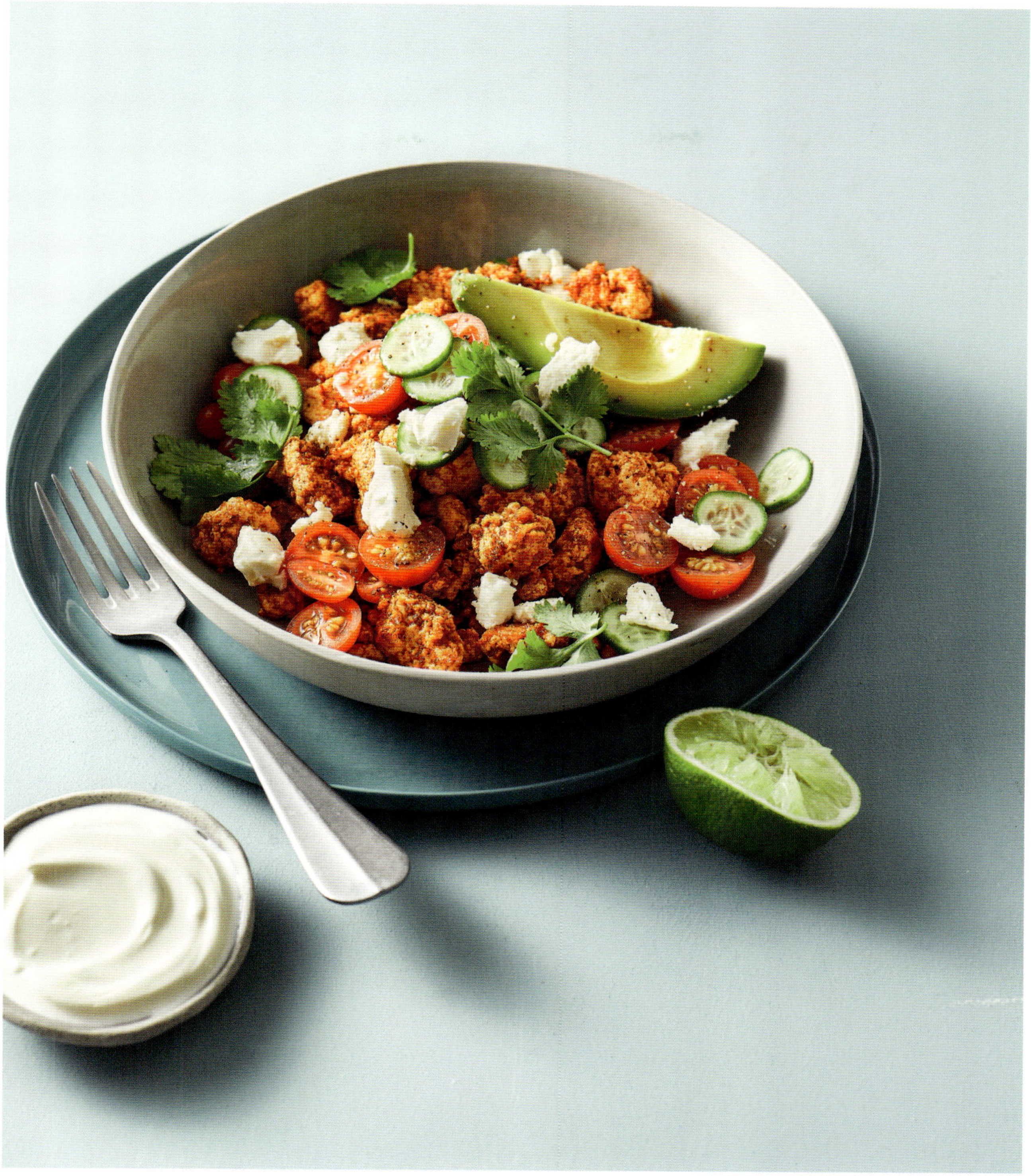

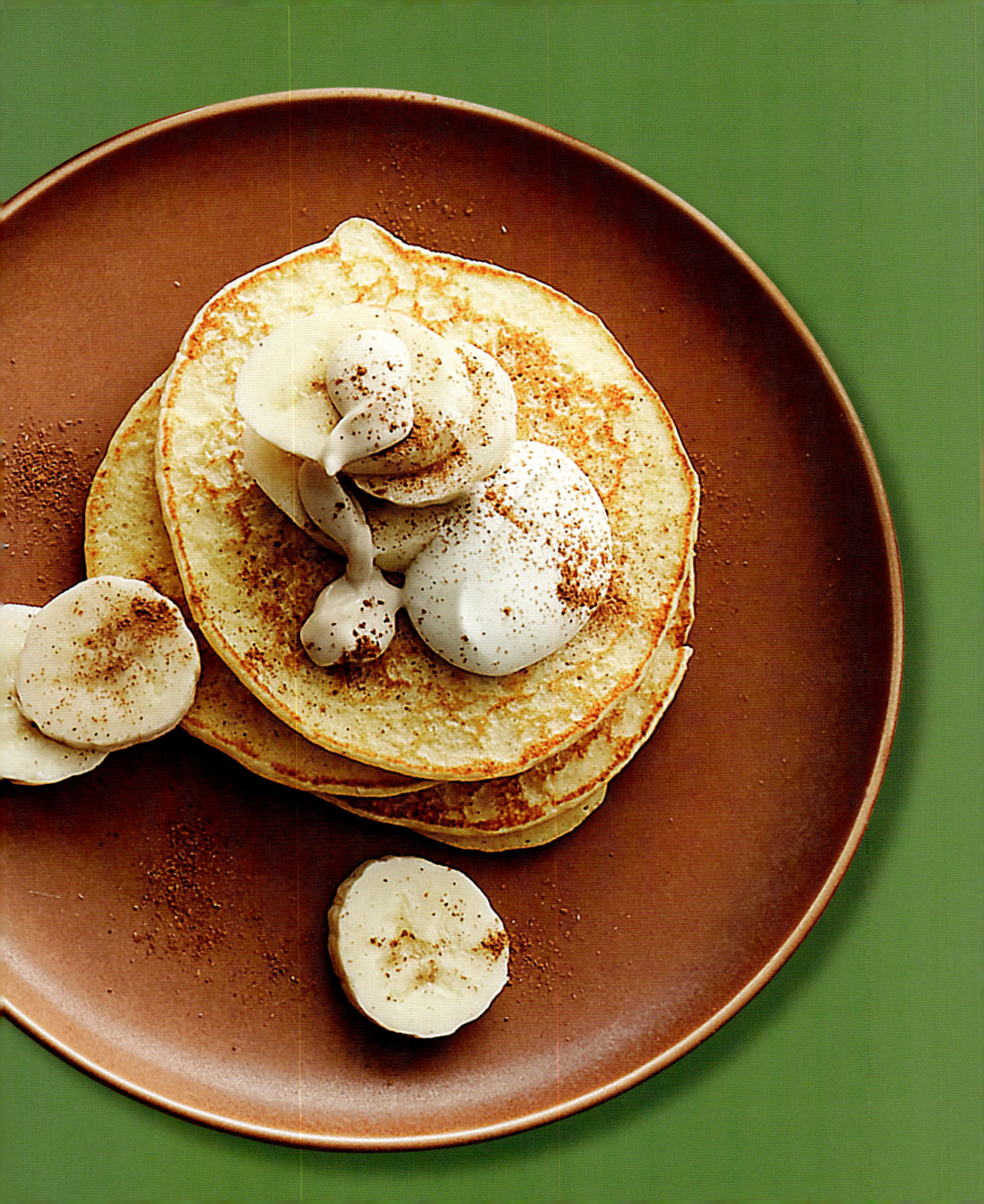

05.

Homemade Staples

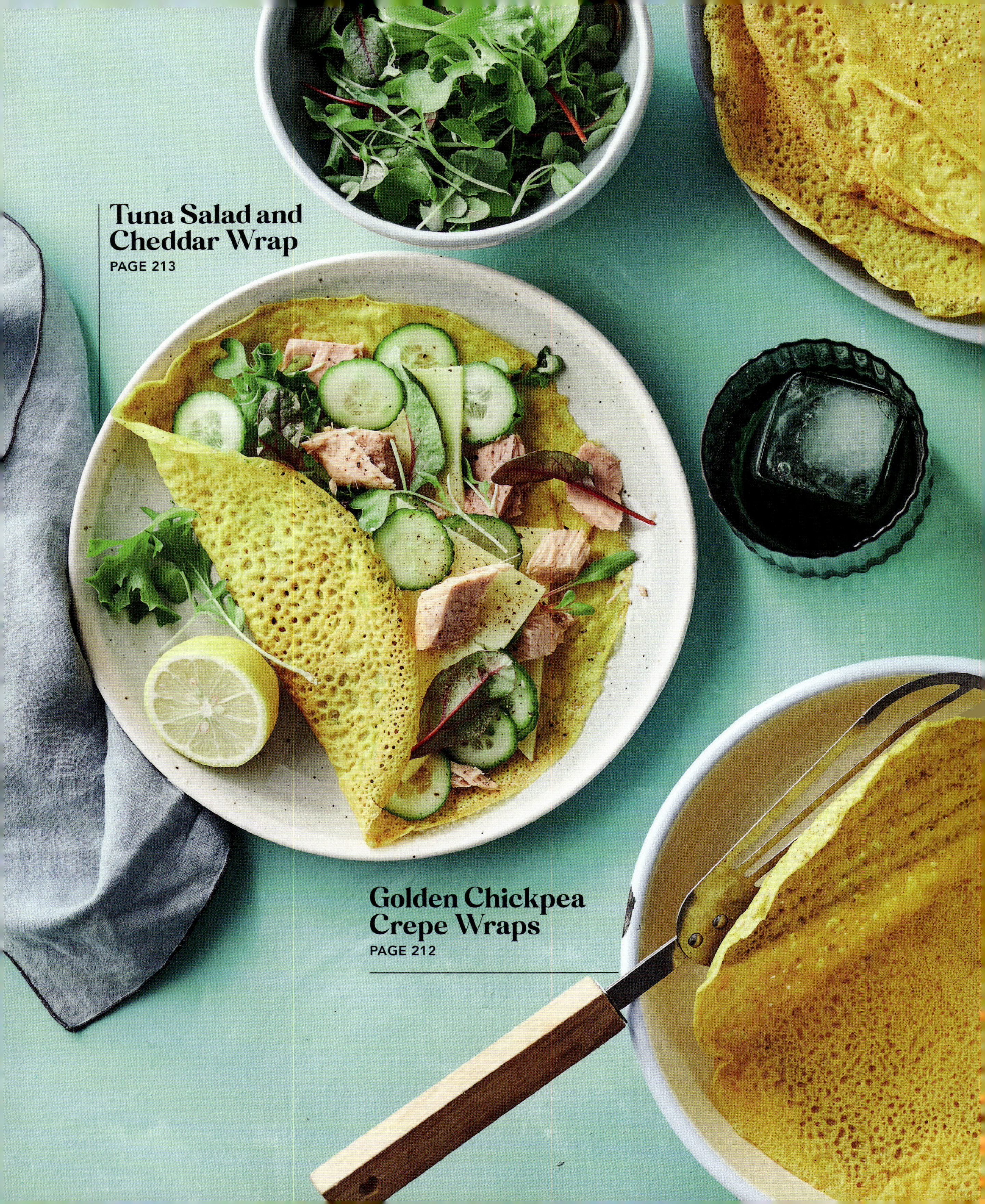

Tuna Salad and Cheddar Wrap
PAGE 213

Golden Chickpea Crepe Wraps
PAGE 212

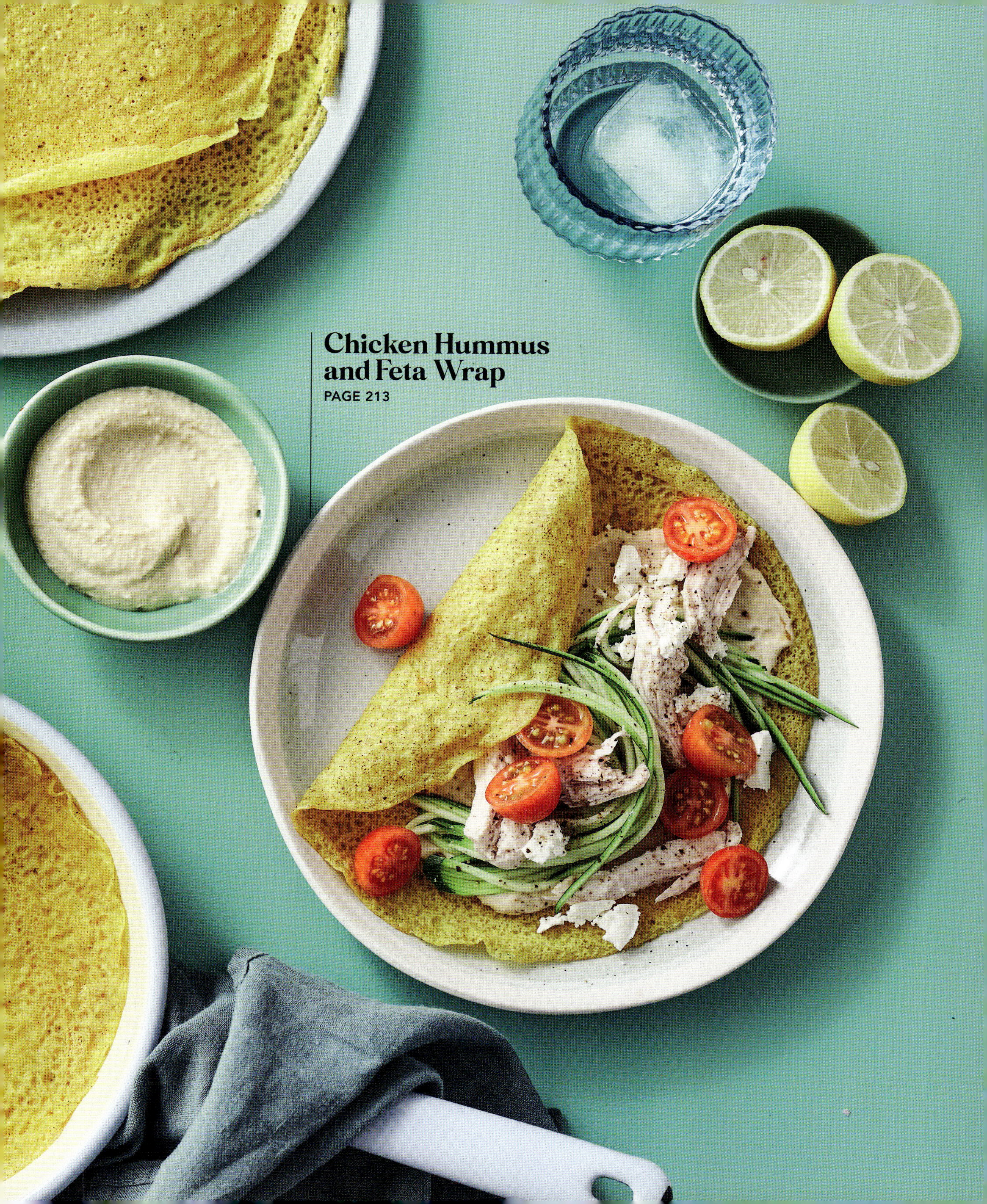

Chicken Hummus and Feta Wrap

PAGE 213

UNITS PER SERVE:	
Breads, Cereals, Legumes, Starchy Veg	1
Dairy	0
Lean Meat, Fish, Poultry, Eggs, Tofu	0
Low–Moderate Carbohydrate Veg	0
Healthy Fats	0.5

Golden Chickpea Crepe Wraps

CARBS **7g** PER SERVE

MAKES: 4 | PREPARATION: 10 MINUTES + 30 MINUTES STANDING | COOKING: 17 MINUTES

100 g chickpea flour (besan)
½ teaspoon ground turmeric
Pinch freshly ground black pepper
1 cup (250 ml) water
1 teaspoon olive oil

1. Place all the ingredients, except the olive oil, in a large bowl and whisk until combined with no lumps. Allow to stand, covered, at room temperature for 30 minutes.
2. Heat a non-stick 28 cm frying pan over medium–high heat. Using a paper towel, rub a little of the olive oil over the surface of the pan. Once the pan is hot, pour in ½ cup (125 ml) of the batter, tilting the pan to ensure the batter covers the surface evenly. Cook for 2 minutes until there are bubbles around the edge and the bottom is browned and crisp. Use a spatula to carefully lift the crepe and flip. Cook for another 1–2 minutes until golden brown. Set aside and repeat with the remaining batter.
3. These wraps can be stored wrapped in a tea towel in the fridge for up to 3 days. Gently warm in a frying pan to make them flexible before using.

UNITS PER SERVE:	
Breads, Cereals, Legumes, Starchy Veg	1
Dairy	1
Lean Meat, Fish, Poultry, Eggs, Tofu	1
Low–Moderate Carbohydrate Veg	3
Healthy Fats	0.5

Tuna Salad and Cheddar Wrap

CARBS 13 g PER SERVE

SERVES: 1 | PREPARATION: 2 MINUTES | COOKING: NIL

1 × Golden Chickpea Crepe (opposite)
90 g tinned tuna in spring water, drained
1½ cups mixed lettuce leaves
½ Lebanese cucumber, finely sliced
20 g slice cheddar

Place all the ingredients onto the golden chickpea crepe and roll up to serve.

UNITS PER SERVE:	
Breads, Cereals, Legumes, Starchy Veg	1
Dairy	1
Lean Meat, Fish, Poultry, Eggs, Tofu	1
Low–Moderate Carbohydrate Veg	1
Healthy Fats	1

Chicken Hummus and Feta Wrap

CARBS 12 g PER SERVE

SERVES: 1 | PREPARATION: 2 MINUTES | COOKING: NIL

1 × Golden Chickpea Crepe (opposite)
2 tablespoons hummus
100 g poached chicken breast, skin removed, sliced (see note)
½ zucchini, sliced into ribbons
1 roma tomato, sliced
20 g reduced-fat Danish feta, crumbled

Place all the ingredients onto the golden chickpea crepe and roll up to serve.

Note

If you are not cooking your own, you can use a purchased pre-roasted chicken or chicken breast. You can find these in the refrigerator section of the supermarket.

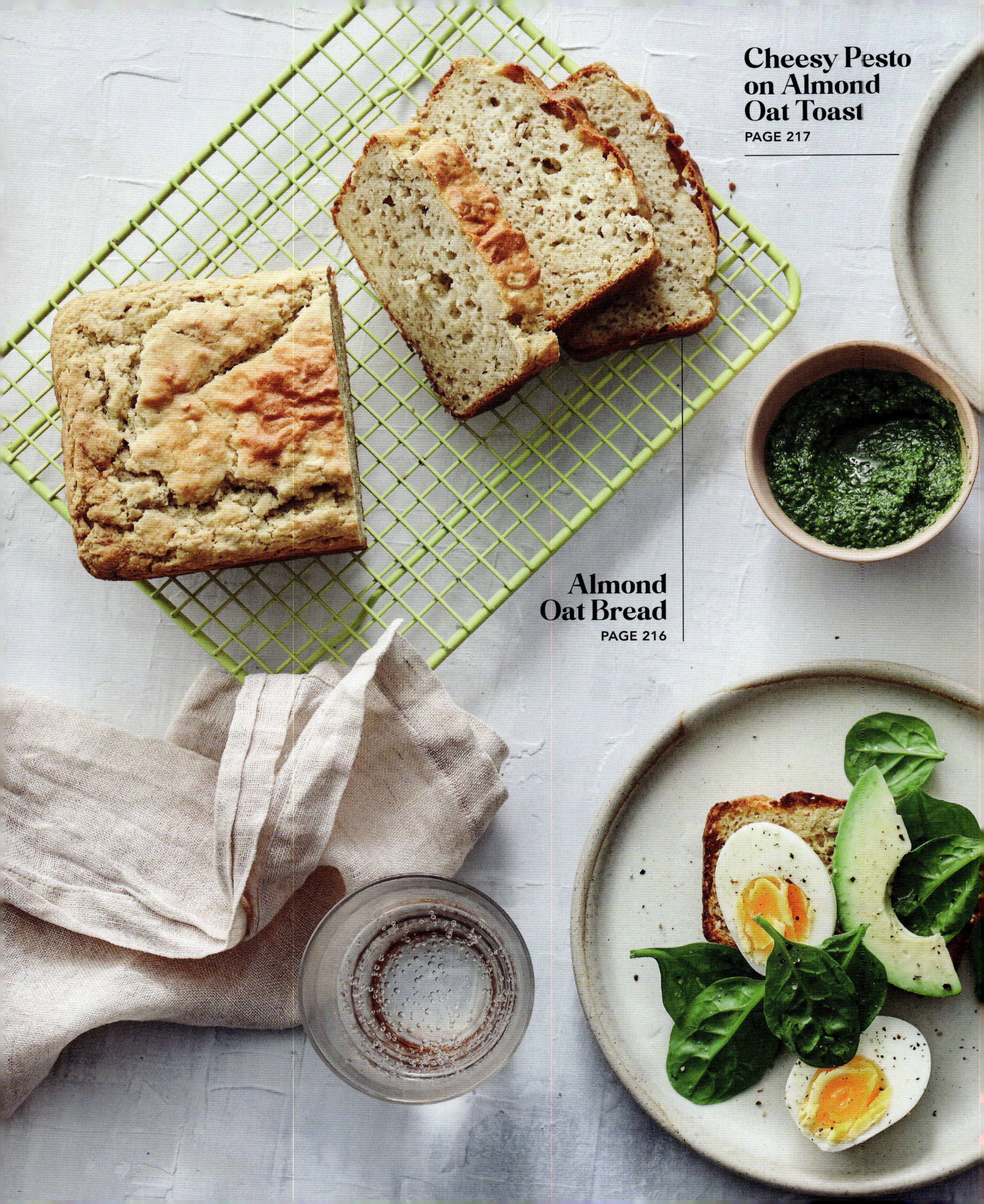

Cheesy Pesto on Almond Oat Toast
PAGE 217

Almond Oat Bread
PAGE 216

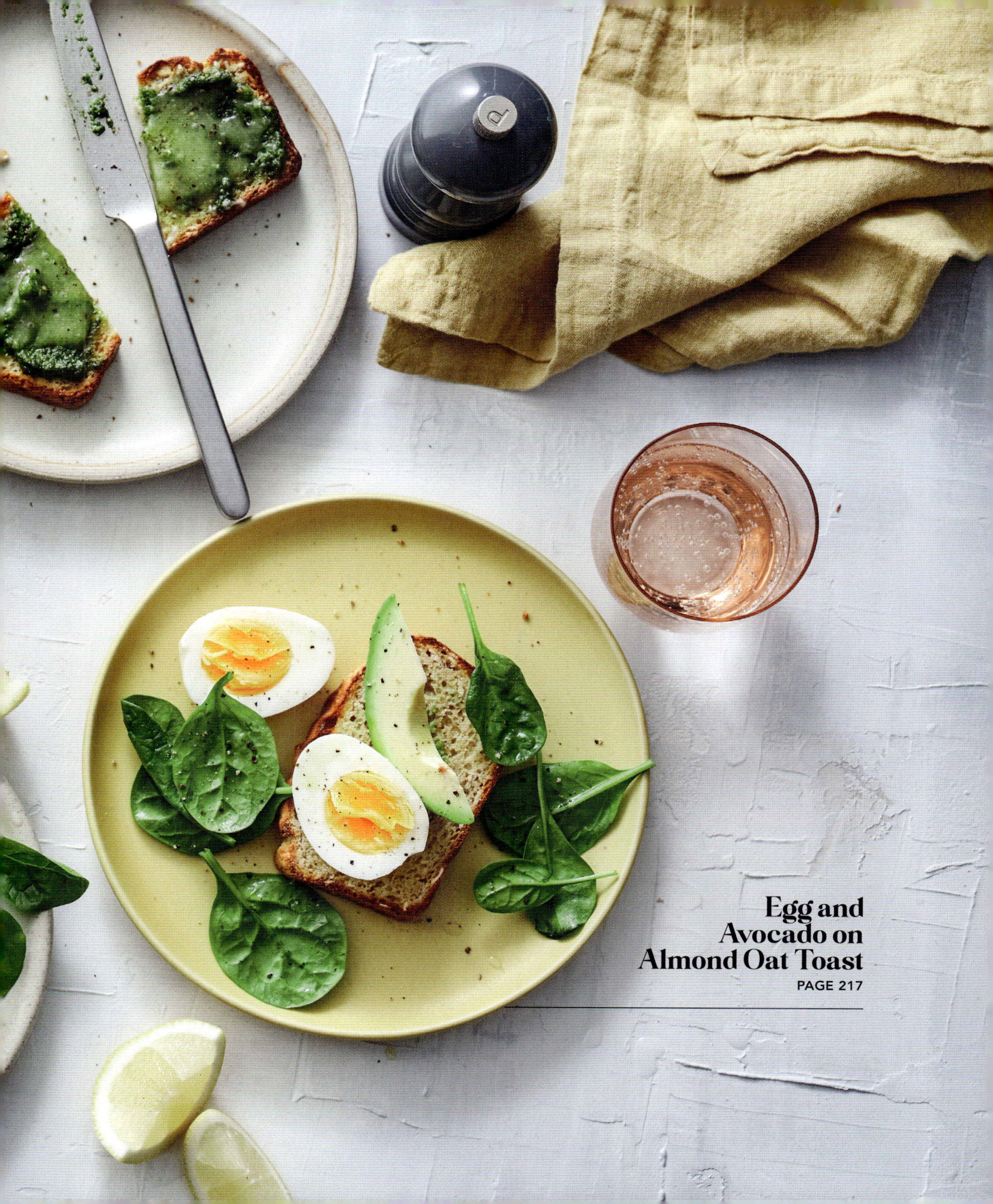

Egg and Avocado on Almond Oat Toast

PAGE 217

UNITS PER SERVE:	
Breads, Cereals, Legumes, Starchy Veg	0.5
Dairy	0
Lean Meat, Fish, Poultry, Eggs, Tofu	0
Low–Moderate Carbohydrate Veg	0
Healthy Fats	1

Almond Oat Bread

CARBS 3g PER SERVE

MAKES: 12 SLICES (1 SERVE = 1 SLICE) | PREPARATION: 10 MINUTES | COOKING: 45 MINUTES

1¼ cups (125 g) almond meal
130 g gluten-free plain flour (or regular plain flour)
60 g rolled oats
3 teaspoons baking powder
¼ teaspoon bicarbonate of soda
2 × 55 g free-range eggs
1 cup (250 ml) full-fat milk, or milk of your choice (when choosing alternative milks, ensure you select those with added calcium for good bone health)
2 teaspoons apple cider vinegar

1. Preheat the oven to 200°C (180°C fan-forced) and grease a standard loaf tin and line with baking paper.
2. Place the almond meal, flour, oats, baking powder and bicarbonate of soda in a large bowl. Mix together with a wooden spoon until well combined.
3. Place the eggs, milk and vinegar in a jug and whisk to combine. Pour the wet mixture into the dry ingredients and mix with a wooden spoon until combined into a thick dough. Transfer to the loaf tin and smooth over the top. Bake in the oven on the middle shelf for 45 minutes, or until an inserted skewer comes out clean.
4. Remove the loaf from the tin, using the baking paper to help, and place on a wire rack to cool completely before cutting into 12 slices.

UNITS PER SERVE:	
Breads, Cereals, Legumes, Starchy Veg	0.5
Dairy	0
Lean Meat, Fish, Poultry, Eggs, Tofu	0.5
Low–Moderate Carbohydrate Veg	1
Healthy Fats	2

Egg and Avocado on Almond Oat Toast

CARBS 3g PER SERVE

SERVES: 1 | PREPARATION: 5 MINUTES | COOKING: 4 MINUTES

1 slice Almond Oat Bread (opposite)
1 × 20 g slice avocado
1 × 55 g free-range egg, hard-boiled and sliced in half
½ cup baby spinach leaves
Wedge of lemon

1. Heat a frying pan over medium–high heat. Add the almond oat bread and toast for 1–2 minutes on each side until lightly golden and warmed through.
2. Place the toast on a plate with the avocado, boiled egg, spinach and the lemon wedge to squeeze over the spinach.

UNITS PER SERVE:	
Breads, Cereals, Legumes, Starchy Veg	0.5
Dairy	1
Lean Meat, Fish, Poultry, Eggs, Tofu	0
Low–Moderate Carbohydrate Veg	0
Healthy Fats	1

Cheesy Pesto on Almond Oat Toast

CARBS 3g PER SERVE

SERVES: 1 | PREPARATION: 5 MINUTES | COOKING: 6 MINUTES

1 slice Almond Oat Bread (opposite)
1 teaspoon pesto
20 g shredded cheddar

1. Heat a frying pan over medium–high heat. Add the almond oat bread and toast for 1–2 minutes on each side until lightly golden and warmed through.
2. Preheat the oven to 220°C (200°C fan-forced).
3. Place the toast on a plate and spread with the pesto. Sprinkle the cheese on top, then place under the oven grill until the cheese is melted.

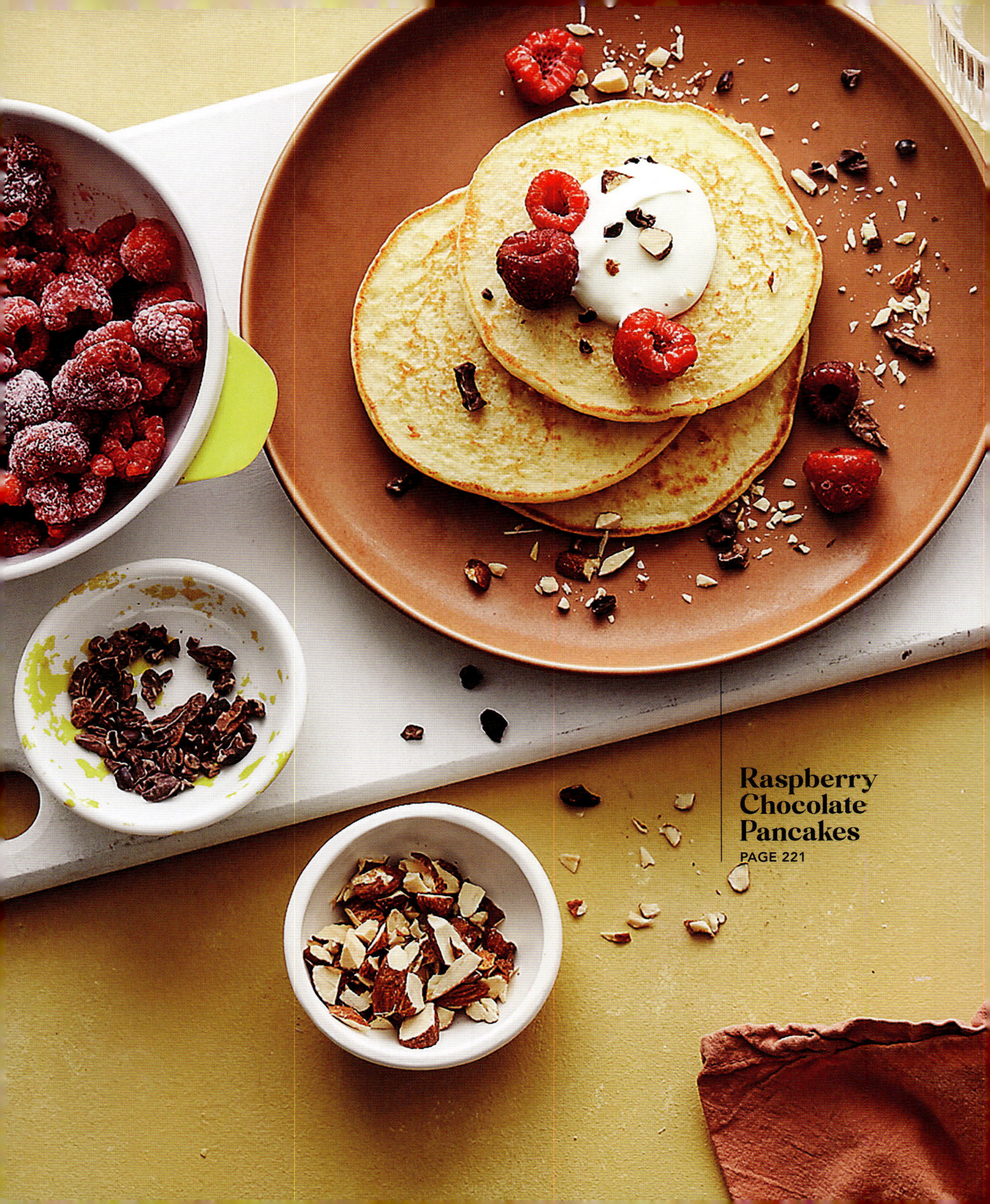

Raspberry Chocolate Pancakes

PAGE 221

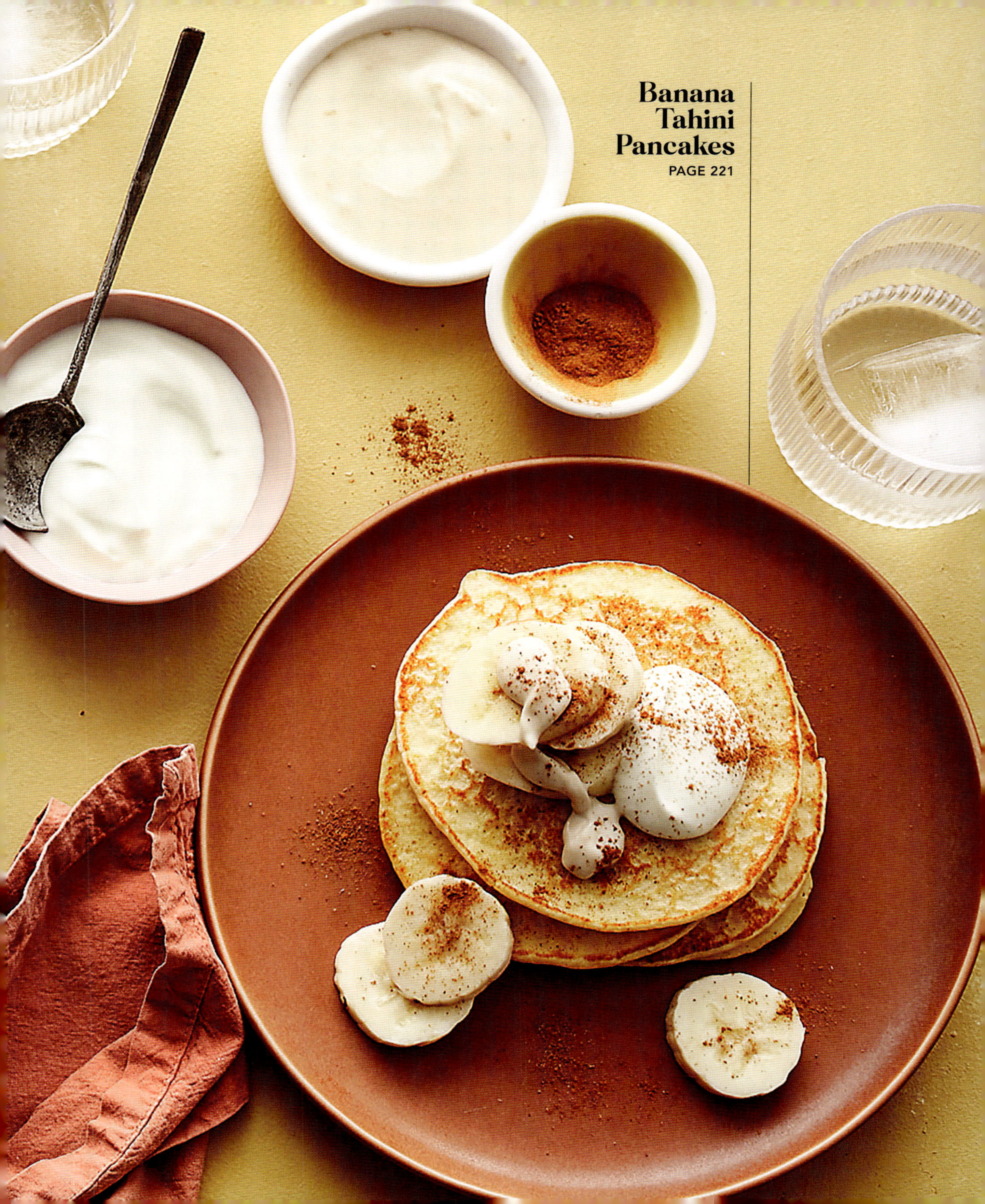

Banana Tahini Pancakes

PAGE 221

UNITS PER SERVE:	
Breads, Cereals, Legumes, Starchy Veg	0.5
Dairy	1
Lean Meat, Fish, Poultry, Eggs, Tofu	0.5
Low–Moderate Carbohydrate Veg	0
Healthy Fats	1

Low-carb Ricotta Pancakes

CARBS 16g PER SERVE

SERVES: 2 (MAKES 6 SMALL PANCAKES) | PREPARATION: 5 MINUTES | COOKING: 10 MINUTES

½ cup (50 g) rolled oats
2 × 55 g free-range eggs
110 g low-fat ricotta
2 teaspoons Nuttelex or canola margarine

1. Add the oats to a blender and pulse until ground to a flour. Add the eggs, ricotta and Nuttelex and process until combined.
2. Heat a large non-stick frying pan over medium heat. Pour in ¼ cupfuls of the batter to make three small pancakes. Cook for 2 minutes until you can see quite a few bubbles popping through, then carefully flip to cook the other side for 1 minute until golden. Set aside and repeat with the remaining batter – you should make six small pancakes.
3. Divide the pancakes between two plates and serve with your chosen toppings.

UNITS PER SERVE:	
Breads, Cereals, Legumes, Starchy Veg	0.5
Dairy	1
Lean Meat, Fish, Poultry, Eggs, Tofu	0.5
Low–Moderate Carbohydrate Veg	1
Healthy Fats	3

Raspberry Chocolate Pancakes

CARBS 20g PER SERVE

SERVES: 2 | PREPARATION: 2 MINUTES | COOKING: NIL

- 1 quantity Low-carb Ricotta Pancakes (opposite)
- 1 cup (125 g) frozen raspberries
- 1 teaspoon raw cacao nibs
- 2 tablespoons chopped roasted unsalted almonds
- 1 tablespoon natural yoghurt

Divide the pancakes between two plates and top with the remaining ingredients.

UNITS PER SERVE:	
Breads, Cereals, Legumes, Starchy Veg	0.5
Dairy	1
Lean Meat, Fish, Poultry, Eggs, Tofu	0.5
Low–Moderate Carbohydrate Veg	0
Healthy Fats	3

Banana Tahini Pancakes (weeks 7–12)

CARBS 20g PER SERVE

SERVES: 2 | PREPARATION: 2 MINUTES | COOKING: NIL

- 1 quantity Low-carb Ricotta Pancakes (opposite)
- 1 banana, sliced into rounds
- 2 teaspoons tahini
- 1 tablespoon natural yoghurt
- Ground cinnamon, to sprinkle

Divide the pancakes between two plates and top with the remaining ingredients.

Note

This recipe includes 2 carbohydrate extras (bananas). Carbohydrate extras are optional and best used if you are needing greater flexibility in your daily intake. In our research trials, carbohydrate extras were requested around week 7. Therefore, the CSIRO Low-carb Diet recommends that you add 2 carb extras or 20 g carb daily if you are looking to maintain weight, increasing exercise or are just wanting a little more in your day. Please refer to page 32 for a list of carb extras and remember these are optional.

Low-carb Pizza Bases

CARBS 10 g PER SERVE

SERVES: 4 (MAKES 2 PIZZA BASES) | PREPARATION: 10 MINUTES | COOKING: 25 MINUTES

600 g cauliflower florets, roughly chopped
60 g almond meal
2 tablespoons tapioca starch, arrowroot flour or cornflour
¼ cup (30 g) finely grated parmesan
3 × 55 g free-range eggs

1. Preheat the oven to 200°C (180°C fan-forced) and line two large baking trays with baking paper.
2. Place the cauliflower florets in a food processor and blitz until smaller than grains of rice. Transfer to a large bowl, add the remaining ingredients and blitz until well incorporated.
3. Spoon half the mixture onto the first baking tray and shape it into a 25 cm circle about 5 mm thick. Repeat with the remaining mixture on the second baking tray. Bake in the oven for 25 minutes or golden and firm. Your bases are now ready for topping.

UNITS PER SERVE (SEE NOTES):	
Breads, Cereals, Legumes, Starchy Veg	0.5
Dairy	0.5
Lean Meat, Fish, Poultry, Eggs, Tofu	0.5
Low–Moderate Carbohydrate Veg	1
Healthy Fats	1.5

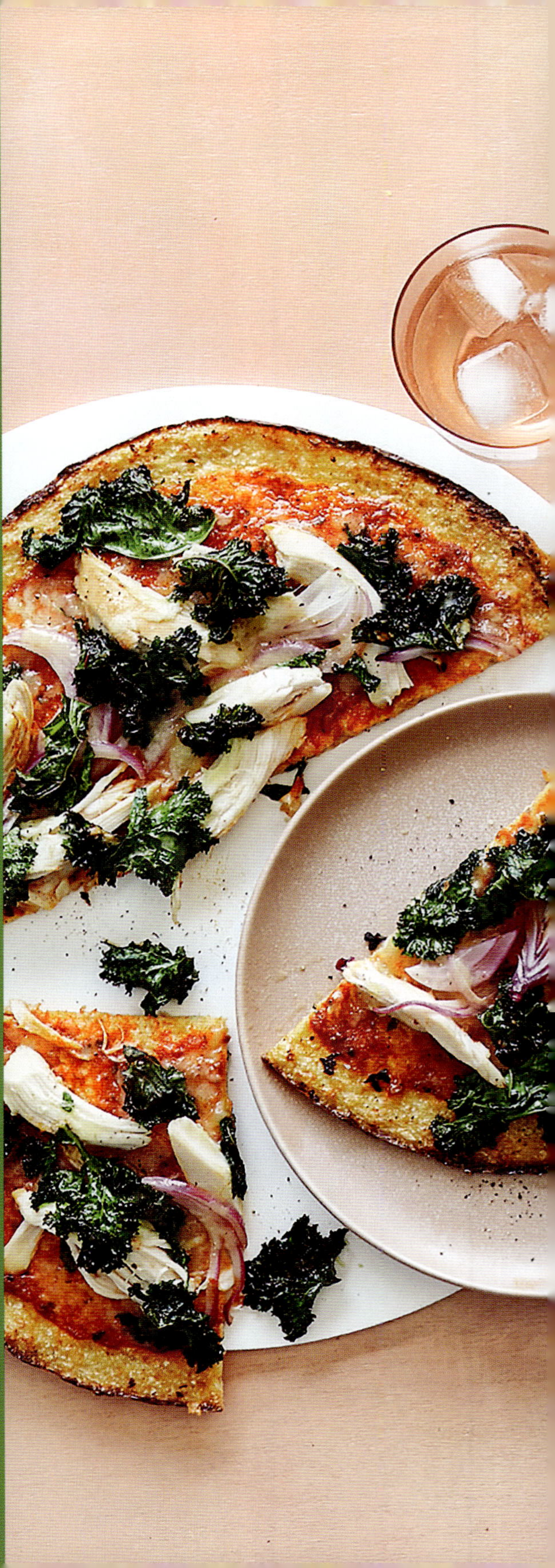

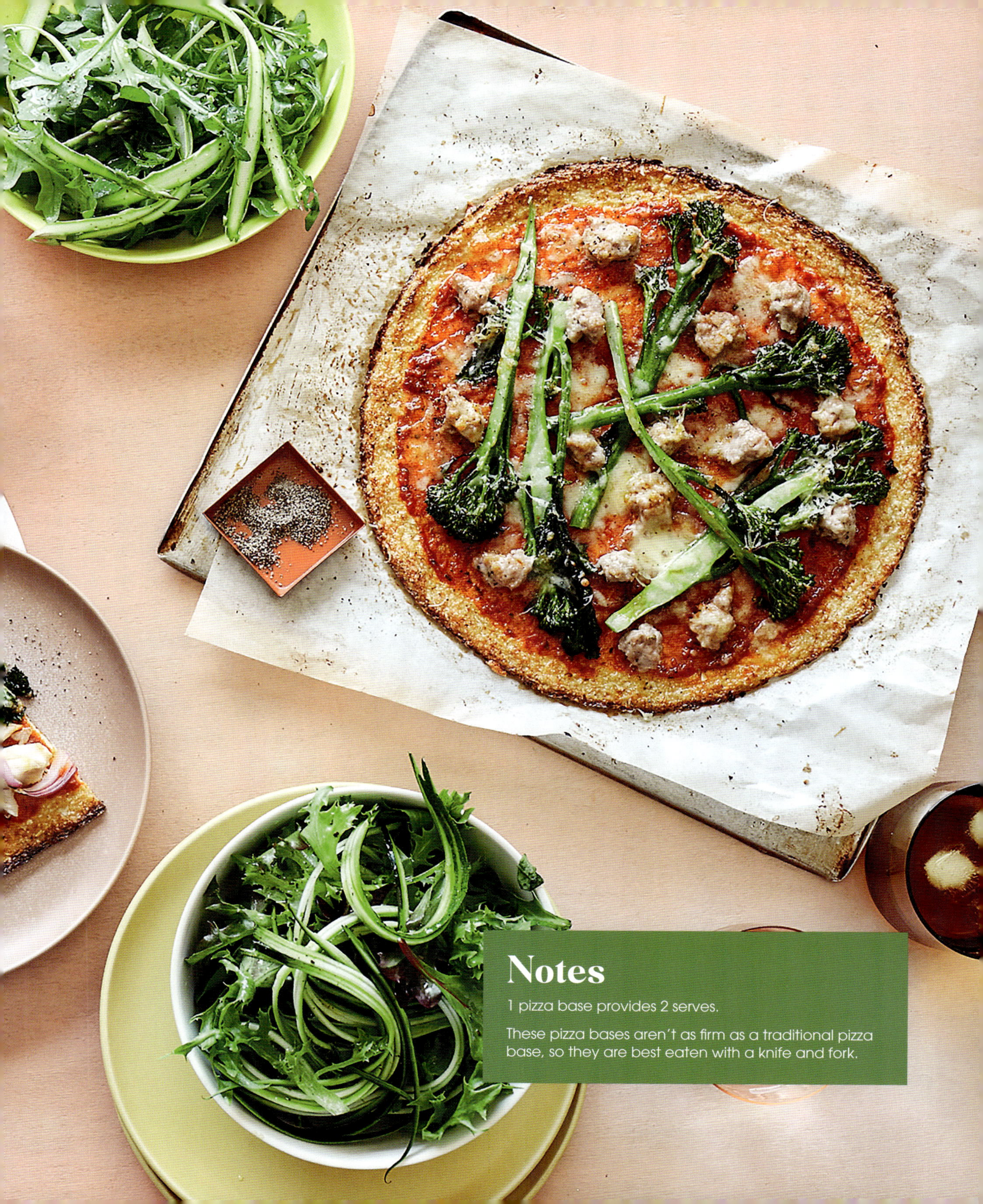

Notes

1 pizza base provides 2 serves.

These pizza bases aren't as firm as a traditional pizza base, so they are best eaten with a knife and fork.

UNITS PER SERVE:	
Breads, Cereals, Legumes, Starchy Veg	0.5
Dairy	1
Lean Meat, Fish, Poultry, Eggs, Tofu	1
Low–Moderate Carbohydrate Veg	3
Healthy Fats	2

Fennel Pork Pizza with Broccolini

CARBS 16 g PER SERVE

SERVES: 4 | PREPARATION: 20 MINUTES | COOKING TIME: 10 MINUTES

⅔ cup (170 ml) tomato passata (no added sugar or salt)
1 teaspoon dried oregano
2 × Low-carb Pizza Bases (page 222), baked and ready to top
1 bunch (520 g) broccolini, stalks sliced in half lengthways
20 g grated parmesan
70 g grated mozzarella
2 teaspoons chilli oil

PORK MEATBALLS

200 g pork mince
2 cloves garlic, crushed
½ teaspoon fennel seeds
¼ teaspoon freshly ground black pepper

ZUCCHINI SALAD

Juice of ½ lemon
2 teaspoons extra virgin olive oil
4 cups mixed lettuce leaves
1 zucchini, shredded

1. Preheat the oven to 200°C (180°C fan-forced).
2. To make the pork meatballs, place all the ingredients in a large bowl and mix with your hands to combine well.
3. Mix the passata and dried oregano together in a bowl, then spread on top of the pizza bases. Top with the broccolini. Break off 1–2 cm pieces of the pork meatball mixture, roll into balls and place on the pizzas. Sprinkle on the cheeses and drizzle on the chilli oil.
4. Cook the pizzas in the oven for 10 minutes until the cheese has melted and the pork has cooked through.
5. To make the zucchini salad, place the lemon juice and olive oil in a large bowl, then add the salad leaves and zucchini. Toss gently to coat the greens in the dressing. Season with freshly ground black pepper.
6. Slice each pizza into quarters and divide between four plates. Serve with the zucchini salad.

UNITS PER SERVE:	
Breads, Cereals, Legumes, Starchy Veg	0.5
Dairy	1
Lean Meat, Fish, Poultry, Eggs, Tofu	1.5
Low–Moderate Carbohydrate Veg	3
Healthy Fats	2.5

Chicken and Crispy Garlic Kale Pizza

CARBS 16 g PER SERVE

SERVES: 4 | PREPARATION: 10 MINUTES | COOKING: 10 MINUTES

⅔ cup (170 ml) tomato passata (no added sugar or salt)
1 teaspoon dried oregano
2 × Low-carb Pizza Bases (page 222), baked and ready to top
¼ small red onion, sliced
250 g shredded roast chicken breast, skin removed (see note)
90 g grated cheddar
2 cups (230 g) kale leaves, stalks removed and roughly torn
1 clove garlic, crushed
2 teaspoons extra-virgin olive oil

ROCKET AND ASPARAGUS SALAD

Juice of ½ lemon
2 teaspoons extra virgin olive oil
1 bunch asparagus, woody ends trimmed, spears peeled with a vegetable peeler, then finely sliced diagonally
4 cups (230 g) rocket leaves

1. Preheat the oven to 200°C (180°C fan-forced).
2. Mix the passata and dried oregano together in a bowl, then spread on top of the pizza bases. Top with the onion, chicken and cheese.
3. Place the kale, garlic and olive oil in a bowl. Massage the oil and garlic into the kale leaves with your fingers until nicely coated in the oil. Scatter the kale over the pizza bases.
4. Cook the pizzas in the oven for 10 minutes until the cheese has melted and the kale is crisp.
5. To make the rocket and asparagus salad, place the lemon juice, olive oil, asparagus and rocket in a large bowl, then toss gently to coat the greens in the dressing. Season with ¼ teaspoon freshly ground black pepper.
6. Slice each pizza into four pieces and divide between four plates. Serve with the rocket and asparagus salad.

Note

If you are not cooking your own, you can use a purchased pre-roasted chicken or chicken breast. You can find these in the refrigerator section of the supermarket.

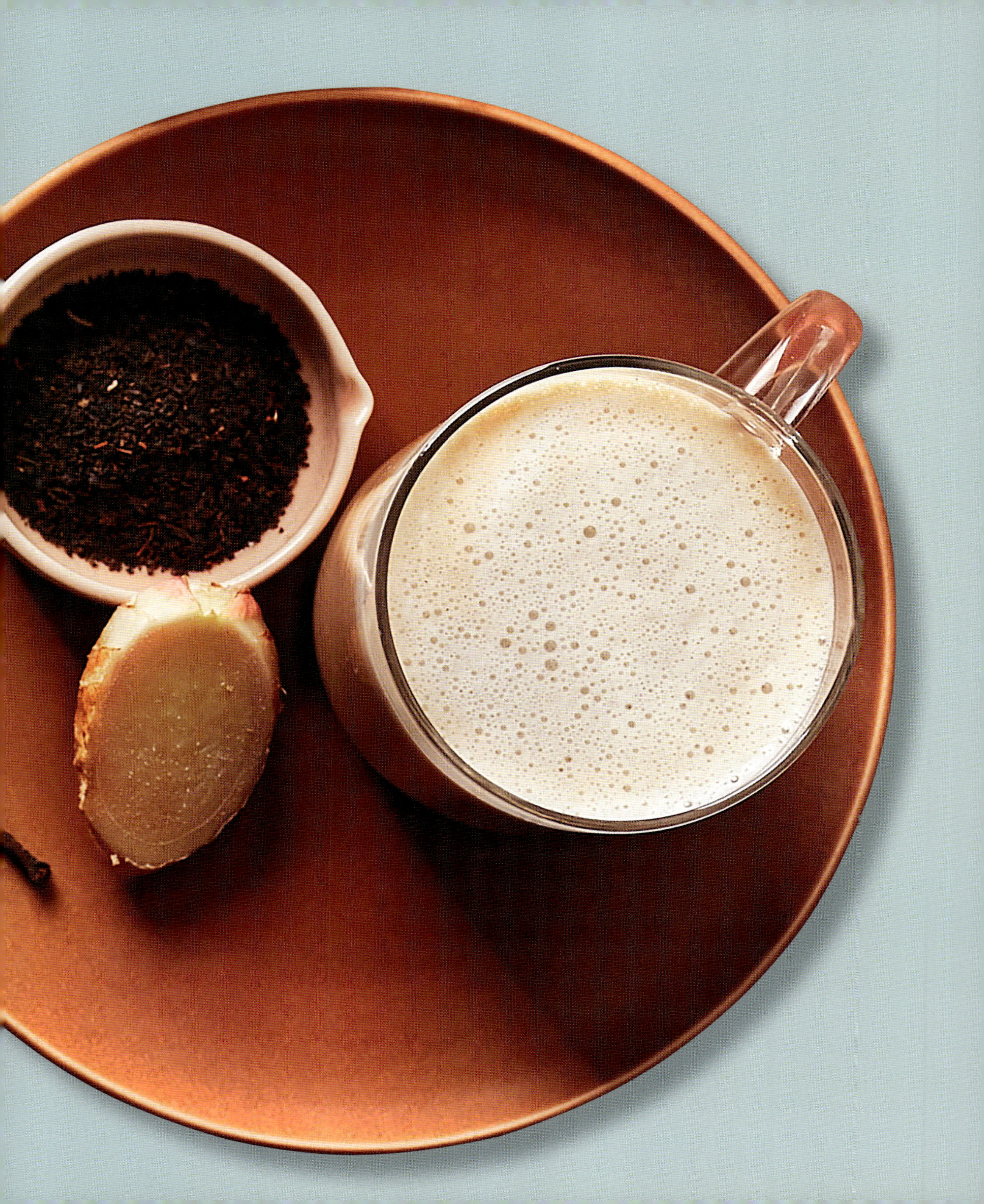

06.

Drinks

UNITS PER SERVE:	
Breads, Cereals, Legumes, Starchy Veg	0
Dairy	1
Lean Meat, Fish, Poultry, Eggs, Tofu	0
Low–Moderate Carbohydrate Veg	0
Healthy Fats	2

Espresso Banana Smoothie (weeks 7–12)

CARBS 15 g PER SERVE

SERVES: 2 | PREPARATION: 5 MINUTES, PLUS FREEZING | COOKING: NIL

- ¾ cup (185 ml) macadamia milk, frozen into ice cubes
- ¾ cup (200 ml) macadamia milk
- 1 tablespoon cashew butter (see notes)
- 1 small banana, chopped and frozen
- 2 teaspoons pure vanilla extract
- 2 shots (80 ml) espresso

1. Place all the ingredients in a blender and blitz to combine. Add a few tablespoons of water and blitz again if you want a thinner smoothie.
2. Divide between two glasses and serve.

Notes

This recipe includes 1.5 carbohydrate extras (banana). Carbohydrate extras are optional and best used if you are needing greater flexibility in your daily intake. In our research trials, carbohydrate extras were requested around week 7. Therefore, the CSIRO Low-carb Diet recommends that you add 2 carb extras or 20 g carb daily if you are looking to maintain weight, increasing exercise or are just wanting a little more in your day. Please refer to page 32 for a list of carb extras and remember these are optional.

When purchasing nut butters, it is important to look at the food label. Ensure your nut butter has no added sugar or salt.

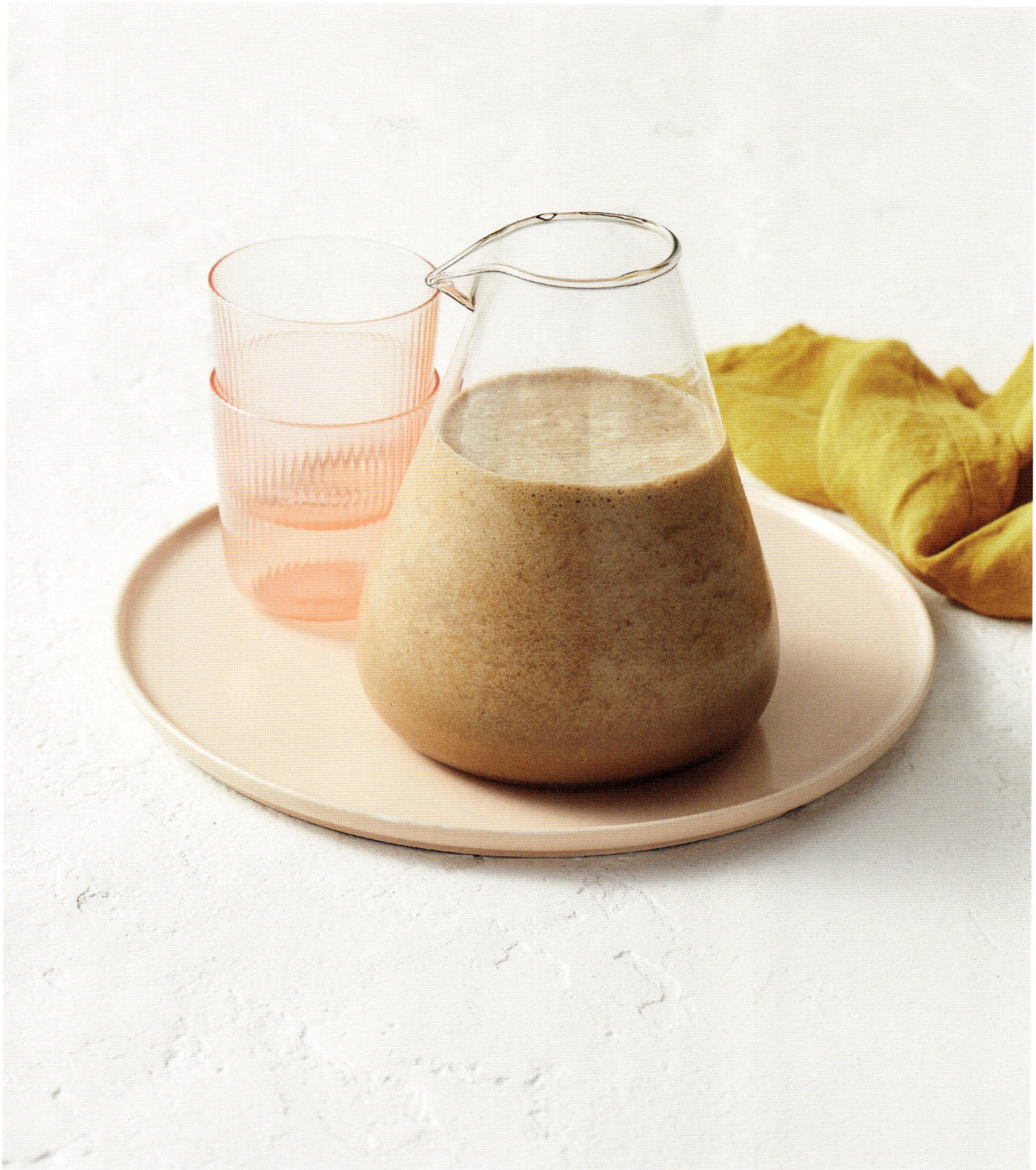

UNITS PER SERVE:	
Breads, Cereals, Legumes, Starchy Veg	0
Dairy	1
Lean Meat, Fish, Poultry, Eggs, Tofu	0
Low–Moderate Carbohydrate Veg	0.5
Healthy Fats	0

French Strawberry Soda

CARBS 9g PER SERVE

SERVES: 2 | PREPARATION: 5 MINUTES | COOKING: NIL

½ cup (100 g) strawberries, diced
2 cups (500 ml) soda water
1 cup (250 ml) full-fat milk

Divide the strawberries between two glasses and mash lightly with a fork, then pour the soda water over the top. Allow to sit for a minute to infuse, then pour in the milk and serve.

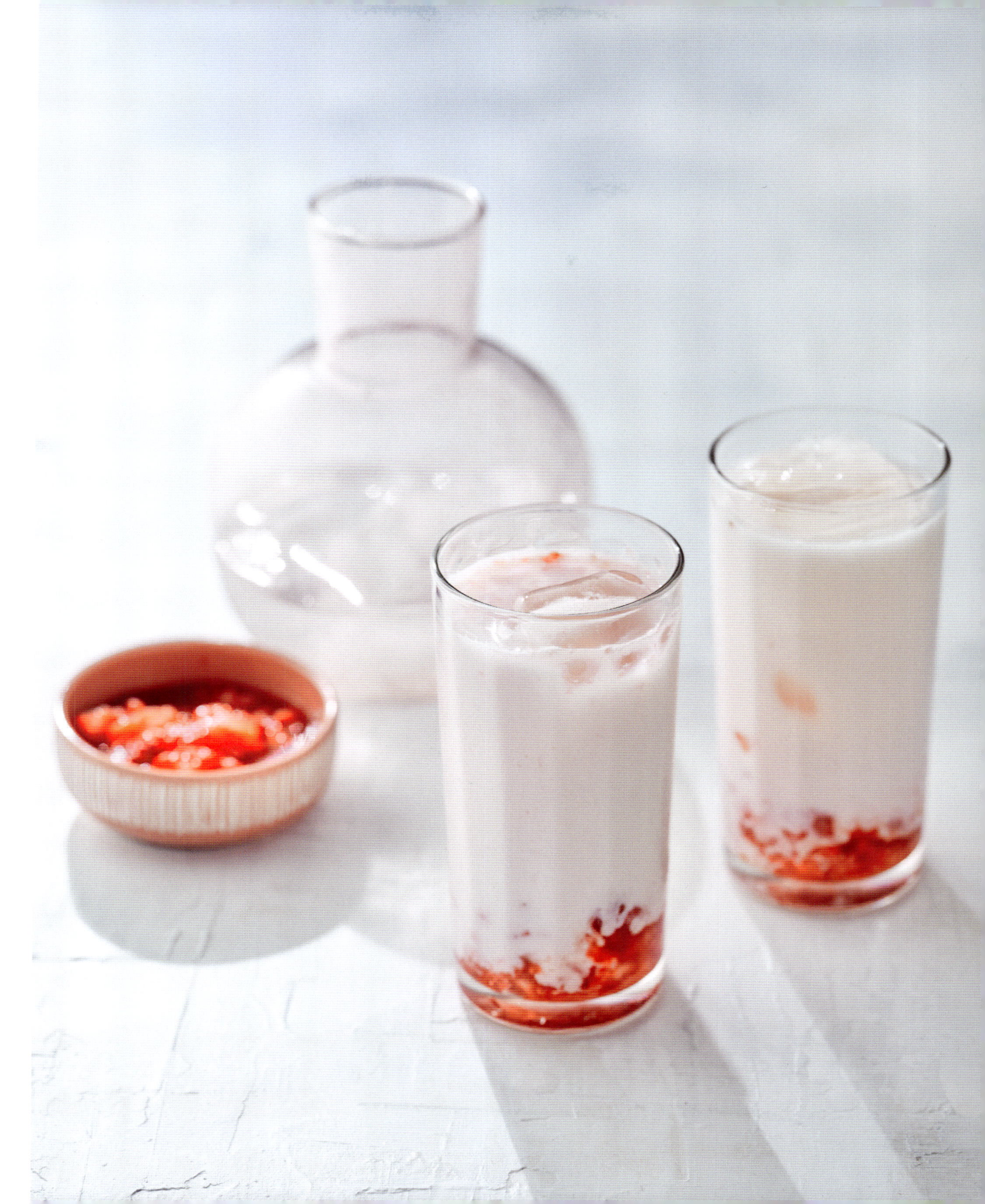

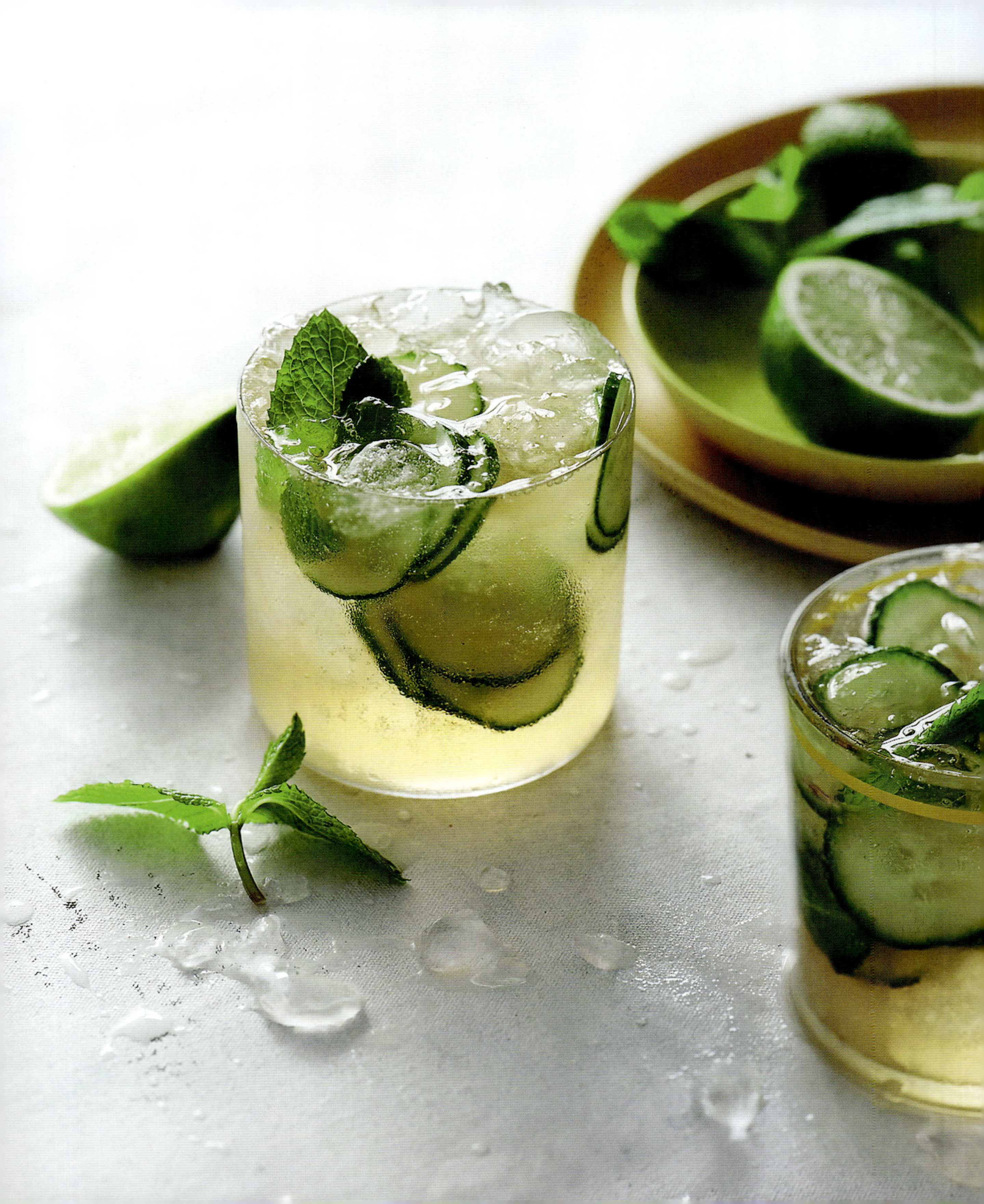

UNITS PER SERVE:	
Breads, Cereals, Legumes, Starchy Veg	0
Dairy	0
Lean Meat, Fish, Poultry, Eggs, Tofu	0
Low–Moderate Carbohydrate Veg	0.5
Healthy Fats	0

Mojito Kombucha Mocktail

CARBS 5g PER SERVE

SERVES: 2 | PREPARATION: 5 MINUTES | COOKING: NIL

- Ice cubes
- 2 cups (500 ml) unflavoured sugar-free kombucha (see note)
- Juice of 1 lime, plus a few lime slices for garnish
- ½ small cucumber, finely sliced
- ½ cup mint leaves

1. Fill two glasses with ice. Divide the kombucha between the glasses, then squeeze in the lime juice and stir to combine.
2. Top with the cucumber slices, mint leaves and a slice of lime to serve.

Note

Ensure you are purchasing sugar-free kombucha with 0 g of sugar. Brands such as Remedy Kombucha ferment their sugar out in processing and sweeten slightly with stevia, which is acceptable.

UNITS PER SERVE:	
Breads, Cereals, Legumes, Starchy Veg	0
Dairy	1
Lean Meat, Fish, Poultry, Eggs, Tofu	0
Low–Moderate Carbohydrate Veg	0
Healthy Fats	0

Chai Latte

SERVES: 2 | PREPARATION: 2 MINUTES | COOKING: 8 MINUTES

CARBS 7g PER SERVE

- 1 cinnamon stick
- 2 cardamom pods
- 2 whole cloves
- 2 star anise
- 4 whole black peppercorns
- 1 cm slice fresh ginger
- 2 teaspoons black tea leaves
- 1½ cups (375 ml) low-fat milk or calcium-enriched soy milk (see note)

Place the cinnamon, cardamom, cloves, star anise and peppercorns in a small saucepan over medium heat. Toast in the dry saucepan for 2–3 minutes until fragrant. Add the ginger, tea leaves and milk and gently simmer for 4–5 minutes. Strain the milk through a sieve into two mugs to serve.

Note

If you have a milk frother, reserve ¼ cup (60 ml) of the warm strained milk, then froth and pour on top of the lattes.

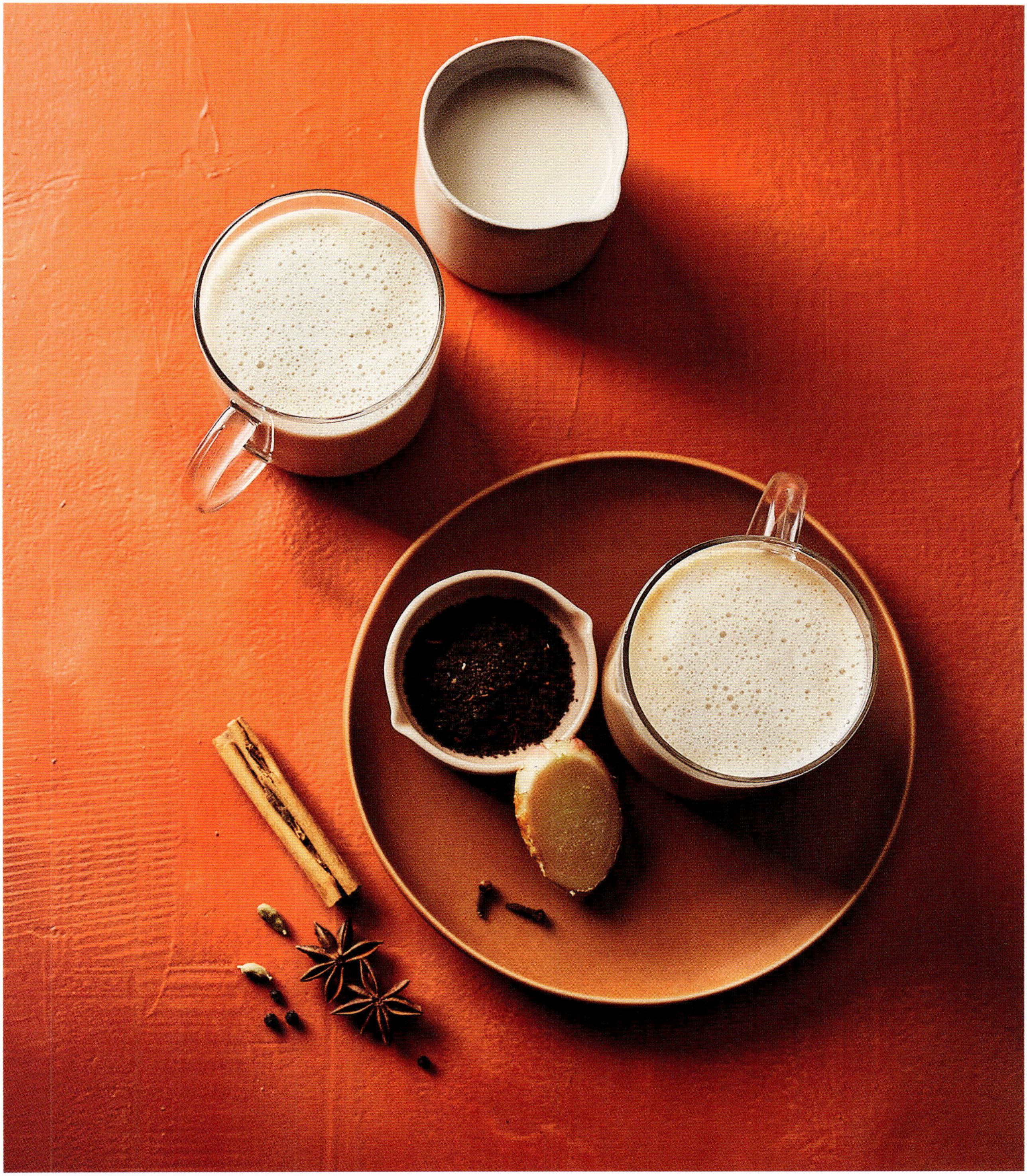

UNITS PER SERVE:	
Breads, Cereals, Legumes, Starchy Veg	0
Dairy	0
Lean Meat, Fish, Poultry, Eggs, Tofu	0
Low–Moderate Carbohydrate Veg	0
Healthy Fats	0

Chamomile Lemonade

CARBS **1g** PER SERVE

SERVES: 2 | PREPARATION: 1 HOUR 10 MINUTES | COOKING: NIL

1 chamomile teabag
2 cups (500 ml) boiling water
Ice cubes
1 cup (250 ml) soda water
Juice of ½ lemon
Lemon slices, to serve

1. Place the chamomile teabag in a mug with 1 cup (250 ml) boiling water. Allow to steep for 5 minutes, then remove the teabag. Allow the tea to cool completely, then place in the fridge for 1 hour or until chilled.
2. Divide the chilled chamomile tea between two glasses filled with ice. Pour the soda water in, then add the lemon juice. Mix to combine and serve with the lemon slices.

Note

You can freeze any leftover chamomile lemonade in an ice-cube tray and use the cubes to flavour your water.

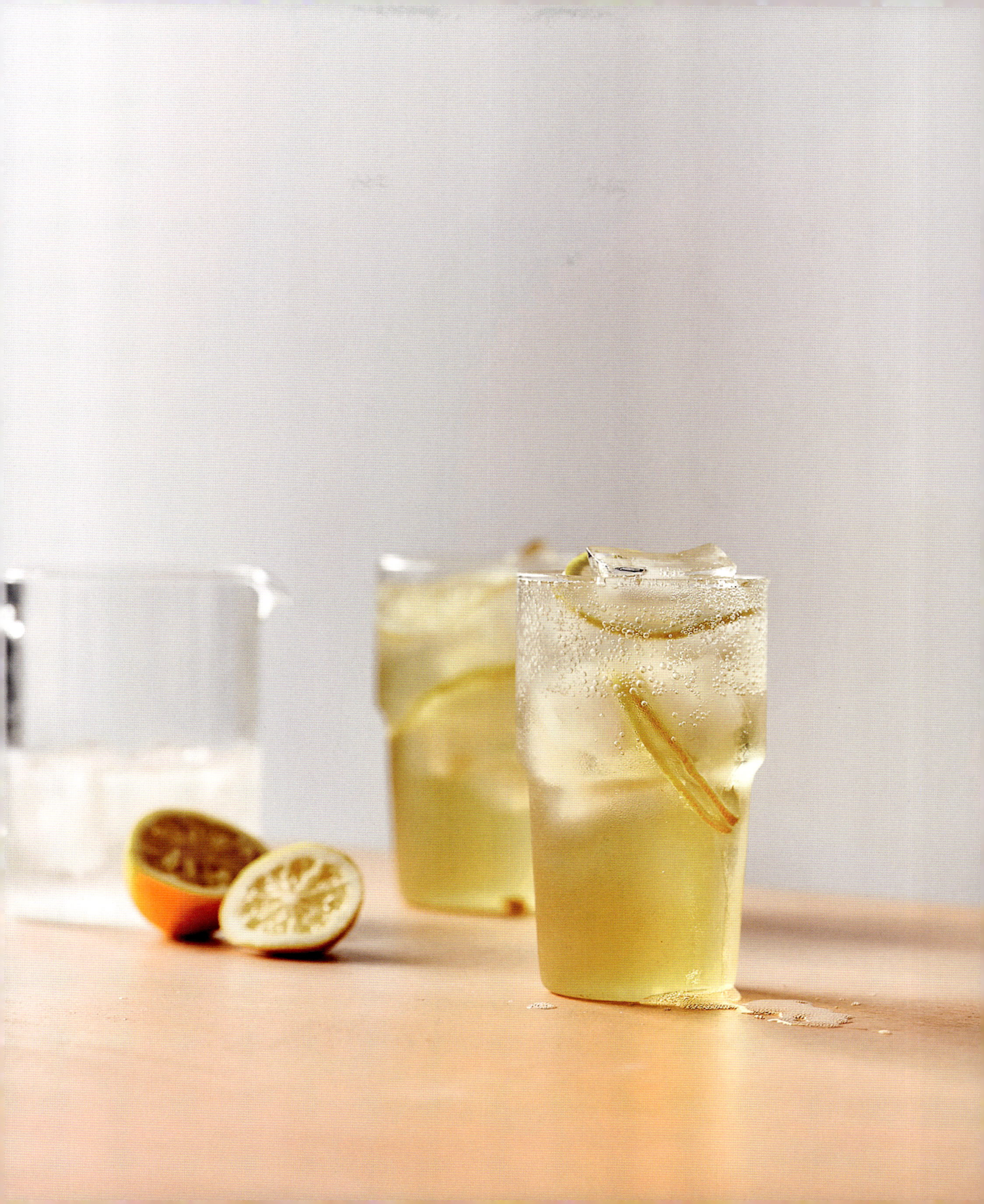

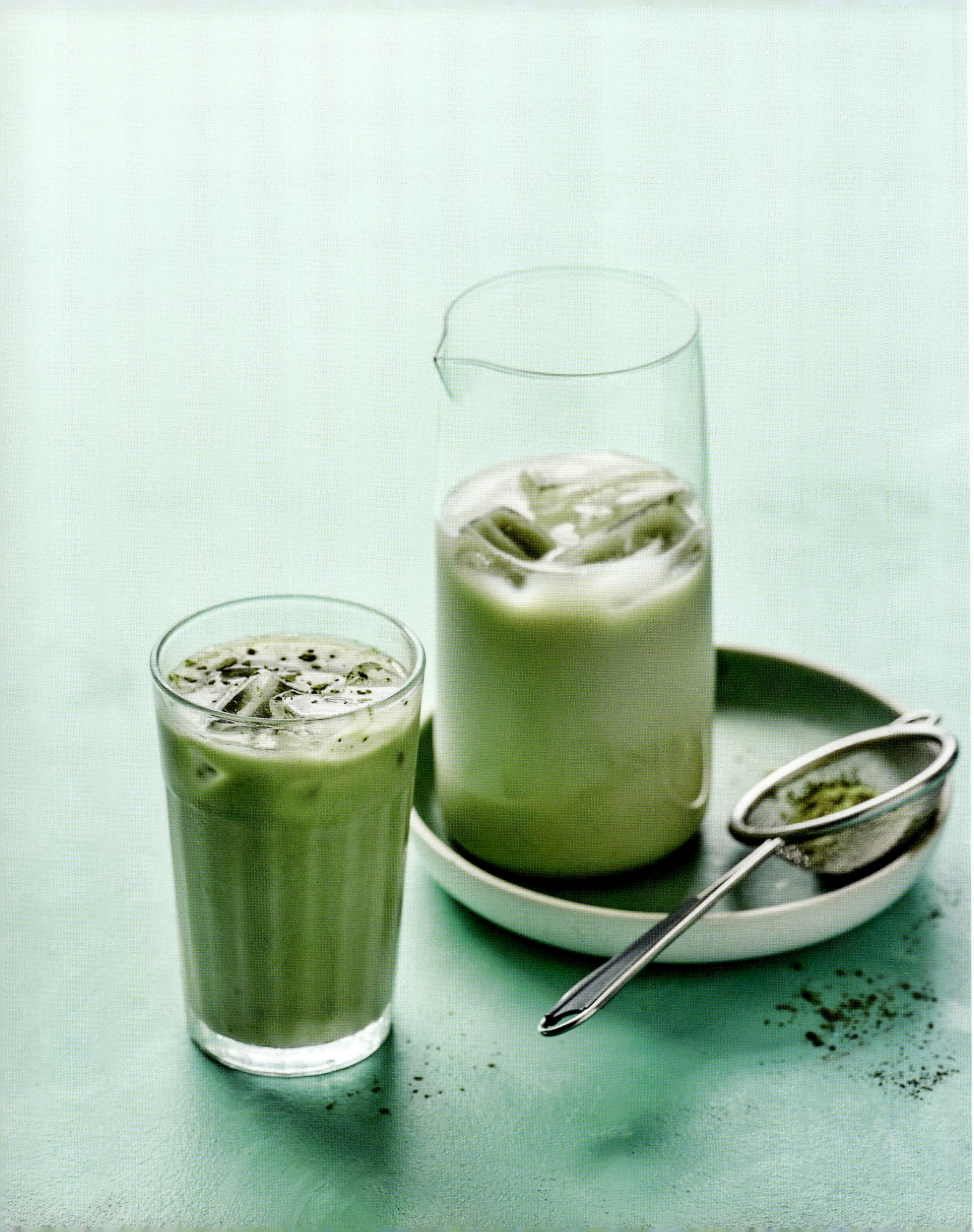

UNITS PER SERVE:	
Breads, Cereals, Legumes, Starchy Veg	0
Dairy	1
Lean Meat, Fish, Poultry, Eggs, Tofu	0
Low–Moderate Carbohydrate Veg	0
Healthy Fats	0

Matcha Latte

CARBS 5g PER SERVE

SERVES: 1 | PREPARATION: 5 MINUTES | COOKING: NIL

1 teaspoon matcha (sugar-free)
1 tablespoon hot water
1 drop pure liquid stevia
¾ cup (170 ml) almond milk
Ice cubes (if making iced latte)

1. Sift the matcha into a mug. Add the hot water and stevia and whisk with a fork or matcha whisk until combined.
2. For a warm latte, warm the milk in a small saucepan over low–medium heat for 2 minutes, or heat in the microwave on High for 30 seconds. Froth with a milk frother if you have one, then pour into the mug to serve.
3. For an iced latte, place the combined matcha and stevia mixture into a glass filled with ice. Pour in the almond milk and serve.

UNITS PER SERVE:	
Breads, Cereals, Legumes, Starchy Veg	0
Dairy	1
Lean Meat, Fish, Poultry, Eggs, Tofu	0
Low–Moderate Carbohydrate Veg	0.5
Healthy Fats	2

Blueberry Tahini Smoothie

CARBS 10g PER SERVE

SERVES: 2 | PREPARATION: 5 MINUTES + FREEZING | COOKING: NIL

100 g low-fat natural yoghurt
¾ cup (185 ml) almond milk
1 tablespoon tahini
80 g blueberries, fresh or frozen
Juice of ¼ lemon
2 teaspoons pure vanilla extract

1. Freeze the yoghurt in an ice-cube tray. (Doing this will thicken and cool your smoothie.)
2. Place the frozen yoghurt cubes, almond milk, tahini, blueberries, lemon and vanilla in a blender and blitz until smooth. Add a dash of water if you'd like a thinner smoothie.
3. Divide between two glasses and serve.

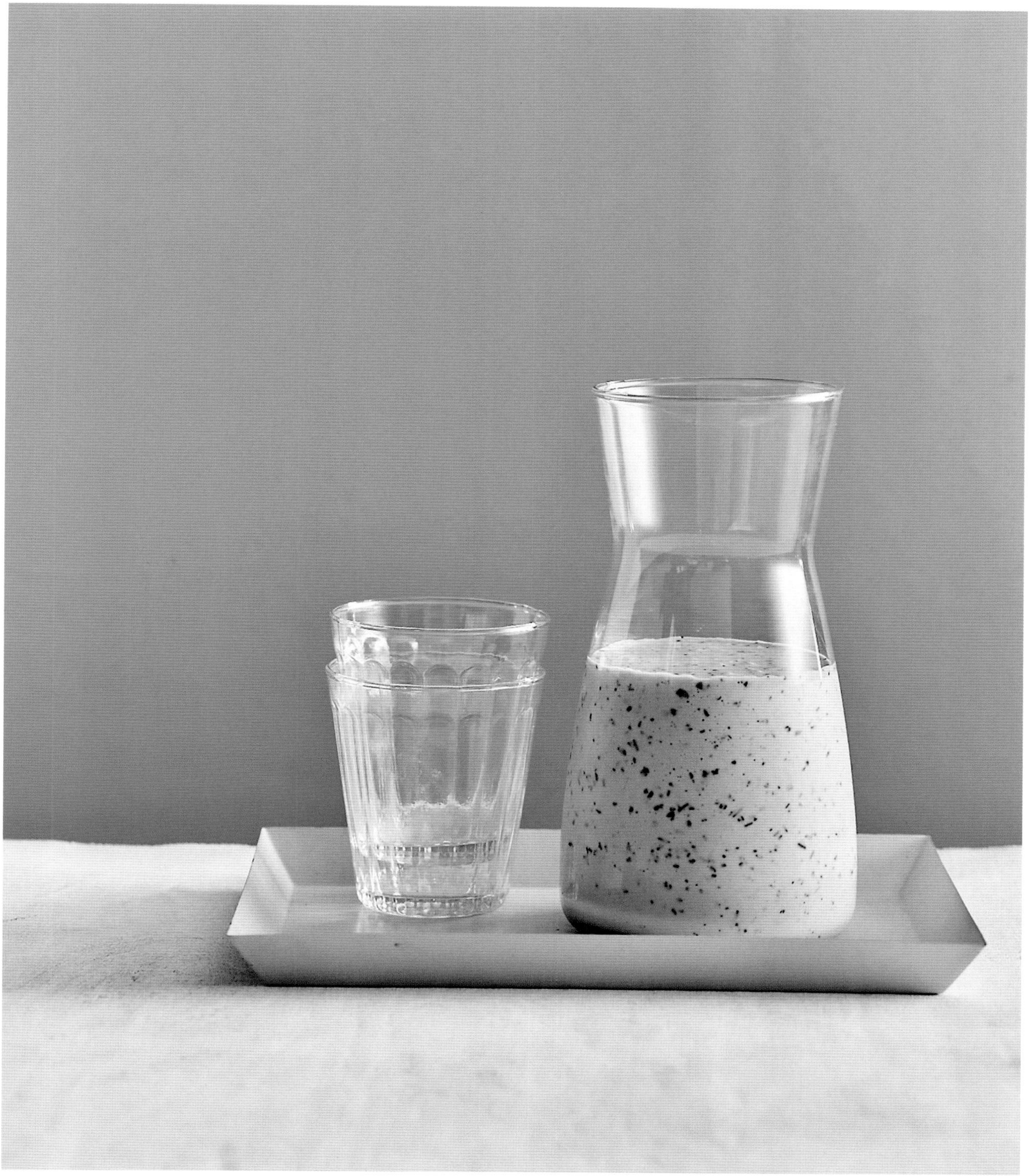

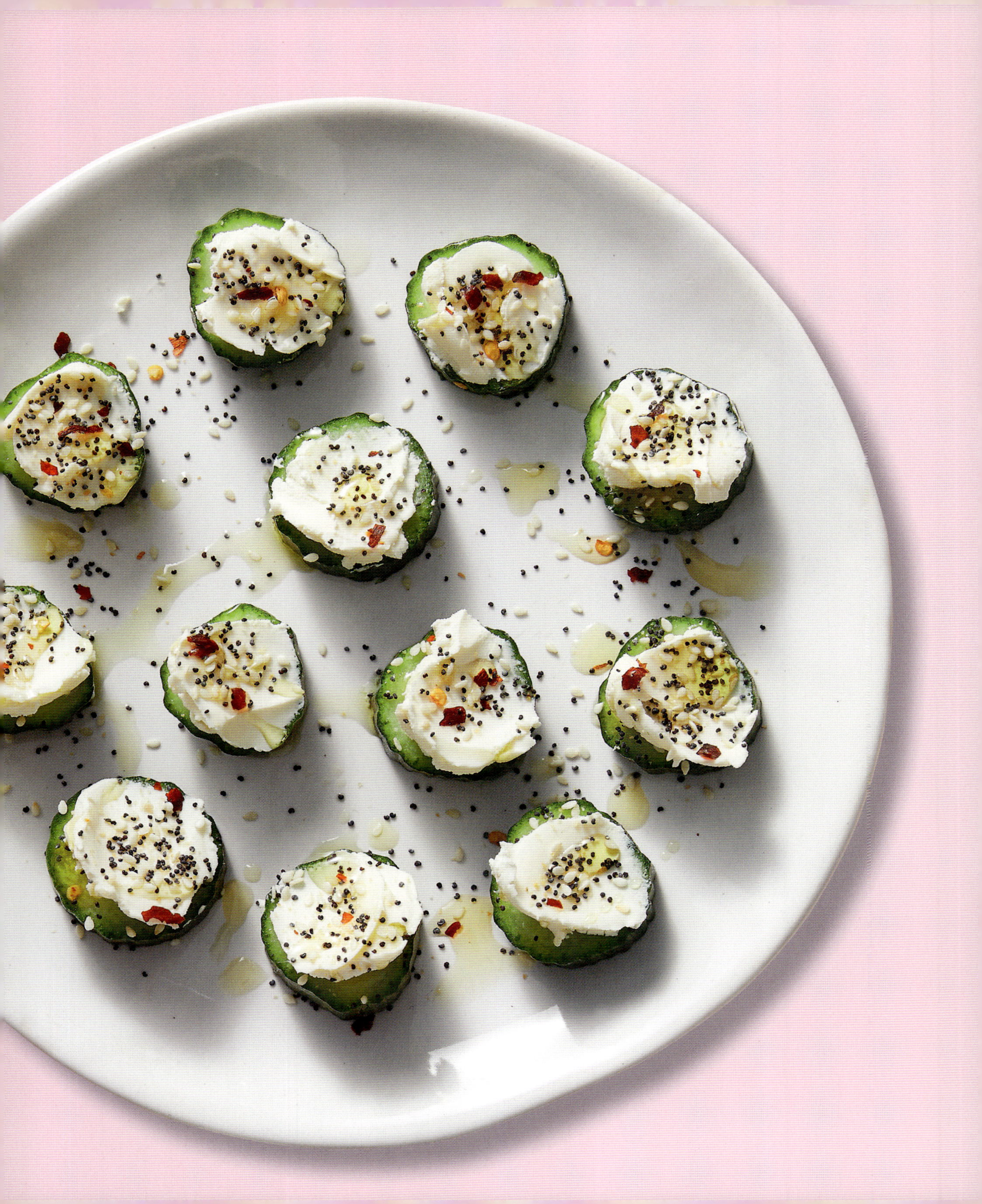

07.

Snacks

UNITS PER SERVE:	
Breads, Cereals, Legumes, Starchy Veg	0
Dairy	1
Lean Meat, Fish, Poultry, Eggs, Tofu	0
Low–Moderate Carbohydrate Veg	1
Healthy Fats	2

Low-carb Snack Platter

CARBS 4g PER SERVE

SERVES: 4 | PREPARATION: 5 MINUTES | COOKING: NIL

⅓ cup (75 g) hummus
80 g sliced cheddar
12 cherry tomatoes
8 pitted green olives
1 small Lebanese cucumber, cut into batons
2 tablespoons roasted unsalted almonds

Place the hummus in a small ramekin on a serving platter. Arrange the remaining ingredients on the platter around the ramekin and serve.

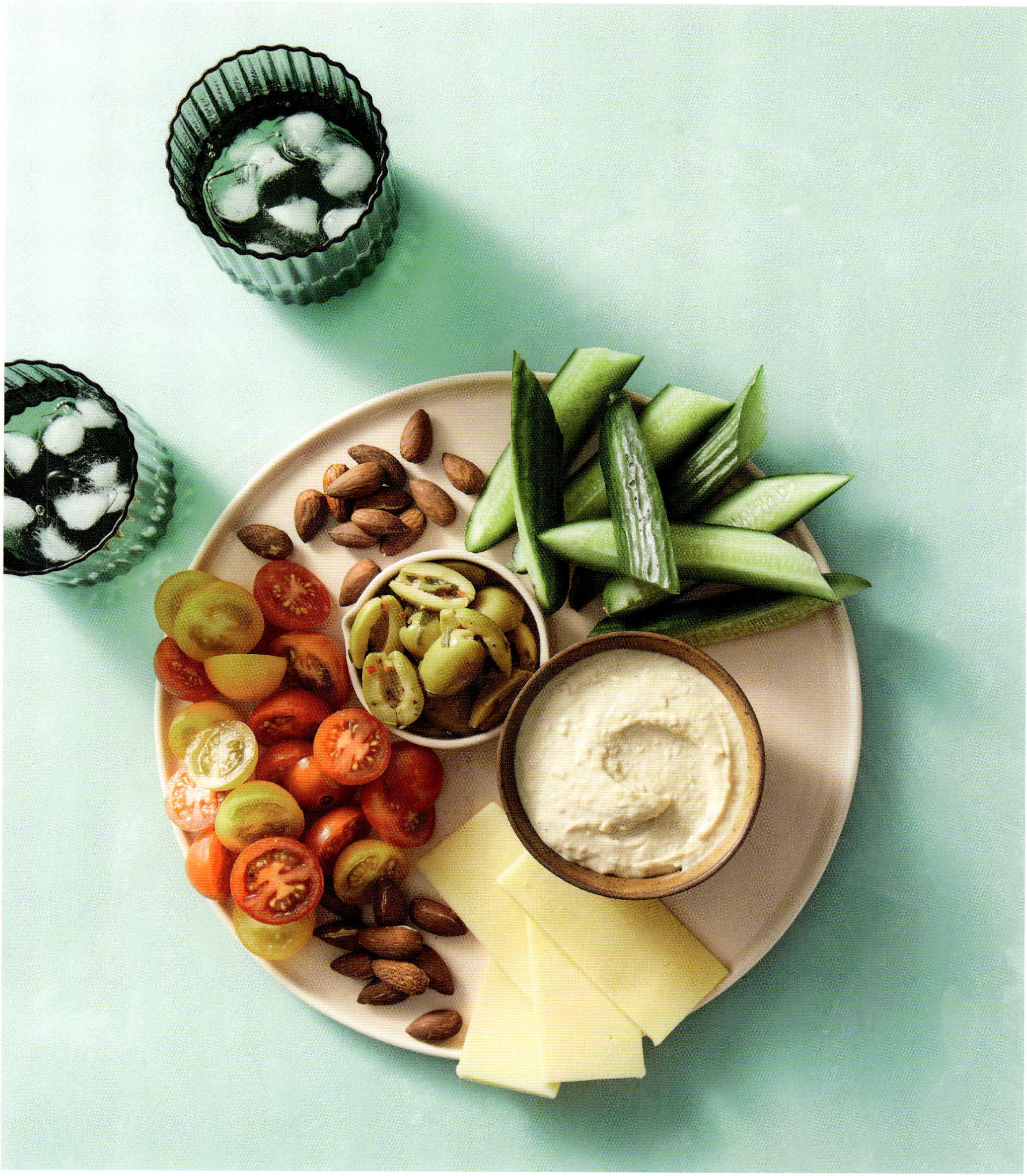

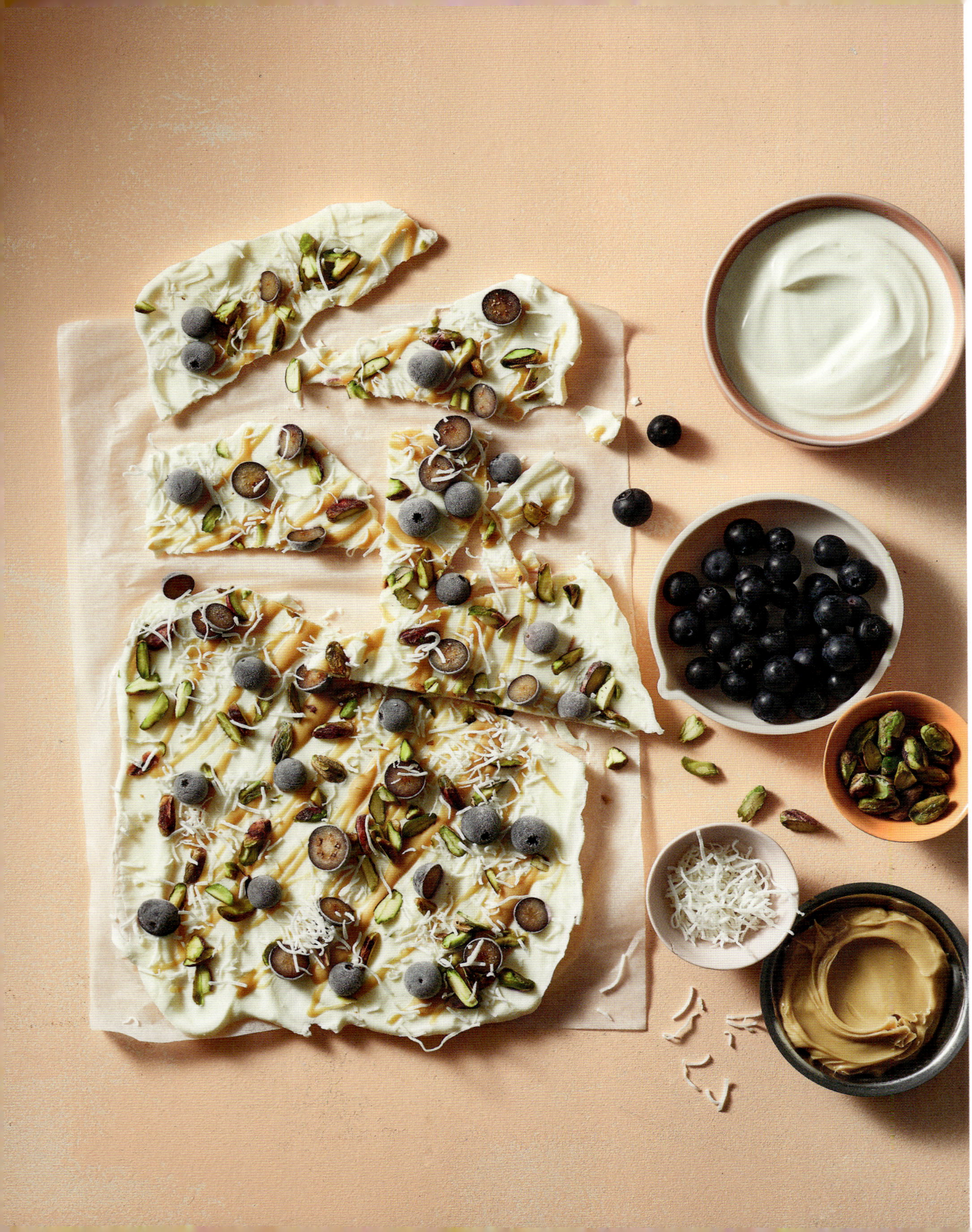

UNITS PER SERVE:	
Breads, Cereals, Legumes, Starchy Veg	0
Dairy	1
Lean Meat, Fish, Poultry, Eggs, Tofu	0
Low–Moderate Carbohydrate Veg	0
Healthy Fats	2

Frozen Yoghurt Bark with Pistachio and Blueberries

CARBS 11g PER SERVE

SERVES: 4 | PREPARATION: 5 MINUTES + 2 HOURS FREEZING | COOKING: NIL

- 1 tablespoon cashew butter (see note)
- 1½ cups (390 g) natural yoghurt
- 1 cup (155 g) blueberries
- 2 tablespoons roughly chopped pistachios
- 2 teaspoons shredded coconut

1. Place the cashew butter in a small microwave-safe bowl and heat it in the microwave for 10 seconds on High.
2. Line a small tray with baking paper. Drizzle the yoghurt across the paper, then drizzle with the warmed cashew butter. Scatter the blueberries, pistachios and shredded coconut over the top. Freeze for 2 hours or until set.
3. Slice into shards to serve. Store in an airtight container in the freezer for up to 1 month.

Note

When purchasing nut butters, it is important to look at the food label. Ensure your nut butter has no added sugar or salt.

UNITS PER SERVE:	
Breads, Cereals, Legumes, Starchy Veg	0
Dairy	1
Lean Meat, Fish, Poultry, Eggs, Tofu	0
Low–Moderate Carbohydrate Veg	1
Healthy Fats	1

Cucumber Cream Cheese Bites

CARBS 2g PER SERVE

SERVES: 4 | PREPARATION: 5 MINUTES | COOKING: NIL

2 teaspoons poppy seeds
2 teaspoons sesame seeds
1 teaspoon garlic granules
Pinch chilli flakes
1 telegraph cucumber, cut into 5 mm thick slices
⅓ cup (85 g) reduced-fat cream cheese
2 teaspoons extra virgin olive oil

1. Place the poppy seeds, sesame seeds, garlic granules and chilli flakes in a small bowl and mix to combine.
2. Place the cucumber slices on a serving plate. Spread the cream cheese over the top, then sprinkle with the seed mix. Drizzle the olive oil over the top and serve.

Note

These snacks are ideal for 'bring a plate' social occasions.

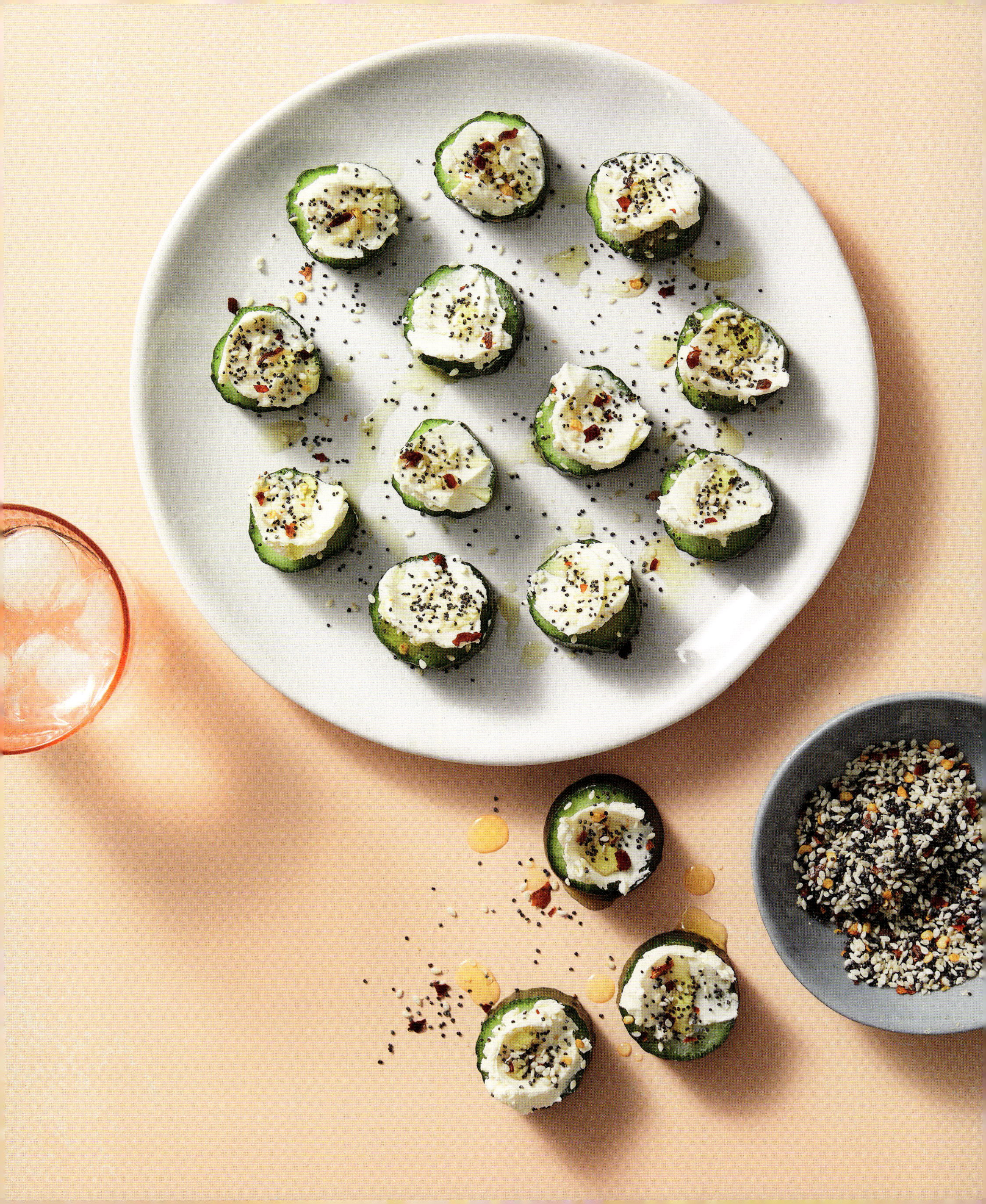

UNITS PER SERVE:	
Breads, Cereals, Legumes, Starchy Veg	0
Dairy	0
Lean Meat, Fish, Poultry, Eggs, Tofu	0
Low–Moderate Carbohydrate Veg	0
Healthy Fats	2

Turmeric Poppy Seed Cashews

CARBS 5g PER SERVE

SERVES: 4 | PREPARATION: 5 MINUTES | COOKING: 14 MINUTES

½ cup (75 g) raw unsalted cashews
¼ teaspoon poppy seeds
¼ teaspoon ground turmeric
1 teaspoon pure vanilla extract
½ teaspoon extra virgin olive oil (or use olive oil spray)

1. Preheat the oven to 200°C (180°C fan-forced).
2. Place the cashews on a baking tray, then sprinkle the poppy seeds, turmeric and vanilla over the top. Drizzle with the olive oil (or use olive oil spray), then toss the mixture with your hands to coat the cashews. Bake in the centre of the oven for 12–14 minutes, tossing the nuts halfway through cooking time, until golden brown and crisp.
3. Divide between four plates to serve. The nuts will keep for up to 1 week in an airtight container.

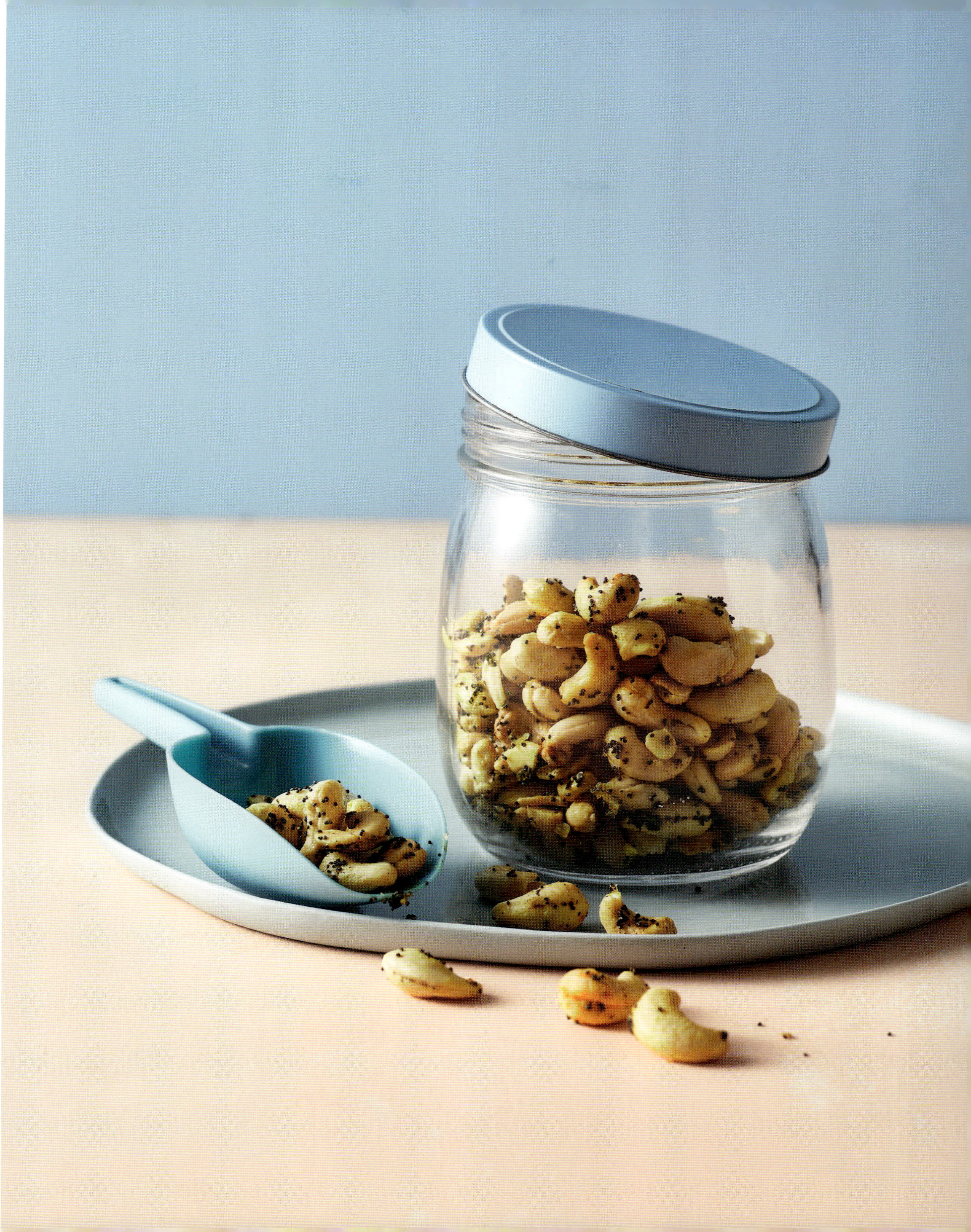

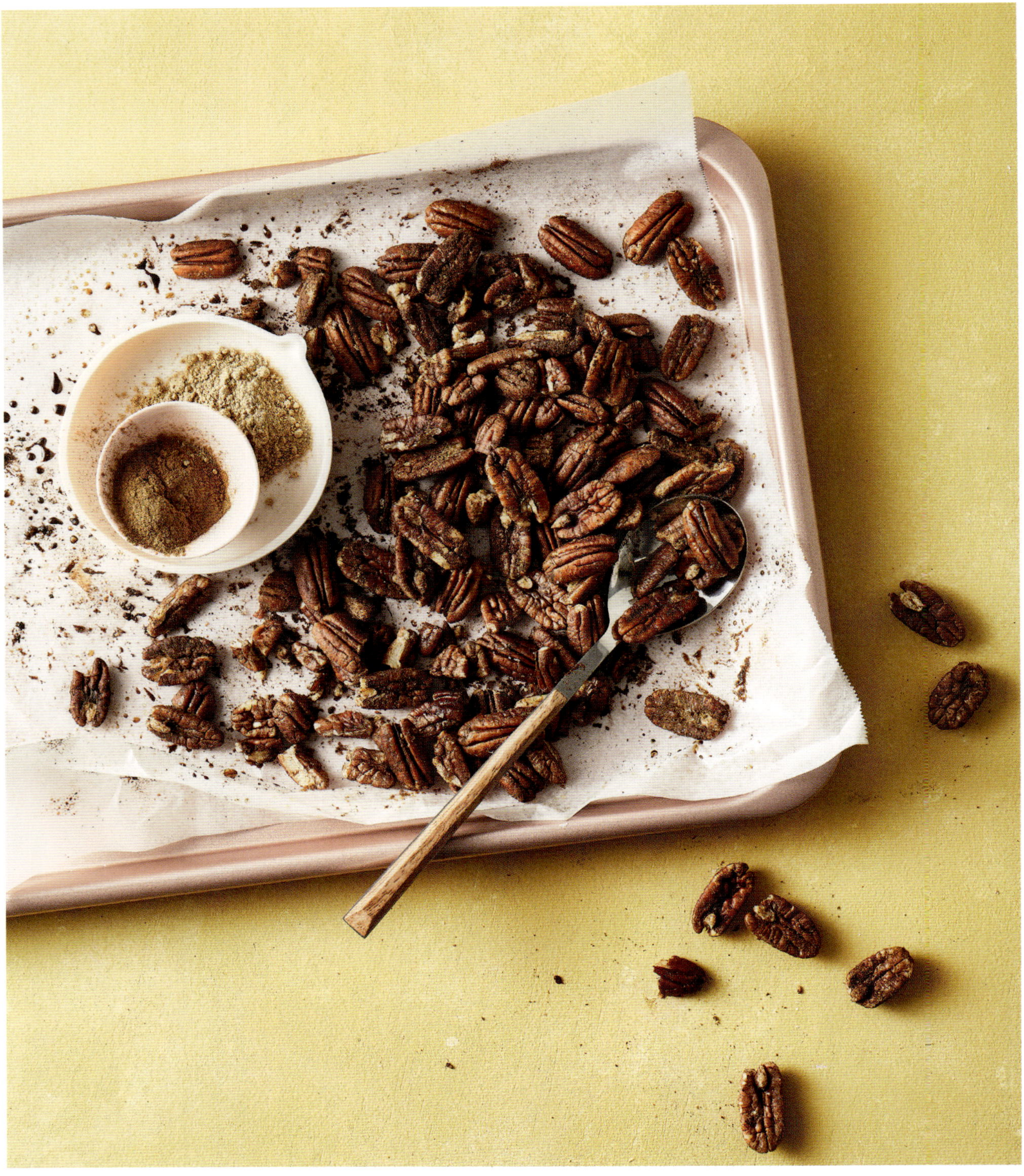

UNITS PER SERVE:	
Breads, Cereals, Legumes, Starchy Veg	0
Dairy	0
Lean Meat, Fish, Poultry, Eggs, Tofu	0
Low–Moderate Carbohydrate Veg	0
Healthy Fats	2

Pumpkin Pie Spiced Pecans

CARBS 2g PER SERVE

SERVES: 4 | PREPARATION: 5 MINUTES | COOKING: 13 MINUTES

¾ cup (75 g) pecans
¼ teaspoon ground cinnamon
Pinch ground ginger
Pinch allspice
½ teaspoon extra virgin olive oil (or use olive oil spray)

1. Preheat the oven to 200°C (180°C fan-forced).
2. Place the pecans on a baking tray and sprinkle the spices over the top. Drizzle with the olive oil (or use olive oil spray), then toss the mixture with your hands to coat the pecans. Bake in the centre of the oven for 8–10 minutes until golden brown and crisp.
3. Divide between four plates to serve. The nuts will keep for up to 1 week in an airtight container.

UNITS PER SERVE:	
Breads, Cereals, Legumes, Starchy Veg	0
Dairy	0
Lean Meat, Fish, Poultry, Eggs, Tofu	0
Low–Moderate Carbohydrate Veg	0
Healthy Fats	2

Middle Eastern Roasted Almonds with Za'atar

CARBS 2g PER SERVE

SERVES: 4 | PREPARATION: 5 MINUTES | COOKING: 14 MINUTES

75 g raw unsalted almonds
2 teaspoons za'atar
½ teaspoon extra virgin olive oil (or use olive oil spray)

1. Preheat the oven to 200°C (180°C fan-forced).
2. Place the almonds on a baking tray and sprinkle with the za'atar. Drizzle with the olive oil (or use olive oil spray), then toss the mixture with your hands to coat the almonds. Bake in the centre of the oven for 12–14 minutes, tossing the nuts halfway through cooking time, until golden brown and crisp.
3. Divide between four plates to serve. The nuts will keep for up to 1 week in an airtight container.

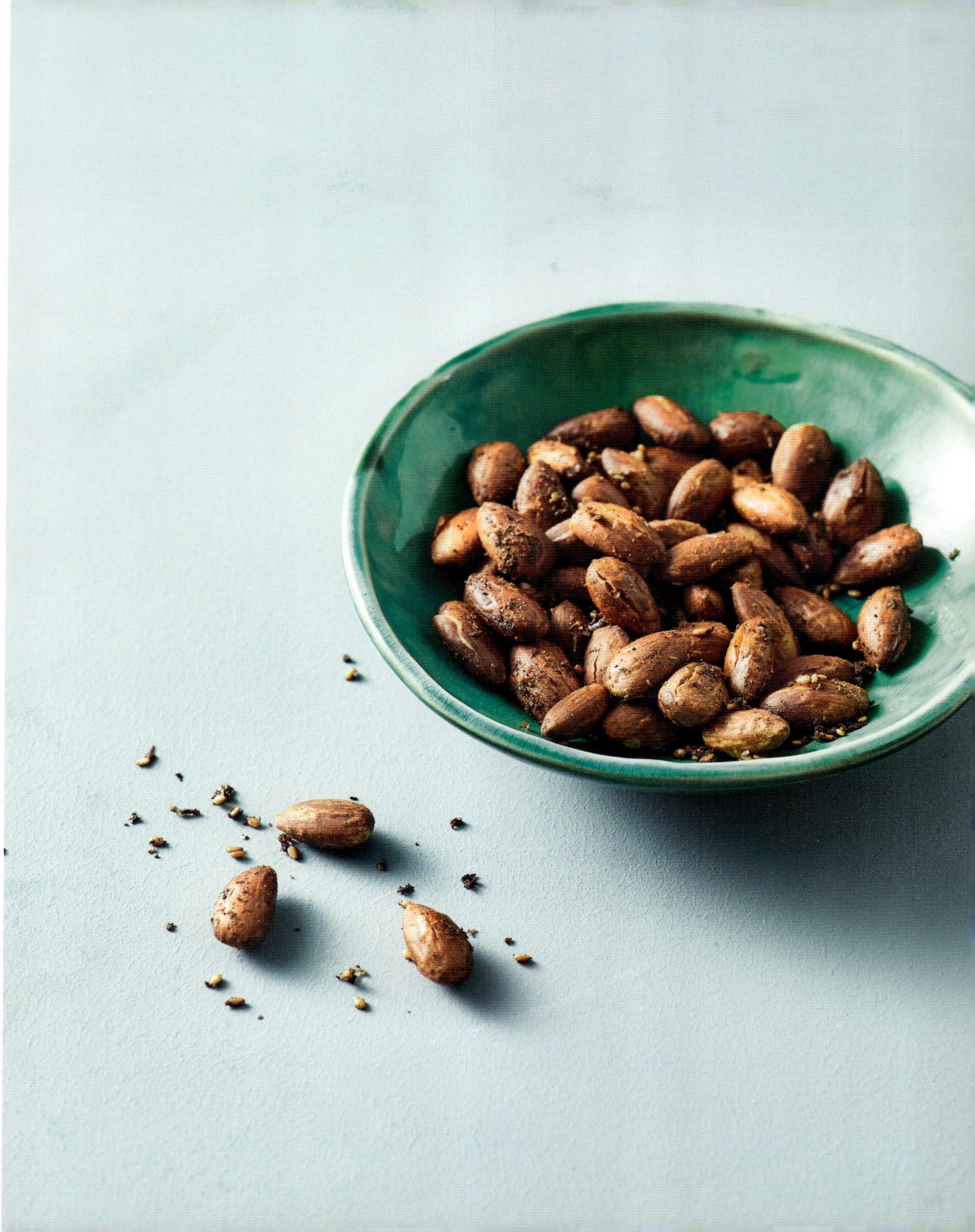

UNITS PER SERVE:	
Breads, Cereals, Legumes, Starchy Veg	0
Dairy	1
Lean Meat, Fish, Poultry, Eggs, Tofu	0
Low–Moderate Carbohydrate Veg	0.5
Healthy Fats	0.5

Raspberries with Vanilla Ricotta

CARBS 4g PER SERVE

SERVES: 4 | PREPARATION: 5 MINUTES | COOKING: NIL

¾ cup (185 g) reduced-fat ricotta
1 teaspoon pure vanilla extract
1 cup (125 g) raspberries
1 tablespoon toasted coconut flakes

1. Place the ricotta and vanilla in a bowl and whip briskly with a fork until smooth.
2. Divide the ricotta between small bowls, top with the raspberries and coconut flakes and serve.

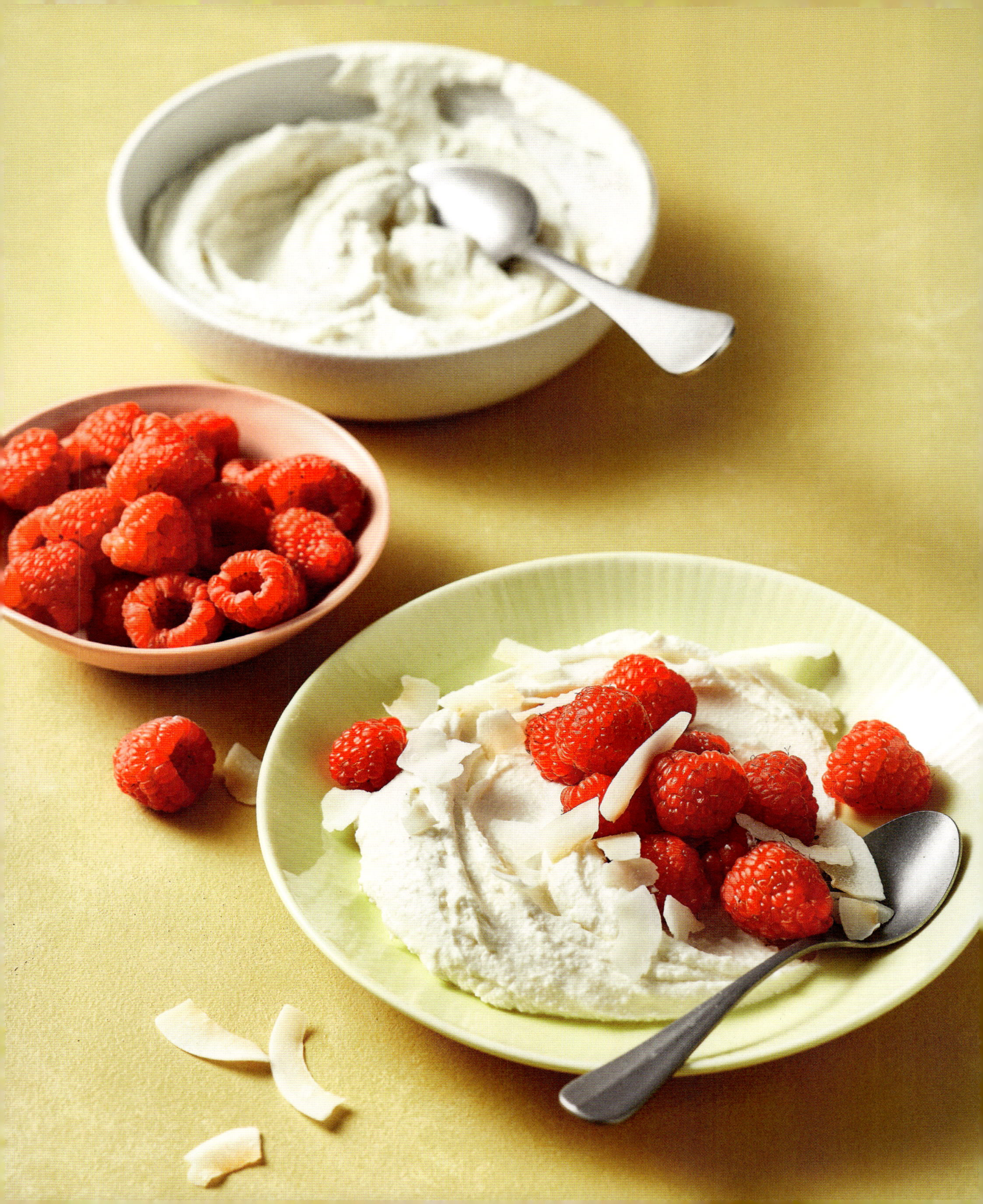

Appendix A: How to assess your body weight status

To determine your weight status and assess whether you are overweight or obese and have an increased risk of metabolic disease you will need to calculate your body mass index (BMI), then measure your waist circumference.

HOW TO CALCULATE YOUR BODY MASS INDEX (BMI)

To determine whether you are overweight or obese, calculate your body mass index (BMI) using the equation below and then compare it with the values in the Check your metabolic disease risk table, opposite. If you would prefer to use an online tool to calculate your BMI, visit https://www.health.gov.au/health-topics/overweight-and-obesity/bmi-and-waist.

SAMPLE BMI CALCULATION

Gary is 1.81 metres (i.e. 181 centimetres) tall and weighs 105 kilograms. His BMI is therefore:

$$\text{BMI (kg/m}^2\text{)} = \text{weight (kg)} / (\text{height (m)} \times \text{height (m)})$$

$$= 105 / (1.81 \times 1.81)$$

$$= 32 \text{ (rounded down)}$$

Comparing this value to those in the table opposite, Gary can see he's in the obese class 1 category and would benefit from losing weight.

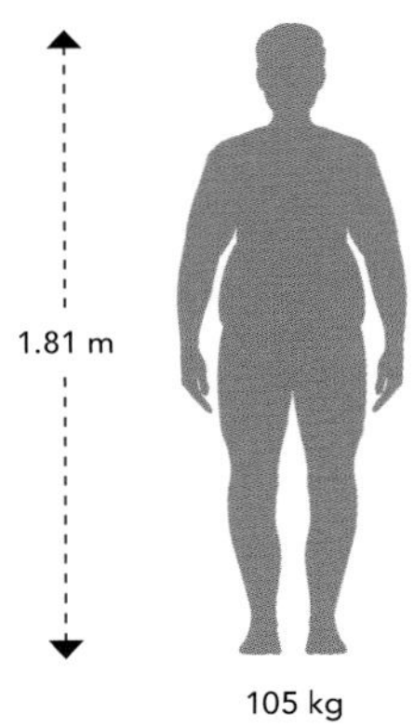

How to measure your waist circumference

- find the top of your hip bone and take the measurement just above this
- ensure the tape measure is level with your belly button and parallel to the floor
- don't hold your breath, and take the measurement at the end of a breath out
- aim to have the tape snug (but not tight) around your waist.

Check your metabolic disease risk

Weight classification	BMI (kg/m^{2})	Metabolic disease risk	
		Waist circumference less than 88 cm (women) or 102 cm (men)	**Waist circumference greater than 88 cm (women) or 102 cm (men)**
Underweight	Less than 18.49	–	–
Healthy (normal)	18.50–24.99	–	–
Overweight (pre-obese)	25.00–29.99	Increased	High
Obese class I	30.00–34.99	High	Very high
Obese class II	35.00–39.99	Very high	Very high
Obese class III	40.00 or more	Extremely high	Extremely high

Source: Adapted from WHO, apps.who.int/bmi/index.jsp?introPage=intro_3.html

There's some debate about the most appropriate cut-offs of BMI and waist circumference measurements for different ethnic groups, including Aboriginal and Torres Strait Islander people, and people of Asian and Pacific heritage. The World Health Organization (WHO) estimates that in different Asian populations the risk of developing type 2 diabetes and heart disease increases with a BMI of 22–25 and a waist circumference of more than 80 centimetres for women and 90 centimetres for men. Whatever your ethnicity, BMI can't take into account your individual body composition – how much body fat or muscle you have – so you should always use your BMI and/or waist circumference as a guide only. If your BMI and metabolic disease risk do seem high, though, start with a visit to your GP as soon as you can for blood glucose tests.

References

American Diabetes Association. 'Facilitating behavior change and well-being to improve health outcomes: standards of medical care in diabetes – 2020.' *Diabetes Care.* 2000; 43(Supplement 1):S48-S65.
Australian National Diabetes Strategy 2021-2030: Australian Government Department of Health; 2021 [Available from: https://www.health.gov.au/resources/publications/australian-national-diabetes-strategy-2021-2030]

British Dietetic Association (2018). 'Low carbohydrate diets for the management of Type 2 Diabetes in adults.' [Available from: https://www.bda.uk.com/improvinghealth/healthprofessionals/policy_statements/policy_statement_-_low_carbohydrate_diets_t2_diabetes]

Brinkworth GD, Buckley JD, Noakes M, Clifton PM. 'Renal function following long-term weight loss in individuals with abdominal obesity on a very-low-carbohydrate diet vs high-carbohydrate diet.' *J Am Diet Assoc.* 2010; 110(4):633-8.

Brinkworth GD, Luscombe-Marsh ND, Thompson CH, Noakes M, Buckley JD, Wittert G, Wilson CJ. 'Long-term effects of very low-carbohydrate and high-carbohydrate weight-loss diets on psychological health in obese adults with type 2 diabetes: randomized controlled trial.' *J Intern Med.* 2016; 280(4):388-97.

Brinkworth GD, Noakes M, Buckley JD, Keogh JB, Clifton PM. 'Long-term effects of a very-low-carbohydrate weight loss diet compared with an isocaloric low-fat diet after 12 mo.' *Am J Clin Nutr.* 2009; 90(1):23-32.

Brinkworth GD, Wycherley TP, Noakes M, Buckley JD, Clifton PM. 'Long-term effects of a very-low-carbohydrate weight-loss diet and an isocaloric low-fat diet on bone health in obese adults.' *Nutrition.* 2016; 32(9):1033-6.

Diabetes Australia (2018). 'Position Statement: Low carbohydrate eating for people with diabetes.' [Available from: https://static.diabetesaustralia.com.au/s/fileassets/diabetes-australia/dbd70857-a834-45b0-b6f1-ea2582bbe5c7.pdf]

Diabetes Canada (2020). 'Position Statement on Low-Carbohydrate Diets for Adults with Diabetes: A Rapid Review.' *Can J Diabetes.* 2020; 44:295-299.

Diabetes UK (2017). 'Position statement: Low-carb diets for people living with diabetes.' [Avaliable from: https://www.diabetes.org.uk/resources-s3/2017-09/low-carb-diets-position-statement-May-2017.pdf]

Evert AB, Dennison M, Gardner CD. et al. 'Nutrition Therapy for Adults with Diabetes or Prediabetes: A Consensus Report.' *Diabetes Care.* 2019; 42(5):731-754.

Feinman RD, Pogozelski WK, Astrup A, Bernstein RK, Fine EJ, Westman EC, et al. 'Dietary carbohydrate restriction as the first approach in diabetes management: Critical review and evidence base.' *Nutrition.* 2015; 31:1–13.

Goldenberg J, Day A, Brinkworth G, Sato J. Yamada S. Jonsson T. Beardsley J, Johnson J, Thabane L, Johnston B. 'Efficacy and safety of low and very low carbohydrate diets for type 2 diabetes remission: a systematic review and meta-analysis of published and unpublished randomized trial data.' BMJ. 2021; 372:m4743.

Huntriss R, Campbell M, Bedwell C. 'The interpretation and effect of a low-carbohydrate diet in the management of type 2 diabetes: a systematic review and meta- analysis of randomised controlled trials.' *European Journal of Clinical Nutrition*, 2018; 72:311-325.

Jesudason DR, Pedersen E, Clifton PM. 'Weight-loss diets in people with type 2 diabetes and renal disease: a randomized controlled trial of the effect of different dietary protein amounts.' *Am J Clin Nutr.* 2013; 98(2):494-501.

Kakoschke N, Zajac IT, Tay J, Luscombe-Marsh ND, Thompson CH, Noakes M, Buckley JD, Wittert G, Brinkworth GD. 'Effects of very low-carbohydrate vs. high-carbohydrate weight loss diets on psychological health in adults with obesity and type 2 diabetes: a 2-year randomized controlled trial. *European Journal of Nutrition*. 2021; 608):4251-4262.

Krauss RM, Blanche PJ, Rawlings RS, Fernstrom HS, Williams PT. 'Separate effects of reduced carbohydrate intake and weight loss on atherogenic dyslipidemia.' *Am J Clin Nutr.* 2006; 83(5):1025-31.

Li S, Ding L, Xiao X. 'Comparing the Efficacy and Safety of Low-Carbohydrate Diets with Low-Fat Diets for Type 2 Diabetes Mellitus Patients: A Systematic Review and Meta-Analysis of Randomized Clinical Trials.' *International Journal of Endocrinology*, 2021; 2021, Article ID 8521756; doi.org/10.1155/2021/8521756

Look ARG, Pi-Sunyer X, Blackburn G, Brancati FL, Bray GA, Bright R, Clark JM, Curtis JM, Espeland MA, Foreyt JP, Graves K, et al. 'Reduction in weight and cardiovascular disease risk factors in individuals with type 2 diabetes: one-year results of the look AHEAD trial.' *Diabetes Care.* 2007; 30(6):1374-83.

Meng Y, Bai H, Wang S, Li Z, Wang Q, Chen L. 'Efficacy of low carbohydrate diet for type 2 diabetes mellitus management: A systematic review and meta-analysis of randomized controlled trials.' *Diabetes Res Clin Pract.* 2017; 131:124-131.

Murdoch C, Unwin D, Cavan D, Cucuzzella M, Patel M. 'Adapting diabetes medication for low carbohydrate management of type 2 diabetes: a practical guide.' *Br J Gen Pract.* Jul 2019; 69(684):360-361.

Pan B, Ge L, Xun YQ, Chen YJ, Gao CY, Han X, Zuo LQ, Shan HQ, Yang KH, Ding GW, Tian JH. 'Exercise training modalities in patients with type 2 diabetes mellitus: a systematic review and network meta-analysis.' *Int J Behav Nutr Phys Act.* 2018; 15(1):72.

The Scientific Advisory Committee on Nutrition. 'SACN report. Lower carbohydrate diets for type 2 diabetes.' [Available from: https://www.gov.uk/government/publications/sacn-report-lower-carbohydrate-diets-for-type-2-diabetes]

Sainsbury E, Kizirian NV, Partridge SR, Gill T, Colagiuri S, Gibson AA. 'Effect of dietary carbohydrate restriction on glycemic control in adults with diabetes: A systematic review and meta-analysis.' *Diabetes Res Clin Pract.* 2018; 139:239-252.

Snorgaard O, Poulsen GM, Andersen HK, Astrup A. 'Systematic review and meta-analysis of dietary carbohydrate restriction in patients with type 2 diabetes.' *BMJ Open Diabetes Res Care.* 2017; 5(1):e000354.

Struik NA, Brinkworth GD, Thompson CH, Buckley JD, Wittert G, Luscombe-Marsh ND. 'Very Low and Higher Carbohydrate Diets Promote Differential Appetite Responses in Adults with Type 2 Diabetes: A Randomized Trial.' *J Nutr*. 2020; 150:800-805.

Suyoto PST. 'Effect of low-carbohydrate diet on markers of renal function in patients with type 2 diabetes: A meta-analysis.' *Diabetes Metab Res Rev.* 2018; 34(7):e3032.

Tay J, Luscombe-Marsh ND, Thompson CH, Noakes M, Buckley JD, Wittert GA, Yancy WS, Jr., Brinkworth GD. 'A very low-carbohydrate, low-saturated fat diet for type 2 diabetes management: a randomized trial.' *Diabetes Care.* 2014; 37:2909-18.

Tay J, Luscombe-Marsh ND, Thompson CH, Noakes M, Buckley JD, Wittert GA, Yancy WS, Jr., Brinkworth GD. 'Comparison of low- and high-carbohydrate diets for type 2 diabetes management: a randomized trial.' *Am J Clin Nutr.* 2015; 102:780-90.

Tay J, Thompson CH, Brinkworth GD. 'Glycemic variability: assessing glycemia differently and the implications for dietary management of diabetes.' *Annu Rev Nutr.* 2015; 35:389-424.

Tay J, Thompson CH, Luscombe-Marsh ND, Noakes M, Buckley JD, Wittert GA, Brinkworth GD. 'Long-term effects of a very low carbohydrate compared with a high carbohydrate diet on renal function in individuals with type 2 diabetes: a randomized trial.' *Medicine (Baltimore).* 2015; 94(47):e2181.

Tay J, Thompson CH, Luscombe-Marsh ND, Wycherley TP, Noakes M, Buckley JD, Wittert GA, Yancy WS, Jr., Brinkworth GD. 'Effects of an energy-restricted low-carbohydrate, high unsaturated fat/low saturated fat diet versus a high-carbohydrate, low-fat diet in type 2 diabetes: A 2-year randomized clinical trial.' *Diabetes Obes Metab.* 2018; 20(4):858-871.

Tay J, Zajac IT, Thompson CH, Luscombe-Marsh ND, Danthiir V, Noakes M, Buckley JD, Wittert GA, Brinkworth GD. 'A randomised-controlled trial of the effects of very low-carbohydrate and high-carbohydrate diets on cognitive performance in patients with type 2 diabetes.' *Br J Nutr.* 2016; 116:1745-1753.

Tay J, Thompson CH, Luscombe-Marsh ND, Noakes M, Buckley JD, Wittert GA, Brinkworth GD. 'Nutritional adequacy of very low- and high-carbohydrate, low saturated fat diets in adults with type 2 diabetes: A secondary analysis of a 2-year randomised controlled trial.' *Diabetes Res Clin Pract*. 2020; 170:108501. doi: 10.1016/j.diabres.2020.108501.

Taylor PJ, Thompson CH, Luscombe-Marsh ND, Wycherley TP, Wittert G, Brinkworth GD. "Efficacy of real-time continuous glucose monitoring to improve effects of a prescriptive lifestyle intervention in type 2 diabetes: a pilot study.' *Diabetes Ther.* 2019; 10(2):509-522.

Taylor PJ, Thompson CH, Luscombe-Marsh ND, Wycherley TP, Wittert G, Brinkworth GD, Zajac I. 'Tolerability and acceptability of real-time continuous glucose monitoring and its impact on diabetes management behaviours in individuals with type 2 diabetes – a pilot study.' *Diabetes Res Clin Pract.* 2019; 155:107814.

Turton J, Brinkworth GD, Field R, Parker H, Rooney K. 'An evidence-based approach to developing low-carbohydrate diets for type 2 diabetes management: A systematic review of interventions and methods.' *Diabetes Obes Metab*. 2019; 21:2513-2525.

van Zuuren EJ, Fedorowicz Z, Kuijpers T, Pijl H. 'Effects of low-carbohydrate - compared with low-fat-diet interventions on metabolic control in people with type 2 diabetes: a systematic review including GRADE assessments.' *Am J Clin Nutr.* 2018; 108:300-331.

Wycherley TP, Thompson CH, Buckley JD, Luscombe-Marsh ND, Noakes M, Wittert GA, Brinkworth GD. 'Long-term effects of weight loss with a very-low carbohydrate, low saturated fat diet on flow mediated dilatation in patients with type 2 diabetes: A randomised controlled trial.' *Atherosclerosis.* 2016; 252:28-31.

Recipe conversion chart

Measuring cups and spoons may vary slightly from one country to another, but the difference is generally not enough to affect a recipe. All cup and spoon measures are level.

One Australian metric measuring cup holds 250 ml (8 fl oz), one Australian tablespoon holds 20 ml (4 teaspoons) and one Australian metric teaspoon holds 5 ml. North America, New Zealand and the UK use a 15 ml (3 teaspoon) tablespoon.

LENGTH

METRIC	IMPERIAL
3 mm	⅛ inch
6 mm	¼ inch
1 cm	½ inch
2.5 cm	1 inch
5 cm	2 inches
18 cm	7 inches
20 cm	8 inches
23 cm	9 inches
25 cm	10 inches
30 cm	12 inches

LIQUID MEASURES

ONE AMERICAN PINT	ONE IMPERIAL PINT
500 ml (16 fl oz)	600 ml (20 fl oz)

cup	metric	imperial
⅛ cup	30 ml	[illegible] fl oz
¼ cup	60 ml	2 fl oz
⅓ cup	80 ml	2½ fl oz
½ cup	125 ml	4 fl oz
⅔ cup	160 ml	5 fl oz
¾ cup	180 ml	6 fl oz
1 cup	250 ml	8 fl oz
2 cups	500 ml	16 fl oz
2¼ cups	560 ml	20 fl oz
4 cups	1 litre	32 fl oz

DRY MEASURES

The most accurate way to measure dry ingredients is to weigh them. However, if using a cup, add the ingredient loosely to the cup and level with a knife; don't compact the ingredient unless the recipe requests 'firmly packed'.

METRIC	IMPERIAL
15 g	½ oz
30 g	1 oz
60 g	2 oz
125 g	4 oz (¼ lb)
185 g	6 oz
250 g	8 oz (½ lb)
375 g	12 oz (¾ lb)
500 g	16 oz (1 lb)
1 kg	32 oz (2 lb)

OVEN TEMPERATURES

CELSIUS	FAHRENHEIT	CELSIUS	GAS MARK
100°C	200°F	110°C	¼
120°C	250°F	130°C	½
150°C	300°F	140°C	1
160°C	325°F	150°C	2
180°C	350°F	170°C	3
200°C	400°F	180°C	4
220°C	425°F	190°C	5
		200°C	6
		220°C	7
		230°C	8
		240°C	9
		250°C	10

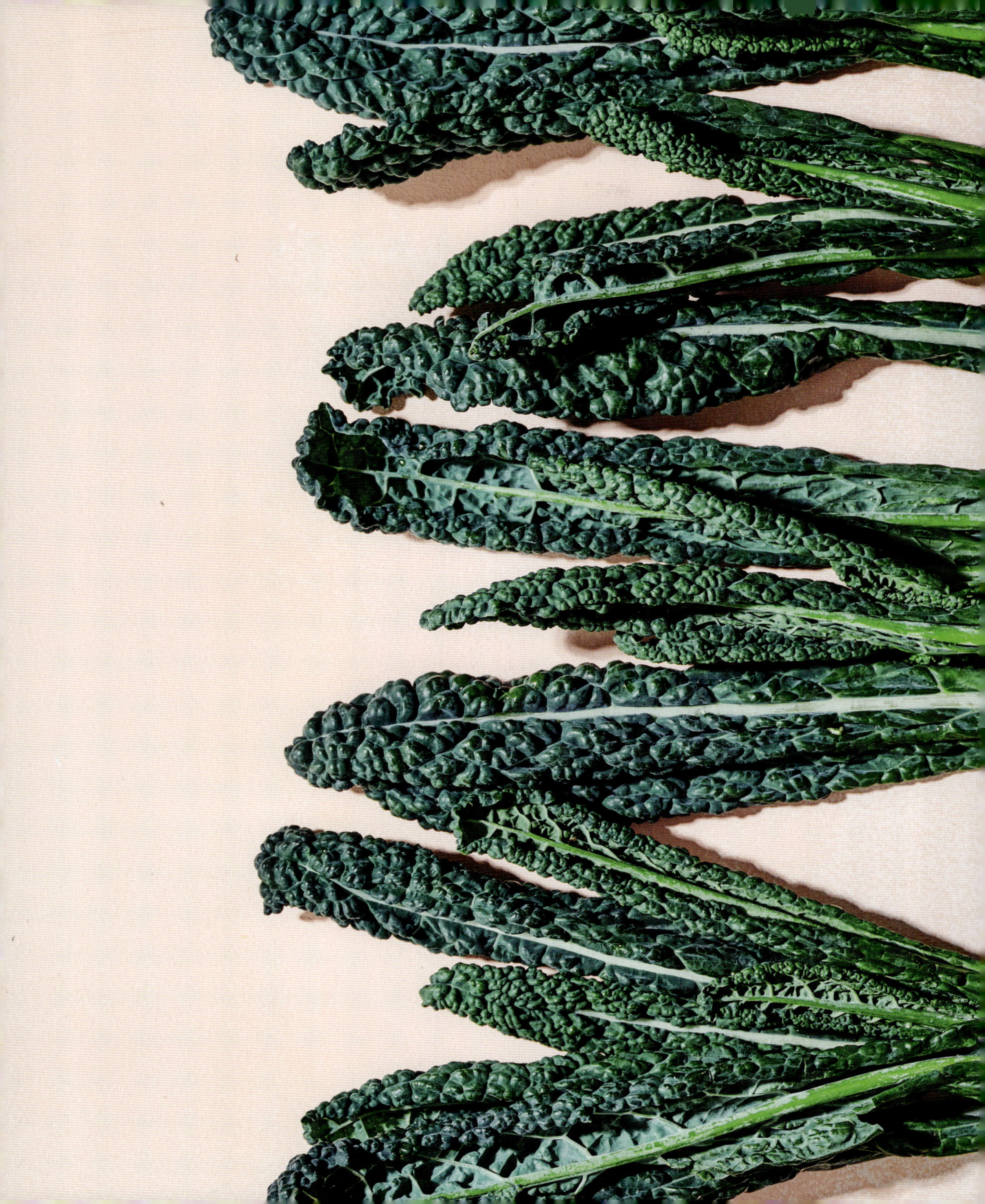

Acknowledgements

The authors would like to highlight the significant contributions of Meg Yonson and Kim Anastasiou, who helped us to prepare the content of this book. Meg, thank you for your inspiring and creative food design, and for creating a collection of delicious and flavoursome recipes consistent with the food and nutrient specifications of the CSIRO Low-carb Diet. Kim, thank you for your unwavering commitment to meticulously reviewing the recipes for scientific compliance, updating recipe protocols, and reviewing the food supply to identify and update the food and ingredient lists for this edition.

Deep thanks to Dr Natalie Luscombe-Marsh (Diabetes SA), Dr Tom Wycherley (University of South Australia) and Professor Campbell Thompson (University of Adelaide). Your contribution to the scientific advancements, content and design of the information across the entire CSIRO Low-carb Diet book series has been invaluable in translating the science into an evidence-based, practical guide that is helping many Australians.

Special thanks to our scientific co-investigators and collaborators for their contributions to our scientific ideas and their guidance and commitment to this important research topic: Professor Manny Noakes (formerly CSIRO), Dr Jeannie Tay (Agency for Science Technology and Research (A*Star), Singapore, Professor Jon Buckley (University of South Australia), Professor Gary Wittert (University of Adelaide), Professor William Yancy Jr (Duke University, USA), Professor Carlene Wilson (Flinders University), Dr Vanessa Danthiir (formerly CSIRO), Dr Ian Zajac (CSIRO), Dr Naomi Kakoschke (CSIRO), Noor Struik (The Nourishing State, Netherlands), and Professor Peter Clifton (University of South Australia).

Thanks to Dr Malcolm Riley (CSIRO) and Erica Kneipp (CSIRO), who provided their professional expertise in reviewing and advising on the book content.

Thanks to the following individuals at the Clinical Research Team at CSIRO Health and Biosecurity for their tireless work in conducting the clinical research activities that underpin the contents of this book: Anne McGuffin, Julia Weaver and Vanessa Courage for coordinating the research trials; Janna Lutze, Dr Paul Foster, Xenia Cleanthous, Gemma Williams, Hannah Gilbert and Fiona Barr for assisting in designing and implementing the dietary interventions; Lindy Lawson, Theresa McKinnon, Rosemary McArthur and Heather Webb for their nursing expertise and clinical patient management; Vanessa Russell, Cathryn Pape, Candita Dang, Andre Nikolic and Sylvia Usher for performing biochemical assays and for other laboratory expertise; Julie Syrette and Kathryn Bastiaans for data management; Kylie Lange and Mary Barnes for assisting with statistical analyses; Bianca Frew for brand management and coordinating and promoting communication opportunities; our external fitness partners and health coaches for implementing the exercise interventions, including Luke Johnston and Annie Hastwell of Fit for Success; Kelly French, Jason Delfos, Kristi Lacey-Powell, Marilyn Woods, John Perrin, Simon Pane and Annette Beckette of South Australian Aquatic and Leisure Centre; and Angie Mondello and Josh Gniadek of Boot Camp Plus. This would not have been possible without your efforts and contributions in conducting this ground-breaking research.

Many thanks to the team at Pan Macmillan Australia: Ingrid Ohlsson, Ariane Durkin, Naomi van Groll and Lucinda Thompson, for their tireless work and support through the publishing process. Special thanks to editor Ariana Klepac and designer Andy Warren. Thanks also to photographers Rob Palmer and Jeremy Simons, stylist Emma Knowles and home economist Kerrie Ray. Lastly, thanks to Adrik Kemp in marketing, and Ellen Kirkness and Clare Keighery in publicity.

Finally, and most importantly, we'd like to thank the research volunteers for their participation in our research trials. It's only through their contributions that our research and these scientific discoveries and significant advancements in clinical practices have been made possible. Your efforts are invaluable and are going a long way to helping many across the world!

Index

A

B

C

D

E

F

N

O

P

Q

R

S

T

U

V

W

Y

Z

Pan Macmillan acknowledges the Traditional Custodians of Country throughout Australia and their connections to lands, waters and communities. We pay our respect to Elders past and present and extend that respect to all Aboriginal and Torres Strait Islander peoples today. We honour more than sixty thousand years of storytelling, art and culture.

First published 2022 in Macmillan
by Pan Macmillan Australia Pty Limited
Level 25, 1 Market Street, Sydney, New South Wales
Australia 2000

NATIONAL LIBRARY OF AUSTRALIA

A catalogue record for this book is available from the National Library of Australia

Design by Andy Warren
Recipe development by Meg Yonson
Edited by Ariana Klepac
Index by Jenny Brown
Prop and food styling by Emma Knowles
Food preparation by Kerrie Ray
Colour + reproduction by Splitting Image Colour Studio
Printed in China by 1010 Printing International Limited

We advise that the information contained in this book does not negate personal responsibility on the part of the reader for their own health and safety. It is recommended that individually tailored advice is sought from your healthcare or medical professional. The publishers and their respective employees, agents and authors, are not liable for injuries or damage occasioned to any person as a result of reading or following the information contained in this book.

10 9 8 7 6 5 4 3